SO-ARO-438

European Observatory on Health Systems and Policies Series

The European Observatory on Health Systems and Policies is a unique project that builds on the commitment of all its partners to improving health care systems:

- World Health Organization Regional Office for Europe
- Government of Belgium
- Government of Finland
- Government of Greece
- Government of Norway
- Government of Spain
- Government of Sweden
- European Investment Bank
- Open Society Institute
- World Bank
- London School of Economics and Political Science
- London School of Hygiene & Tropical Medicine

Series Editors

Josep Figueras is Head of the Secretariat and Research Director of the European Observatory on Health Systems and Policies and Head of the European Centre for Health Policy, World Health Organization Regional Office for Europe.

Martin McKee is Research Director of the European Observatory on Health Systems and Policies and Professor of European Public Health at the London School of Hygiene & Tropical Medicine as well as a co-director of the School's European Centre on Health of Societies in Transition.

Elias Mossialos is Research Director of the European Observatory on Health Systems and Policies and Brian Abel-Smith Reader in Health Policy, Department of Social Policy, London School of Economics and Political Science and Co-Director of LSE Health and Social Care.

Richard B. Saltman is Research Director of the European Observatory on Health Systems and Policies and Professor of Health Policy and Management at the Rollins School of Public Health, Emory University in Atlanta, Georgia.

The series

The volumes in this series focus on key issues for health policy-making in Europe. Each study explores the conceptual background, outcomes and lessons learned about the development of more equitable, more efficient and more effective health systems in Europe. With this focus, the series seeks to contribute to the evolution of a more evidence-based approach to policy formulation in the health sector.

These studies will be important to all those involved in formulating or evaluating national health care policies and, in particular, will be of use to health policy-makers and advisers, who are under increasing pressure to rationalize the structure and funding of their health systems. Academics and students in the field of health policy will also find this series valuable in seeking to understand better the complex choices that confront the health systems of Europe.

The Observatory supports and promotes evidence-based health policy-making through comprehensive and rigorous analysis of the dynamics of health care systems in Europe.

European Observatory on Health Systems and Policies Series

Series Editors: Josep Figueras, Martin McKee, Elias Mossialos and Richard B. Saltman

Published titles

Funding health care: options for Europe
Elias Mossialos, Anna Dixon, Josep Figueras, Joe Kutzin (eds)

Health care in central Asia
Martin McKee, Judith Healy and Jane Falkingham (eds)

Health policy and European Union enlargement
Martin McKee, Laura MacLehose and Ellen Nolte (eds)

Hospitals in a changing Europe
Martin McKee and Judith Healy (eds)

Regulating entrepreneurial behaviour in European health care systems
Richard B. Saltman, Reinhard Busse and Elias Mossialos (eds)

Forthcoming titles

Effective purchasing for health gain
Josep Figueras, Ray Robinson and Elke Jakubowski (eds)

Regulating pharmaceuticals in Europe: striving for efficiency, equity and quality
Elias Mossialos, Monique Mrazek and Tom Walley (eds)

Social health insurance systems in western Europe
Richard B. Saltman, Reinhard Busse and Josep Figueras (eds)

European Observatory on Health Systems and Policies Series

Edited by Josep Figueras, Martin McKee, Elias Mossialos and Richard B. Saltman

Health policy and European Union enlargement

Edited by
Martin McKee,
Laura MacLehose and
Ellen Nolte

Open University Press

Open University Press
McGraw-Hill Education
McGraw-Hill House
Shoppenhangers Road
Maidenhead
Berkshire
England
SL6 2QL

email: enquiries@openup.co.uk
world wide web: www.openup.co.uk

and Two Penn Plaza, New York, NY 10121-2289, USA

First published 2004
Reprinted 2004

A catalogue record of this book is available from the British Library

ISBN 0 335 21353 7 (pb)   0 335 21354 5 (hb)

Library of Congress Cataloging-in-Publication Data
CIP data applied for

Typeset by RefineCatch Limited, Bungay, Suffolk
Printed in Great Britain by MPG Books Ltd, Bodmin, Cornwall

Contents

List of contributors

Tit Albreht is Head of the Centre for Healthcare Organisation, Economics and Informatics at the Institute of Public Health of the Republic of Slovenia in Ljubljana

Roza Adany is Professor of Public Health and Director of the Hungarian School of Public Health in Debrecen, Hungary

Ivana Bozicevic is a lecturer at the Andrija Štampar School of Public Health in Zagreb, Croatia

James Buchan is Professor of Health Care Employment Policy at Queen Margaret University College, Edinburgh, Scotland

Richard Coker is a senior lecturer in public health at the London School of Hygiene & Tropical Medicine

Evgenia Delcheva is Head of the Department of Financial and Economic Analysis and Prognosis at the National Health Insurance Fund in Sofia, Bulgaria

Carl-Ardy Dubois is a Research Fellow at the European Observatory on Health Systems and policies

Anna B. Gilmore is a clinical lecturer at the London School of Hygiene & Tropical Medicine

Antero Heloma is a public health physician at the Provincial Government of Uusimaa in Finland

Rainer Hess is Managing Director, Federal Association of Social Health Insurance Physicians, Germany ("Kassenärztliche Bundesvereinigung")

Elke Jakubowski is Acting Regional Adviser, Futures Fora, WHO Regional Office for Europe

Nicholas Jennett is a Senior Health Economist at the European Investment Bank

Panos Kanavos is a Lecturer in International Health Policy at the London School of Economics and Political Science, London, UK

Manuel Lobato is Professor of Commercial Law at the Universita Autónoma de Madrid, Spain

Karen Lock is a Research Fellow at the European Observatory on Health Systems and Policies

Martin McKee is Research Director at the European Observatory on Health Systems and Policies and Professor of European Public Health at the London School of Hygiene & Tropical Medicine

Laura MacLehose is a Research Fellow at the European Observatory on Health Systems and Policies

Sallie Nicholas is Head of the International Division of the British Medical Association, London, UK

Ellen Nolte is a Research Fellow at the European Observatory on Health Systems and Policies and Lecturer in Public Health at the London School of Hygiene & Tropical Medicine

Stjepan Oreškovic is Director of the Andrija Štampar School of Public Health in Zagreb, Croatia

Esa Österberg is Senior Researcher at the National Research and Development Centre for Welfare and Health, Finland

Anne Marie Rafferty is Reader in Nursing Policy at the London School of Hygiene & Tropical Medicine

Alison Wright-Reid is a health and safety consultant in the United Kingdom

Magdalene Rosenmöller is a Lecturer at the IESE Business School in Barcelona and Madrid, Spain

Monika Zajac is a public health specialist in Poland

Witold Zatonski is Professor of Medicine in the Department of Cancer Epidemiology and Prevention, M. Sklodowska-Curie Memorial Cancer Centre and Institute of Oncology, Warsaw, Poland

Series editors' introduction

European national policy-makers broadly agree on the core objectives that their health care systems should pursue. The list is strikingly straightforward: universal access for all citizens, effective care for better health outcomes, efficient use of resources, high-quality services and responsiveness to patient concerns. It is a formula that resonates across the political spectrum and which, in various, sometimes inventive configurations, has played a role in most recent European national election campaigns.

Yet this clear consensus can only be observed at the abstract policy level. Once decision-makers seek to translate their objectives into the nuts and bolts of health system organization, common principles rapidly devolve into divergent, occasionally contradictory, approaches. This is, of course, not a new phenomenon in the health sector. Different nations, with different histories, cultures and political experiences, have long since constructed quite different institutional arrangements for funding and delivering health care services.

The diversity of health system configurations that has developed in response to broadly common objectives leads quite naturally to questions about the advantages and disadvantages inherent in different arrangements, and which approach is 'better' or even 'best' given a particular context and set of policy priorities. These concerns have intensified over the last decade as policy-makers have sought to improve health system performance through what has become a European-wide wave of health system reforms. The search for comparative advantage has triggered – in health policy as in clinical medicine – increased attention to its knowledge base, and to the possibility of overcoming at least part of existing institutional divergence through more evidence-based health policy-making.

The volumes published in the European Observatory series are intended to provide precisely this kind of cross-national health policy analysis. Drawing on an extensive network of experts and policy-makers working in a variety of academic and administrative capacities, these studies seek to synthesize the available evidence on key health sector topics using a systematic methodology. Each volume explores the conceptual background, outcomes and lessons learned about the development of more equitable, more efficient and more effective health care systems in Europe. With this focus, the series seeks to contribute to the evolution of a more evidence-based approach to policy formulation in the health sector. While remaining sensitive to cultural, social and normative differences among countries, the studies explore a range of policy alternatives available for future decision-making. By examining closely both the advantages and disadvantages of different policy approaches, these volumes fulfil a central mandates of the Observatory: to serve as a bridge between pure academic research and the needs of policy-makers, and to stimulate the development of strategic responses suited to the real political world in which health sector reform must be implemented.

The European Observatory on Health Systems and Policies is a partnership that brings together three international agencies, three national governments, two research institutions and an international non-governmental organization. The partners are as follows: the World Health Organization Regional Office for Europe, which provides the Observatory secretariat; the governments of Greece, Norway and Spain; the European Investment Bank; the Open Society Institute; the World Bank; the London School of Hygiene & Tropical Medicine and the London School of Economics and Political Science.

In addition to the analytical and cross-national comparative studies published in this Open University Press series, the Observatory produces Health Care Systems in Transition (HiTs) profiles for the countries of Europe, the journal *EuroHealth* and the newsletter *EuroObserver*. Further information about Observatory publications and activities can be found on its website *www.observatory.dk*.

Josep Figueras, Martin McKee, Ellias Mossialos and Richard B. Saltman

Foreword

At the time of publication of this book, the process of enlargement – with the accession of ten new Member States to the European Union – is apparently reaching a conclusion. In reality, this is just the end of the beginning.

In particular, the integration of the new Members will pose major challenges to their health systems. These systems have come from a different setting than for the majority of the existing Members. They spend much less than the EU yet face greater problems. And the new countries are joining an EU which is itself seeing significant changes in public health and health care delivery.

Of particular interest to the European Investment Bank – as a founder member of the European Observatory on Health Systems and Policies, and as a policy-driven public bank funding the enlargement process – is the extent to which good health and high quality health care are just consumption goods (the cost of which is borne today mainly by the public sector) or investments for the future. We believe that they are both. This study helps identify the issues that will need to be addressed to achieve efficiently the goal of better health across the enlarged Union, and to maximize the future economic and social benefits that will come with this.

We need to be aware that health status and its drivers vary greatly across the accession states, and their health care delivery systems also differ. We should not expect that there will be easy answers to the question of the impact of enlargement on health. But we should want to base health policy on relevant evidence. This book records the diversity and, by a rigorous analysis of various dimensions of health, provides policy-makers with much of the needed evidence.

Philippe Maystadt
President, European Investment Bank

Acknowledgements

This volume is one of a series of books produced by the European Observatory on Health Care Systems. We are very grateful to all our authors, who responded promptly both in producing and later amending their chapters in the light of ongoing discussions.

We particularly appreciate the valuable input of those reviewers who participated at various stages in the process. These included our steering committee who commented on the original proposal, in particular Roxanna Bonnell, Anca Dumitrescu, Armin Fidler, Isabella de la Mata, Ali McGuire, Charles Normand, Nina Schwalbe, Aris Sissouras, Olav Slaattebrekk and Steve Wright. They also included those who participated in a workshop to discuss a draft of the book, in Warsaw in July 2003. In addition to most of the authors, who helpfully commented on each others' chapters, were Carlos Artundo, John Cacchia, Jennifer Cain, Yves Charpak, Rene Christensen, Marc Danzon, Maggie Davies, Esteban de Manuel Keenoy, Rotislava Dimitrova, Armin Fidler, Josep Figueras, Laslo Gulasci, Jarno Habicht, Mihály Kökény, Marzena Kulis, Suszy Lessof, Miroslaw Manicki, John Martin, Viktoras Meizis, Bernie Merkel, Paulina Miskiewicz, Natasha Muscat, Liuba Negru, Toomas Palu, Robertas Petkevicius, Andreas Polynikis, Mariana Postolache, Aiga Rurane, Katrin Saluvere, Monika Strozik, Boguslav Suskis and Cristian Vladescu. We are also grateful to those individuals who contributed to the other output from this project, the special edition of *EuroHealth* on EU enlargement, which contains many case studies on which we were able to draw.

We would also like to thank all our colleagues in the Observatory for their continuing support. In particular we want to thank Caroline White, who has managed the overall production of the text, a description that does less than justice to the many tasks this involves, and to Sue Gammerman, who with Caroline organized the workshops in Warsaw. We are also grateful to Jeffrey Lazarus for managing the manuscript delivery and production and to Jo Woodhead for copy-editing some chapters.

Finally, we are grateful to the WHO Regional Office for Europe and DG Sanco of the European Commission for financial support for the book workshop.

Martin McKee, Laura MacLehose and Ellen Nolte

chapter one

Health and enlargement

Martin McKee, Laura MacLehose and Ellen Nolte

A historic enlargement

Just after 7 pm on 9 November 1989, Günter Schabowski, a member of the Communist Party *Politbüro* in Berlin, announced to a startled press conference that, for the first time since his city had been divided by the wall in 1961, private visits to the west would be permitted. When asked when this would happen he replied: "As far as I know, immediately" (Hilton 2001). Within a few hours, thousands of East German citizens had passed through the wall that had not just served as a barrier to them but which had symbolized the division of post-war Europe. Those events, along with others in Prague, Warsaw, Budapest, Sofia and Bucharest, led to a seismic shift in the political geography of Europe. Just over three months later, Lithuania declared its independence from the Soviet Union. This independence, along with that of its neighbours, became a reality in the aftermath of the coup against Mikhail Gorbachev on 18 August 1991.

Yet the political geography was also changing in western Europe. The original six members of the European Economic Community, brought together by the Treaty of Rome in 1957, had already undergone a series of expansions. The year 1973 saw the accession of Denmark, Ireland and the United Kingdom. In 1981 they were joined by Greece and then, in 1986 by Spain and Portugal, all countries that had recently made a successful transition to democracy. In 1993 the European Community became the European Union, with the passage into law of the Maastricht Treaty. Citizens of individual Member States became citizens of the European Union. Their governments began to move towards European Monetary Union, with most adopting a single currency, which went into circulation in January 2002. And they agreed to pursue a common foreign and security policy. The borders of the European Union also changed, with agreement on a further expansion, in 1995, bringing in three countries, Finland, Sweden and Austria, whose neutrality during the Cold War had led them to remain apart from the major blocs.

Taken together, these events in both parts of Europe made it inevitable that further change would occur. The Member States of the European Union indicated their willingness to welcome the newly democratic countries of central and eastern Europe, with one former communist state, the German Democratic Republic, becoming part of the European Union almost at once as it acceded to the Federal Republic of Germany. The countries of central and eastern Europe, and some others in southern Europe that had long been associated with the Union, indicated their willingness to join.

The process of European Union enlargement will have major implications for health and health care policy in all parts of Europe. This book looks at what these implications are and what responses are needed. It is one of a series of products on this topic arising from a study conducted by the European Observatory on Health Care Systems. Other products include a special edition of the journal *EuroHealth*, containing a series of detailed case studies on specific issues related to enlargement, many of which have been used to inform the writing of this book. In addition, this book is accompanied by a policy brief that examines concisely many of the key issues.

Health and enlargement

This book examines the relationship between health and enlargement. As the previous sections show, the relationship between European law and health and health policy is complex and multifaceted. In part this is because of the nature of the determinants of health and disease. The European Union has stated that it is pursuing a high level of health protection and public health, however, the policies that can contribute to these goals span almost the entire breadth of European Union activities. The situation with regard to health services is even more complex and dynamic, in part because of the failure to create a meaningful demarcation of the competence of the Member States and the European institutions. The process of enlargement is also complex, not least because of the diversity of candidate countries and the rapidity with which change is taking place.

No book on this subject can hope to be comprehensive, not least because so much of the pathway to accession and beyond is through uncharted territory. Instead, what we have tried to do is to take a series of issues in the area of health policy where accession to the European Union is likely to have an impact. Where possible we have looked at how particular candidate countries are adapting to the new circumstances but this can give only a partial picture. Consequently, we have also invited those who have gone through the process of accession to relate their experiences.

The book begins with three chapters that set the broad context for the remaining chapters. Chapter 2 first describes the political process of EU enlargement before looking at the complex and often confusing position of health and health services within the European system. It then reports on a survey undertaken for this book that seeks to identify the concerns of some of those most intimately involved in the health aspects of enlargement, and then, recognizing the dynamic nature of this process, reviews some of the things that have been happening as this book was being prepared.

Chapters 3 and 4 provide more background, looking at health and health systems within the candidate countries. The main message from these chapters is one that will be repeated throughout the book, that is the diversity of countries involved in this process and the variety of challenges they face. In particular, as Chapter 4 (on health systems) shows, that although there are many factors promoting convergence in the candidate countries, there are also many differences in the paths they are following.

In Chapter 5 we step back from the detailed process of accession to look at the case for investment in health in the candidate countries. Noting the large gap in economic performance between the current Member States and the candidate countries, Jennett draws on a growing body of evidence about the determinants of growth to show why it will be essential for the governments concerned, and for the European Union as a whole, to invest in activities that promote health in the candidate countries. Health and wealth are inextricably linked.

In Chapter 6 Nolte looks at the experience of the one former communist state so far to have joined the European Union, the former German Democratic Republic. Although in many ways unique, as it was essentially absorbed within the legal and constitutional framework of the Federal Republic, supported by a massive financial investment, it provides both examples of success and cautionary tales.

Chapters 7–10 look at the consequences of free movement of health professions. In Chapter 7, Nicholas reviews the current European legal framework within which professional mobility takes place. As in so many other areas where European law impacts on health policy she exposes ambiguities and contradictions, reflecting the absence of a coherent policy. After tracing the historical developments that have led to the current situation, she then looks in detail at the situation facing physicians, in particular the factors that determine how much movement takes place. In Chapter 8, Zajac looks at how one country, Poland, is adapting to the challenges posed by accession, establishing new systems of professional education and registration. Chapters 9 and 10, by Jakubowski and Hess and by Buchan and Rafferty respectively, look at the market for physicians and for nurses within the current European Union, in both cases speculating on the lessons of experience so far for candidate countries post-accession. In Chapter 11 we turn our attention to patients. Again, the situation is extremely fluid, as the problems with the existing legal framework give rise to a stream of cases before the European Court of Justice (ECJ), from which a body of law is emerging in an often confusing and piecemeal fashion.

Chapters 12 and 13 look at two areas where issues of public health have traditionally confronted those of free trade, health and safety and communicable disease surveillance and control. In both cases considerable investment is needed, with enlargement creating particular challenges for the EU as it finds itself bordering countries where there are still substantial health problems, such as Ukraine and the Russian Federation.

Chapter 14 looks at the issue of trade and health, focusing on two products that are lawfully traded but which have important implications for health: alcohol and tobacco. It asks the question, will accession raise or lower standards? It concludes that this will depend on where a country starts from, with evidence that it may weaken existing policies where they are already strong, but can strengthen those that are weak. Chapter 15 also looks beyond the health system to consider the impact of accession on some of the wider determinants of health, in particular through European agricultural policy.

Chapters 16 and 17 look at different aspects of pharmaceutical policy. In Chapter 16 Kanavos describes the results of a survey of how the candidate countries in central and eastern Europe have adopted new policies on pharmaceutical regulation and reimbursement, as well as the further challenges that lie ahead. In Chapter 17, Lobato looks back to the experience of an earlier accession, arguing that the adoption of European standards of patent protection was, contrary to some initial concerns, beneficial to Spain overall.

It is very unlikely that the European Union will stay still. Already several countries in south-east Europe are anxious to join and Chapter 18 looks at the challenges facing the countries in south-east Europe that form part of the Balkan Stability Pact, some of which are likely to be next in line to join the accession process.

Implications

As even this brief overview shows, the range of issues affected by the process of EU enlargement is enormous, each with implications for both acceding and existing Member States. Yet prediction of what the consequences of this complex process will be is fraught with problems. Most obviously, the institutions that the candidate countries are joining will themselves be very different when they have 25 rather than 15 members. The new Member States will have their own agendas to pursue in the Council of Ministers and the European Parliament. Prediction is even more difficult in the area of health policy. The ambiguous position of both public health and health care within the European Treaties has already created a great deal of confusion within the EU, not least because, as is most clearly seen in the area of patient mobility, the failure of Member States to address health issues within the legislative framework of the EU means that decisions are left to the ECJ, which ends up making law on a case-by-case basis. It is almost certain that, in the current ambiguous situation, the process of enlargement will throw up ever more complex cases for the ECJ to deal with.

Shortly after this book is published, the first wave of candidate countries will have taken their place as Member States. It might, therefore, be argued that this book will already be obsolete. Clearly we disagree. Despite the enormous progress so far, there will still be a substantial unfinished agenda. Passing a law is not the same as implementing it. There will be many opportunities for mutual learning, as those countries faced with problems learn from those who have already solved them. There is also a major unfinished agenda in relation to progress in health attainment and health system reform. As we show in this book, especially in the countries of central and eastern Europe, there is still a very long way to go to attain levels of health comparable to those in western Europe. Accession offers opportunities to accelerate progress, but as we show when considering trade and health, it also brings risks. There is a great deal to be done by countries themselves, regardless of their membership of the EU.

However, this book is also aimed at those countries that are not in the first wave or, as in south-east Europe, have yet to join the accession process. It is also aimed at those in countries where EU membership is a long way off, such as Ukraine, but which are already doing much to harmonize their laws with those in the EU.

The act of enlargement will be a momentous occasion for Europe; this book is an attempt to ensure that, in all the excitement, the cause of health is not overlooked.

Reference

Hilton, C. (2001) *The wall: the people's story*. Stroud: Sutton Publishing.

chapter two

The process of enlargement

Martin McKee, Magdalene Rosenmöller,
Laura MacLehose and Monika Zajac

Transition in central eastern Europe:
No choice: Enlargement was a must

Even though the fall of communism in the countries of central and eastern
Europe came as a complete surprise to most people, it very soon became clear
that these countries would, at some point, be joining the EU. This created high
expectations among politicians and populations alike and soon became an
important driver in the process of reform.

Almost at once, the EU started to negotiate Association Agreements with these
newly democratic countries of central Europe, based on existing ones signed
with Turkey (1963), Malta (1970) and Cyprus (1972). In 1993, there was a consensus that it was time to take things further. At the European Council in
Copenhagen, the then Member States explicitly stated that "the associated
countries in central and eastern Europe that so desire shall become members of
the European Union". It continued, saying that "accession will take place as
soon as an applicant is able to assume the obligations of membership by satisfy-
ing the economic and political conditions required". These obligations, subsequently referred to as the "Copenhagen Criteria", required the achievement of:

- stability of institutions guaranteeing *democracy*, the rule of law, human rights
  and respect for and protection of minorities;
- the existence of a *functioning market economy* as well as the capacity to cope
  with competitive pressure and market forces within the Union;
- the ability to *take on the obligations of membership* (the "*acquis communautaire*")
  including adherence to the aims of political, economic and monetary union
  and the creation of conditions for its integration through the adjustment of
  its administrative structures, so that European Community legislation can be
  transposed into national legislations implemented effectively through
  appropriate administrative and judicial structures.

There were many factors favouring enlargement, which was seen as bringing important benefits not only to the acceding states but also for the existing Member States and for the entire continent of Europe. First, using arguments reminiscent of those underlying the original European Economic Community, it enabled the creation of an extended zone of peace, stability and prosperity in a Europe that had, until very recently, been divided by the Cold War. Second, the addition of more than 100 million people, in rapidly growing economies, to the EU's 370 million was expected to boost economic growth and create jobs in both old and new Member States. Third, the adoption by the new Member States of EU policies for protection of the environment and the fight against crime, drugs and illegal migration would lead to a better quality of life overall for citizens throughout Europe. Fourth, the new Member States were expected to enrich the EU through increased cultural diversity, interchange of ideas, and better understanding of other peoples. Last but not least, an enlarged Europe would have a stronger role in world affairs – in foreign and security policy, trade policy, and the other fields of global governance, not least as a counterbalance to the United States in what seemed to be developing into an increasingly unipolar world. However, it should also be noted that some of those pressing for enlargement, in particular the then United Kingdom government, also saw the enlargement of the EU as a means to prevent further integration, given the very different economic situation of many of the potential candidate countries. Put another way, a broader Europe was an obstacle to a deeper Europe.

A key element of the obligations of membership is the adoption and implementation of what is termed the *acquis communautaire*. This is the accumulated body of European legislation that had been agreed throughout the evolution of the European Community and subsequent Union. The *acquis* comprises 31 Chapters, covering the entire range of EU policies. Those of particular relevance to health are Chapter 13, on social policy, and Chapter 23, on consumers and health protection. However, almost all have some implications for health, even if this is not well-recognized by those involved.

In December 1997 the European Council, meeting in Luxembourg, decided that sufficient progress had been made by the countries involved for it to be possible to initiate the enlargement process. The same year, European foreign ministers, meeting in Apeldoorn, agreed that discussions could begin with Turkey, which had applied unsuccessfully to join the EU in 1987, about entering into formal negotiations at some time in the future.

Thus, in March 1998, the EU began negotiations on accession with six countries: Cyprus, the Czech Republic, Estonia, Hungary, Poland and Slovenia. In September 1998 Malta reactivated its 1990 application, which it had frozen in 1996 and, in 1999, negotiations were extended to Bulgaria, Latvia, Lithuania, Romania and Slovakia. While some had considered that the initial six applicants would accede to the EU in a first wave, the 1999 European Council in Helsinki stated that all applicants, including Turkey, would be considered on an equal basis, with accession subject to meeting the entry (Copenhagen) criteria.

In October 2002, the European Commission recommended closing negotiations with ten countries: Cyprus, the Czech Republic, Estonia, Hungary, Latvia, Lithuania, Malta, Poland, Slovakia and Slovenia, on the basis that they now met

Table 2.1   The Chapters of the *acquis communautaire*

Chapter 1	Free Movement of Goods	Chapter 19	Telecommunications and
Chapter 2	Free Movement for Persons		Info
Chapter 3	Freedom to Provide Services	Chapter 20	Culture and Audiovisual
Chapter 4	Free Movement of Capital		Policy
Chapter 5	Company Law	Chapter 21	Regional Policy and
Chapter 6	Competition Policy		Coordination
Chapter 7	Agriculture	Chapter 22	Environment
Chapter 8	Fisheries	**Chapter 23**	**Consumers and Health**
Chapter 9	Transport Policy		**Protection**
Chapter 10	Taxation	Chapter 24	Justice and Home Affairs
Chapter 11	European Monetary Union	Chapter 25	Customs Union
Chapter 12	Statistics	Chapter 26	External Relations
Chapter 13	**Social Policy**	Chapter 27	Common Foreign and
Chapter 14	Energy		Security Policy
Chapter 15	Industrial Policy	Chapter 28	Financial Control
Chapter 16	Small and Medium	Chapter 29	Finance and Budgetary
	Enterprises		Provisions
Chapter 17	Science and Research	Chapter 30	Institutions Negotiations*
Chapter 18	Education and Training	Chapter 31	Other Negotiations*

* and Pre-Accession Coordination

the criteria for admission to the EU. This is now scheduled to take place in May 2004, in time to participate in the 2004 elections to the European Parliament. It is hoped that negotiations will be completed with Romania and Bulgaria soon after, leading to accession in 2007. There is, as yet, no agreed target date for Turkey's accession.

It is apparent that the current enlargement process differs greatly from those that have gone before, both in scale and nature. The number of countries in the EU will increase by 80%. Its surface area will expand by 34% and its population will increase by 28%. However, the greatest difference between this expansion and the earlier ones is the difference between the existing members and many of the new ones. It is the economic gap that has so far attracted most attention, with the 2001 Gross Domestic Product (GDP) per capita less than half of the average of the current Member States, although the gap is less when adjusted for differences in purchasing power. Equally importantly, in view of the current systems of EU funding, the nature of the economies differ. Whereas agriculture accounts for 2.1% of the economy in the existing Member States, it represents 13.8% and 14.4% respectively of the economies in Bulgaria and Romania.

However, the difference between the candidate and existing Member States is equally apparent in many other measures of the progress of nations. Of particular relevance in the present context, life expectancy at birth is below that of Portugal, the lowest among the current Member States, in all candidate countries except Cyprus and Malta. Major differences also exist between the acceding countries themselves, making the writing of this book a difficult endeavour.

There is considerable heterogeneity within the candidate countries. GDP per capita in 2001 varied eight-fold, from €1900 in Bulgaria to €15 100 in Cyprus. Life expectancy at birth is close to the EU average in Malta and Cyprus, but nine years less in Turkey and over eight years less in Latvia. This diversity is especially apparent when one looks at the recent political history of each country. Three candidate countries (Estonia, Latvia and Lithuania) were part of the Soviet Union until 1991. Three others (the Czech Republic, Slovakia and Slovenia), were parts of other larger states until just over a decade ago, two (Cyprus and Malta) have been non-aligned democracies since independence from the United Kingdom in the 1960s, and one (Turkey) has been a long-standing member of NATO, with a period of military rule in the 1980s.

Enlargement will not only affect the candidate countries. As even this brief exploration shows, the EU will change considerably after 2004. Largely in response to the challenges of enlargement, the EU engaged in a wide-ranging process of reform in the late 1990s, entitled Agenda 2000. This involves legislative action in four main areas: the reform of the common agricultural policy, structural policy reform, the development of pre-accession instruments and a new financial framework. The Constitutional Convention, being discussed at the time of writing, will change fundamentally the ways in which the institutions of the EU work together. As a consequence, any consideration of enlargement must also look at the implications for existing Member States, as they become part of a much larger, and more complex entity, and one that is characterized by much greater diversity in both wealth and health.

A shifting target – health and European law

Before exploring health in the enlargement process it might be useful to take a brief look at health in the process of European integration. As described in more detail by some of the authors in other publications (McKee et al. 2002; Mossialos and McKee 2002) considerations of health appeared only slowly during the construction of Europe, while at the same time the scope of European law expanded in areas that impinged on health care. This mutual interaction of health and European law already poses a series of challenges for existing Member States, while enlargement is adding to this complexity.

The EU was founded by the 1957 Treaty of Rome with its political goal being the desire to prevent a future war between France and Germany, which had been the cause of so much suffering three times in the preceding 100 years. But the provisions were nearly exclusively economic, viewing existing tariff barriers as an obstacle to economic growth. As a consequence, the emphasis was on free movement, enshrined in the four fundamental freedoms of movement, of goods, capital, people and services.

As with all international provisions on free movement, dating back at least as far as the introduction of quarantine by the Venetian Republic, opening of borders was counterbalanced in the Treaty of Rome by the ability to block movement on grounds of public health, but otherwise the Treaty had little to say about health. The one exception was always very peripheral; the European Economic Community had inherited from its predecessor Treaties on coal and steel and atomic energy with a responsibility for occupational health services for workers in the coal, steel and nuclear industry in border areas. Consequently, its competence in the broader area of health was considered by most commentators to be extremely limited.

It was, therefore, a surprise to many when, in 1986, the European Community adopted the *Europe against Cancer Programme*. Unlike most other Community actions, where the legal basis for action is set out in considerable detail, in this case it was simply justified on the basis of its compliance with "the Treaty establishing the EC", which listed one objective of the European Community as "accelerated raising of the standard of living". Although several commentators have noted that this legal basis was, at best, dubious, high level political support, in particular from the then French President Mitterand, and a lack of any concerted opposition from other Member States meant that the arguments in favour of it were accepted.

In 1993 an element, albeit somewhat limited, of clarity was introduced by the

---

Box 2.1   A short introduction to the European legislative process

The primary basis for EU legislation is formed by a series of Treaties, agreed by the governments of the Member States, from the 1957 founding Treaty of Rome to the most recent Treaty of Nice. Once ratified, the Treaties determine the competence at EU level and what remains the responsibility of Member States.

The Treaties set out the broad goals of the EU so it is generally necessary for them to be interpreted and applied to specific areas of policy. Although there is a variety of ways in which this can take place, depending on the topic involved, the most common is for the European Commission (a body of international civil servants, headed by a president and commissioners appointed by the Member States) to propose legislation to the Council of Ministers (representing the governments of Member States) and the European Parliament (directly elected by the citizens of Europe). Approval of the legislation is normally subject to agreement by both bodies, with a conciliation mechanism in case of disagreement. Agreement by the Council of Ministers can be either by unanimity or by qualified majority voting.

European legislation, which takes priority over national legislation, can take several forms. *Regulations* are specific measures that have immediate and direct force of law without adaptation to national circumstances, common in areas such as external trade. The most common type of legislation is the *Directive*. This sets out the goals to be achieved but leaves it to each Member State to determine how to achieve them. Once passed, a Directive must be passed into national law within a designated period. Other instruments include *Decisions*, which are also legally binding but which do not have general effect, and *Recommendations* and *Opinions*, which are not legally binding.

Inevitably there will be circumstances in which the precise applicability of a piece of legislation is unclear. It then will fall to the European Court of Justice (ECJ) to decide. The ECJ interprets the law on the basis of the fundamental goals of the EU, and in particular the pursuit of the fundamental freedoms. As a consequence, in the relative absence of specific legislative activity in the field of health care, it is often the ECJ that has made laws. In particular, it has played an important role in the extension of rights of patients to seek care in other Member States.

Treaty of Maastricht, which stated that the Community will *contribute to a high level of health protection for its citizens* and inserted a new Article, number 129, into the Treaty, giving force to this new objective. Article 129 made provision for community action to prevent diseases, in particular major health scourges. The only one mentioned specifically was drug dependence, largely to ensure that this issue was not addressed solely within the framework of law enforcement, and so outside the mechanisms of the EU. Importantly it specified that health protection should form a part of the Community's other policies, so generating a long running debate about the provision of subsidies to tobacco production under the Common Agricultural Policy. However, Community institutions were limited to coordination of policies and programmes, but were prevented from harmonizing legislation.

For Community action to take place, four criteria should be fulfilled. First, there is a significant health problem for which *appropriate preventive actions* are possible. Second, the proposed activity must *supplement or promote* other Community policies such as the operation of the internal market. Third, Community actions are to be *consistent* with those of other international organizations, and in particular the World Health Organization. Fourth, the aim of Community action must be such that it cannot be achieved by Member States acting alone. The last of these is an expression of the concept of *subsidiarity*, whereby action at the level of the European Community should go no further than needed to achieve the stated objective.

In practice, Article 129 provided the basis for a programme of action in health promotion, information, education and training in public health. This took a rather broader view of health determinants than the "major scourges", although it did focus mainly on a limited number of topics including cancer, AIDS and other communicable diseases, health data, injuries, pollution-related diseases and rare diseases.

While many public health advocates in Europe welcomed the new Article, there was also a widespread view among them that it did not go far enough. In particular there was concern about the ambiguous position of health services; with some arguing that policies to promote health that ignore the contribution of health services are untenable. Yet health care was an area into which many governments did not wish to stray, for various reasons. This was a view seemingly shared by the then president of the European Commission, Jacques Delors, who had otherwise been a strong advocate of further European integration, when he remarked that this was an "inappropriate" area for the EU (Brown 1995).

Consequently, in the run up to the next Treaty revision, at Amsterdam (1997) there was no clear consensus in favour of changing Article 129. Although it had been a compromise between advocates of a more expansive and more limited Union, it to some extent met all of their concerns, permitting some action but limiting what might be agreed in the future. However, the situation was about to change. A new disease, Bovine Spongiform Encephalopathy (BSE), had emerged in cattle, especially in the United Kingdom, although with smaller numbers of cases across Europe. Belatedly the British Government accepted that the spread of this disease to humans was the reason for a growing number of cases of a rapidly degenerative brain disease in young adults. The response to these new developments was extremely inadequate, characterized by denial, collusion with vested interests, and incompetence (McKee et al. 1996). In a subsequent European Parliament inquiry, British officials were found to have misled their EU counterparts. The EU's health protection arrangements had been tested and found wanting. Similar weaknesses were becoming apparent in other countries, in particular in relation to contamination of blood products in France. Treaty revision became inevitable.

Article 152 of the Treaty of Amsterdam is, however, widely seen as having many of the limitations of Article 129. It was inserted at the last moment, with minimal consultation, and as yet another compromise, it is in places confusing and almost self-contradictory, in marked contrast to, for example, articles on consumer protection or the environment. However, it does introduce greater clarity in some areas. Thus, for the first time, it is stated that Community action shall be directed towards improving public health, although what is meant by public health remains unclear.

A further lack of clarity arises from the indistinct border between public health and policies in many other areas, such as the environment (with the relevant Treaty article again emphasizing the role of community action in promoting public health), and consumer protection. Indeed, it can be argued that health considerations are implicit in many other articles of the Treaty, such as research, agriculture and social policy. Furthermore, any mechanisms to promote free movement of people must ensure that, in moving, they are not subjected to unnecessary threats to their health. Similarly, free movement of goods is only possible if there are mechanisms to ensure that those goods are safe.

Notwithstanding this lack of clarity, it is now apparent that public health is attaining a higher priority within the EU. Developments in health policy at a European level have long been a consequence of "spill-over", being introduced in response to policies in other areas. Thus, free movement of goods was only acceptable if manufacturers were subject to a level playing field in relation to any costs imposed by health and safety requirements. Similar considerations apply to food production, with free movement of food products only acceptable if mechanisms existed to ensure production was safe. However, the EU is now taking action in areas where the principle goal is the promotion of health, most notably action against tobacco, a still lawfully traded good that is one of the leading causes of premature death and disability in Europe. The challenges are made even more evident in the light of enlargement and the significant institutional capacity gaps that may exist in some candidate countries. However, the occasion of enlargement might be seized by the EU as an opportunity to bring forward much needed initiatives to support national actions in a series of health and health care related areas.

Adding to the complexity – health services and European law

The Amsterdam Treaty also seeks to clarify how EU law affects health services, stating that "Community action in the field of public health shall fully respect the responsibilities of the Member States for the organisation and delivery of health services and medical care". The exclusion of health services from the competence of the EU, but solely that of national governments was considered by many of those governments as a definitive statement. However, the true situation soon proved not to be quite so simple and as we will see in subsequent chapters the limited institutional capacity in some candidate countries will add to the complexity of the interaction between internal market and national health systems.

There is now a broad consensus within Europe that health services cannot be regarded simply as another type of service or be left to the market, as those in most need of them are often least likely to be able to afford them, and the interactions between users and providers are characterized by widespread asymmetries of information, placing the user in a potentially vulnerable position.

Following the European principle of "solidarity", all countries in Europe, including the transition countries, have established systems to ensure universal, or near universal coverage (a few countries, such as Germany and the Netherlands, make exceptions for the well-off as they are assumed to be able to take care of themselves). These systems, while configured in many different ways, all involve a complex set of heavily regulated relationships between those collecting and dispersing funds and those providing care. As a consequence, many Member States have had concerns that opening up health care to the single European market could have the consequence of undermining some of these relationships, in particular those using constraints on capacity as a means of cost containment.

Yet even if health services are exempted from the Treaty, on the basis of the wording agreed at Amsterdam, health services can only operate by using many things that are covered by the single market. Free movement embraces goods, such as medical technology and pharmaceuticals, people, such as patients and health professionals, and services, such as some providers of health care or the activities that are required for health care to function. Thus, the process of acquisition of these things is subject to European law, in particular in that it must be transparent and non-discriminatory. As already seen, the EU has developed an extensive body of legislation covering many areas that are directly involved in the provision of health care.

It has long been apparent that a single market, guaranteeing freedom of movement of people, can only function if those people can travel without fear of losing the protection they enjoy in their own countries in respect of health care. Thus, a series of directives in the early 1970s set out mechanisms for various groups of people whose work involved cross-border travel to receive health care in other Member States, with provisions for those abroad temporarily to obtain care in an emergency. In addition, mechanisms were put in place to enable those organizations paying for health care to send patients abroad for treatment. The latter provisions emphasized the central role of the health care payer. Patients wishing to receive treatment elsewhere for a pre-existing condition were required to obtain prior authorization from the payer. An important reason for this restriction was the need to ensure that patient flows did not damage national health care infrastructures, by making some facilities nonviable, or by undermining cost-containment mechanisms.

This situation began to change in 1998 with two rulings by the ECJ in cases where citizens of Luxembourg, which operates on the basis of reimbursement of expenses incurred by patients, sought the right to be reimbursed for the purchase of spectacles and orthodontic treatment in Belgium and Germany respectively. Although several governments argued before the ECJ that free movement of goods and services did not apply to social security systems, the ECJ held that while "Community law does not detract from the powers of the Member States to organise their social security systems" this does not mean that "the social security sector constitutes an island beyond the reach of community law". The right to obtain health care without prior authorization was thus upheld, and rulings in subsequent cases have extended the scope of European law to health care systems in which the patient does not have to pay and then be reimbursed; and to hospital care.

The formal situation in relation to health systems is therefore somewhat confused. Many governments that had previously been reassured that the Treaty provisions put health services beyond the reach of the EU have had their complacency challenged by the rulings of the ECJ. At the same time, some are beginning to see the potential benefits from greater collaboration, in particular where they face shortages of capacity or have identified concrete benefits for cooperating across frontiers. In some cases, as between Northern Ireland and the Republic of Ireland, greater cooperation in the health care sector may even be primarily a mechanism to achieve other goals, in this case peace and reconciliation.

In the absence of a clear legal basis for action in the Treaty, one possibility that is attracting increasing attention is the Open Method of Coordination, established at the 2000 Lisbon European Council. This facilitates exchange of best practice and achieving greater convergence in areas where harmonization of legislation is not possible. It involves agreeing broad goals, establishing indicators and benchmarks of good practice, developing guidelines for policy, with targets to be achieved, that can be adopted where possible, and establishing a system of monitoring that is organized on the basis of mutual learning. The High Level Process on Patient Mobility, established in February 2003 by the health ministers of 14 Member States and coordinated by the European Commission, started to look into these issues. In June 2003 health ministers of the candidate countries were asked to join this process. All these developments seem to indicate a wider recognition that Treaty revision may be necessary. These issues, as they affect both candidate countries and existing Member States, will be explored in later chapters.

Health in the enlargement process and arrangements to facilitate accession

Having seen the complex situation of health within the European system, the next section examines what has been done to facilitate its incorporation in the process of enlargement, with a particular focus on the transition countries of central and eastern Europe. The political changes in these countries at the end of the 1980s triggered a major departure from central planning towards market-based economies and democracy. The simultaneous political and economical transition was compared with "building a ship at sea" (Elster et al. 1998). It was a very painful process, especially in the early phase. All countries witnessed, to some degree, a profound fiscal crisis, increases in inflation and unemployment, widening income gaps and increases in crime. Health sector reform in such a situation was inevitably a difficult endeavour, exacerbated by the challenges to public health and the legacy of failing communist era health systems. Implementation of reform was often less rapid and successful than anticipated. Furthermore, an emphasis on reform in other sectors, coupled with political instability and weak managerial capacity also slowed down the process (Rosenmöller 2002b).

Support for the transition process came from various sources. The European Commission was quick to launch the *Phare programme* in 1989. Phare originally stood for "Poland Hungarian Assistance for the Reconstruction of the Economy" and, as the French word "*phare*" (lighthouse) indicates, was meant to be a sign of hope, a light in the storm. The Phare programme became the single most important source of assistance to the candidate countries. In 1999 it accounted for 36% of total development assistance to central and eastern Europe (CEE) (OECD DAC 2000).

At a time when accession was only an aspiration, Phare responded to the most urgent needs of the transition process. For the first half of the 1990s funding was "demand driven", aimed at systems development, knowledge transfer and human resource development. Health reform projects were initiated in Poland, Hungary and Czechoslovakia (as it then was). Other countries soon followed. From 1990 to 1998 Phare committed a total of €105 million to health sector reform in CEE, supporting health system developments such as: sustainable financing; hospital management; primary care development; information systems; pharmaceutical sector regulation; and human resource management.

The basis of accession, as laid out at the 1993 Copenhagen summit, prompted the redefinition and subsequent reorganization of the Phare programme, taking effect in 1995. At that point it became "accession driven", a tool to support countries in their preparations for joining the EU. The key focus was on transposing the *acquis communautaire* into national legislation. Phare concentrated on the development of institutional capacity and investment in infrastructure. As health care was not a competence at Community level and thus not a central issue in the accession process, Phare health sector support was essentially discontinued. Funds devoted to health dropped from 3% of the total Phare budget in 1990 to 0.5% in 1996, while the need for technical and investment assistance in the health sector remained high, as incomplete reforms left much to be done (Rosenmöller 2001).

Many of the remaining Phare funds went into twinning arrangements (supporting cooperation between similar institutions in candidate countries and Member States). In particular, twinning supported the adoption of health-related acquis such as occupational health, phyto-sanitary control and food safety. Additionally Phare contributed to the participation of candidate countries in EU public health and research programmes. After initial bureaucratic problems facing both the EU and the candidate countries were resolved, all countries participated in both programmes.

Support was also provided by other organizations. The European Investment

Bank (EIB) provides long-term investment for closing the income gap between rich and less advantaged regions in Europe. The EIB started to invest in CEE in the early 1990s with a total of €15 billion, seeing it as a major and growing area for lending. Its increasing focus on the public sector encompasses health, where capital requirements are high, especially in CEE (European Investment Bank 2001). In 1991 the EU established the European Bank for Reconstruction and Development (EBRD) with a mandate to facilitate the development of market economy in CEE. It became the largest single investor in the region, investing a total of €9 billion during the 1990s. Although no direct support was granted to the health sector, the EBRD played an important indirect role by improving the overall economic context within which health systems operated.

The World Bank has also played an important role in supporting health reform in the CEE (Preker and Feachem 1996). Besides the provision of vital technical analysis at the beginning of the transition, World Bank loans supported health services development; hospital restructuring; primary health care; decentralization; and the pharmaceutical sector. The main recipients of the World Bank's US $561 million health portfolio over the 1990s were Romania, Poland, Hungary, Bulgaria, Estonia and Latvia. Projects have taken accession-related issues very seriously, in particular strengthening institutional capacity. A memorandum of understanding signed in 2000 allows for co-financing of accession-related programmes by the Commission and the international financing institutions.

The World Bank's support is likely to continue beyond the official accession date. Its "graduation policy" foresees a review of borrowing countries according to their per capita income. Other countries (for example Italy, Netherlands, Ireland and Portugal) continued to borrow from the World Bank even after becoming EU members, each then relatively wealthier than many present candidate countries (World Bank 2002). The International Finance Corporation (IFC), the private sector arm of the World Bank Group, committed a total of US $40 million over the 1990s for health care projects such as diagnostic imaging, haemodialysis centres, medical services companies and distribution of medical supplies. Other international organizations gave valuable technical assistance: the OECD supported the development of national accounts including health expenditure surveys, often in cooperation with Phare; the WHO Regional Office for Europe with their "liaison officers" in CEE health ministries, supported the policy-making function with the technical resources of the WHO Europe office. The frequently updated WHO HiTs (Health Care Systems in Transition profiles) provide a regular update on each country's reform progress. CEE officials are integrated in the different WHO Europe networks.

EU Member States and others have also provided substantial bilateral support with the aim of transferring know-how, fostering economic development, and creating new opportunities for the donor countries. More specifically, bilateral aid has supported health system development and public health activities as an important factor promoting social sustainability through the period of transition. Aid often followed traditional links; for example, the Scandinavian countries were very active in the Baltic region and France in Romania. Similarly, Germany and Austria have been closely involved in supporting those countries with a pre-Second World War Bismarckian type of health system, such as the Czech Republic, Slovakia and Hungary (Rosenmöller 2002a).

Support from the most recently acceding EU Member States has been of particular interest. Austria has shared its experience of European integration with several countries; Finland has supported health and safety at work initiatives; and Sweden has promoted direct cooperation between research institutions. Other smaller donors have identified niches. Belgium has supported anti-drug policies in Romania and Poland and Ireland has contributed to WHO-Europe managed nursing and midwifery projects (EC Consensus 1998).

Meeting expectations? The views of health policy makers in candidate countries

What do the countries themselves think about accession? The preceding sections have set out an image of "Europe and health" that is frequently one of uncertainty and ambiguity, with many issues unresolved. What do those who are about to join the EU think that membership will bring for their countries? For the purposes of this study, a Delphi study was undertaken among key informants from the departments for European and international affairs of the candidate countries' Ministries of Health (or ministries responsible for health issues such as the Ministry of Social Affairs in Estonia). Each was asked what s/he perceived to be the challenges and benefits arising from EU accession. The iterative, three round process of the Delphi technique, developed by the Rand Corporation in 1948 (Lindeman 1981) had the advantage that key informants could, without geographical constraints, anonymously exchange their opinions, with the final results reflecting the extent of consensus among the entire group. This avoided the discussion being dominated by a few individuals (Fink et al. 1984).

Candidate countries at different stages of accession negotiation have different levels of experience and knowledge about EU health policy. Consequently in the first round they were asked to define the topics of most importance to them, which then were addressed in a second round. The first round contained five open questions (Box 2.2). Respondents were asked to create their own lists of challenges and benefits for the health of their populations and health systems separately and then to propose areas that need further attention. In the second round, responses were grouped using a process of constant comparison. The themes and the topics under each theme were then sent back to the experts for ranking by importance, as a means of clarifying understanding and adding more detail.

The most important challenges to the candidate countries' health systems were perceived to be the process of harmonization of health care legislation, the upward pressure on health care expenditure and the need to improve population health as a means of reducing demand on health services. Other issues were quality standards, health system performance, equity and the pharmaceutical sector. Somewhat surprisingly, issues usually regarded as important, such as increasing professional mobility and enhancing patients' rights, were ranked lowest.

Box 2.2 Open questions in the Round 1 questionnaire

- What are the *5 main challenges* that the accession process will pose for the *health system* of your country?
- What are the *5 main challenges* that the accession process will pose for the *health of your population*?
- What are the *5 main benefits* for your *health system* that you expect as a result of joining the EU?
- What are the *5 main benefits* for the *health of your population* that you foresee as a result of joining the EU?
- What are the *5 main health issues* facing accession countries in general that need further attention at the EU level?

For the potential challenges to the health of the population in candidate countries again some findings were intuitive and others less so. There was a clear identification of the challenge posed by the need to enhance the role of public health and to improve policies on prevention. Similarly improving the population's socioeconomic status was seen as problematic. Perhaps less intuitively, the threat of communicable diseases related to increased free movement (of patients and of professionals) was ranked relatively low.

Potential benefits of EU membership for health care systems were seen in the fact that a European consensus could facilitate improvement in quality of facilities and services. The rankings within themes showed that there were particularly high expectations in relation to topics such as benchmarking and introducing more evidence-based policies. EU membership was also seen as enhancing the scope for public participation in the health system. Once again, any benefits stemming from free movement of patients and professionals ranked low on the list. Potential benefits to the health of the population were seen in the increasing focus on public health, the strengthening of regulations and guidelines and improving quality and access to health services. Again patient rights ranked quite low.

Finally, the greatest priority for more attention at EU level was considered to be the need to address the perceived tension between health policy at EU and national levels, reflecting some continuing confusion about the precise interpretation of subsidiarity. Other concerns largely reflect existing EU competencies in the broad area of health protection, such as environmental health, food safety and communicable disease control. However, improved health care performance, an area that is technically excluded from the competence of the EU, was also ranked relatively highly, while the development of common policies in areas such as mental health and chronic diseases were regarded as relatively less important.

The interpretation of the results is not that straightforward. The study design had some limitations: each country was represented by a single key informant, located in a single ministry. Although those informants were asked to draw on the views of others, doubts remains about the degree of representation, particularly given the large diversity of opinions in each country, which would be extremely difficult to capture.

However, it showed that, in general, there was a considerable consistency across countries, although it also revealed that not all topics that, intuitively, might have been considered as important, were viewed in this way by some of those most involved. It identified concerns about the process of harmonizing European and domestic legislation, with some uncertainty about the balance between national and European health policy-making. EU accession was seen as bringing challenges, but also benefits. However, some of the issues that might otherwise be considered as most important were given a relatively low priority, in particular greater movement of health professionals and patients. Importantly, these issues, not seen as important in health ministries, were the subjects of greatest concern among policy-makers drawn from a wider constituency who attended a workshop to review this project in June 2003.

Recent developments

At the end of the 1990s, it became clear that health should receive a greater emphasis in the enlargement process, in particular in the transition countries. Representatives of Member States participating in the High Level Committee on Health, a six-monthly informal policy meeting between the Commission and policy-makers from the Member States, argued for health and enlargement to be higher on the Commission's agenda. Consequently the Public Health Unit in what was then Directorate-Generale V (DG V) organized a study partially funded by EC Phare Consensus. This led to the publication of the *Commission Staff Working Paper SEC* (1999)713 on health and enlargement (European Commission 1999). Even though the document recognized the differences between accession countries, it outlined a series of key issues present to different degrees in all countries: the lack of well-defined modern public health policy concepts, increases in communicable diseases together with a decline in vaccination coverage, increases in drug use, the need for better emergency facilities, the low social status of health professionals, the lack of involvement of civil society and the negative health impact of environmental degradation.

The document proposes a series of options in response to these challenges. Many have since been put into practice, such as enabling candidate countries to participate in Community programmes, encouraging their involvement in EU health and research activities, and enhanced communication. Country specific studies were undertaken under the health monitoring programme in collaboration with the WHO Regional Office for Europe, producing the *"Highlights on Health in the Candidate Countries"* series (European Commission 2003). However, in some areas such as enhancing institutional capacity, there is still much to be done.

Although the British (1998,1), Austrian (1998,2) and German (1999,1) European Presidencies organized some activities concerning health and enlargement, the topic was first placed formally on the Health Council agenda under the Finnish presidency. The November 1999 Health Council reacted very positively to the Commission's Staff Working Paper, recognizing the "external" dimension of health issues, and highlighted the need to take into account health issues beyond the borders of the EU when developing a health strategy

(Council of the European Union 2002). Since then health and enlargement has been on successive Council agendas. Candidate countries' ministers began to join health council meetings, while their ministerial officials regularly participate at the high level committees. Subsequent EU presidencies organized specific health and enlargement conferences, such as Sweden in June 2001 and Greece in May 2003.

The European Parliament, too, started to place a higher emphasis on this issue. A Public Hearing on Health and Enlargement was organized in November 1998, forming the basis for the Needle report (Needle 1999). The fifth parliamentary term (1999–2004) was the setting for another public hearing (July 2000) resulting in the Bowis report (2000) which again stressed the importance of health in the enlargement process (Bowis and Oomen-Ruijten 2000).

The *Regular Reports* monitoring countries' progress towards accession, published by the European Commission annually in autumn, concentrated mainly on the "hard" acquis, but noted that most countries lagged behind in health care reform, especially with regard to economic sustainability of health systems. The 2000 report on Hungary states that "weak financial structures in the health care system continue to place a heavy burden on public finances" (European Commission 2002).

Most health related chapters in the "hard acquis", were completed by 2001, such as Chapters 13 and 23 covering areas such as health and safety at work, phyto-sanitary health, food safety and consumer protection. But implementation and enforcement were very slow to develop. In particular the tobacco directive was transposed very late. Conditions for the mutual recognition of health care qualifications have remained problematic. In many countries this was largely due to the overlap in responsibilities of different professional organizations. Similarly the creation of networks of epidemiological surveillance and control of communicable diseases was adopted late and has yet to be implemented in most countries. Collaboration with the European Centre for Drug Monitoring in Lisbon has been established but nationally the fight against drugs has often been hindered by a lack of inter-ministerial coordination.

Candidate countries have only slowly begun to participate in Community health programmes in 2000, with the AIDS, Cancer, Drugs and Health Promotion programmes attracting the most active participation. Hesitation on part of the candidate countries has reflected the considerable bureaucratic hurdles and, in many cases, the need for complementary funding. The health monitoring programme, while covering many issues of great importance for candidate countries, has attracted little participation by these countries. Since then the candidate countries have been more actively involved in the preparation and implementation of the new EU Public Health programme, with its three strands: health information, rapid reaction to threats to health and health determinants. The additional "cross cutting" issues included a particular focus on health and enlargement, which apparently attracted great interest in the first call for proposals under the new programme in March 2003.

In November 2002 the first ever recommendations of the European Health Policy Forum (EHPF) dealt with health and enlargement (European Health Policy Forum 2002). The EHPF is part of the European Health Forum, an "information and consultation mechanism of stakeholders in the health field, created to ensure that the European Commission's health strategy is transparent and responds to public concerns". It has a multi-faced structure including three main elements; the wider, *open forum*, to be organized first in spring 2004; a *virtual forum*, an interactive internet page currently in consultation and preparation process and the mentioned *health policy forum*. The latter is formed by 40 permanent members: non-governmental organizations (NGOs) and other not-for-profit organizations in the public health field, patient organizations, representations of health professionals, trade unions, health service providers, health insurances and the health industry. The criterion for participation is being "truly European", that is, operating at the EU level. Since its inception in July 2001 the forum has held regular meetings every six months.

The recommendations by the EHPF on health and enlargement were elaborated by the European Heart Network (EHN), and the European Health Management Association (EHMA) in an iterative consultancy process with EHPF members, starting in April 2002. The final version was adopted in November 2002. The objective was to draw attention to the challenges posed by an increasingly integrated Europe to public health and health systems in the context of enlargement. The study recognizes the differences between candidate countries but draws attention to their common challenges. It sets out some important issues that Europe will have to address such as free movement of patients and professionals (topics such as professional qualifications, potential "brain drain"), pharmaceutical policy, tobacco advertising and food safety. It argues that weak institutional capacity and lack of experience in some candidate countries might inhibit them from participating fully in existing EU programmes, such as the communicable disease network or the new public health programme. It also argues that, given these challenges, the European Commission should assume a more important role in health throughout an enlarged EU. The report notes the imminence of enlargement and thus the necessity that work should begin swiftly, but also that many things currently seen as challenges of enlargement will require longer-term solutions to continue long after accession has occurred. It recommends promoting investment in public health and health systems and building a civil society, in particular supporting development of associations of professionals, health care providers and the public, and more targeted use of the Public Health Programme and of regional and structural funds, EIB investments and the Sixth Framework programme for research.

In the June 2003 meeting of the EHPF the Commission responded to these recommendations. The document has been disseminated among Member States, the European Parliament and others, attracting much interest. The Open Forum meeting planned for early 2004 is expected to focus primarily on the imminent enlargement. "Health and enlargement" will stay on the EHPF agenda – even though a better name will be needed in 2004 when the candidate countries will be Member States.

In conclusion, this chapter highlights the existing complexity of the relationship between health and health services and European law, a complexity that will be accentuated by enlargement. As the Delphi study shows, there is considerable concern about how to respond to this complexity, and its many ambiguities in candidate countries. Yet while the challenges that health and health systems pose to the process of enlargement are increasingly recognized, and while much has already been achieved, much more has still to be done in many areas. Many of these issues will be examined in subsequent chapters of this book.

References

Bowis, J. and Oomen-Ruijten, G.H.C. (2000) Report on public health and consumer protection aspects of enlargement. Brussels: European Parliament, Committee on the Environment, Public Health and Consumer Policy.

Brown, K. (1995) Government to Demand Curb on European Court, *Financial Times*, 2 February.

Council of the European Union (2002) 2219th Meeting of the Council (HEALTH), Brussels, 18 November 1999.

EC Consensus (1998) Technical Assistance to the CEEC by the European Commission, Member States, International Organisations and others. Consensus Internal Document. Brussels: EC Phare Consensus Programme.

Elster, J., Offe, C., Preuss, U.K., et al. (1998) *Institutional Design in Post-communist Societies. Rebuilding a Ship at Sea.* Cambridge: Cambridge University Press.

European Commission (1999) Commission Staff Working Paper on Health and Enlargement. Luxembourg: Commission of the European Communities.

European Commission (2002) Regular Report from the Commission on Progress towards Accession by each of the Candidate Countries. Brussels: European Commission.

European Commission (2003) Highlights on Health in the Candidate Countries. Outcome from a project of the Health Monitoring Programme (1997–2002). Brussels: European Communities and World Health Organisation.

European Health Policy Forum (2002) Recommendation for Community Action on Health and Enlargement. Brussels: European Health Policy Forum, EHMA and EHN.

European Investment Bank (2001) The Bank's Operations in the Accession Countries of Central and Eastern Europe. Review of Current and Future Lending Policy. Luxembourg: EIB.

Fink, A., Kosecoff, J., Chassin, M. and Brook, R. (1984) Consensus methods: characteristics and guidelines for use, *American Journal of Public Health*, 74(9):979–83.

Lindeman, C.A. (1981) Priorities within the health care system: a Delphi survey, *American Nurses' Association*, 5:1–49.

McKee, M., Lang, T. and Roberts, J. (1996) Deregulating Health: Policy Lessons of the BSE Affair, *Journal of the Royal Society of Medicine*, (89):424–6.

McKee, M., Mossialos, E. and Baeten, R. (eds) (2002) *The Impact of EU Law on Health Care Systems*. Brussels: Peter Lang.

Mossialos, E. and McKee, M. (2002) *EU Law and the Social Character of Health Care*. Brussels: Peter Lang.

Needle, C. (1999) Report on the development of public health policy in the European Community European Parliament. Strasbourg: Committee on the Environment, Public Health and Consumer Policy.

OECD DAC (2000) Development Cooperation Report 2000. Paris: OECD Development Assistance Committee.

Preker, A.S. and Feachem, R.G.A. (1996) Facing the Health Challenge of the 21st Century: The Role of the World Bank, *EuroHealth*, 2(3):12–14.

Rosenmöller, M. (2001) Health and Enlargement. Halfway there, *Eurohealth*, 6(5):9–11.

Rosenmöller, M. (2002a) Health and Support for EU accession. Phare and other initiatives, *Eurohealth*, 8(4 Special Issue, Autumn 2002):36–8.

Rosenmöller, M. (2002b) *The Influence of Contextual Factors on the Implementation of*

Health Care Reform in the Countries of Central and Eastern Europe. Draft. London: LSHTM.

World Bank (2002) Review of Bank's activities in the Health Sector in Europe and Central Asia 1990–2000. Draft. Washington: The World Bank.

chapter three

Health status and trends in candidate countries

Martin McKee, Roza Adany and Laura MacLehose

Different countries, different challenges to health

A first step in understanding the consequences of enlargement for health is to describe current patterns and trends in health in the candidate countries. In Chapter 1 it was noted that this poses a challenge. The countries are extremely diverse, ranging from the three Baltic republics, with relatively low levels of life expectancy that have mirrored those in the Russian Federation for most of the 1990s, to Malta and Cyprus, where life expectancy is already close to the current EU average.

It is, however, possible to discern three broad categories among the candidate countries, first in terms of their levels of health and accompanying risk factors and, second, in terms of availability of data. The three categories comprise, first, the countries of central and eastern Europe (CEE), second, Malta and Cyprus, and third, Turkey. These categories will be examined in turn, beginning with the countries of CEE, which face some of the greatest challenges to health.

Central and eastern Europe

The candidate countries of CEE share some common demographic features. All have levels of life expectancy that lag behind those in western Europe, although they are at last improving. They also have experienced marked falls in birth rates, especially since 1990. The combined effect is a rapid ageing of their populations, with important consequences for the future. Yet beyond these general statements, in health as in wealth and in history, these countries exhibit great diversity.

The three Baltic republics were part of the Soviet Union until 1991 while most of the others were nominally independent but were locked into the Soviet bloc during the post-war period and Slovenia was part of Yugoslavia. After more than a decade has passed since the political transition, these divisions continue to be mirrored, to a considerable extent, in patterns of life expectancy (Figure 3.1).

Trends in mortality

The large fluctuations in life expectancy seen in the three Baltic republics since the mid-1980s were almost identical to those experienced in other ex-Soviet

Figure 3.1   Life expectancy at birth (in years) in the Baltic states, other countries of central and south eastern Europe, Slovenia and the European Union

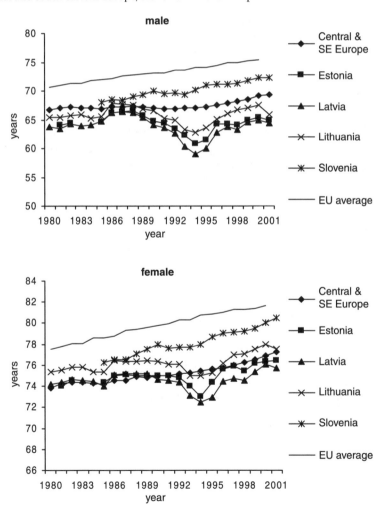

Source: WHO European Health for all database, 2003

countries and, in particular, the Russian Federation and Ukraine until 1998, after which the Baltic republics continued to improve while the gains in the other ex-Soviet states began to reverse.

The situation in the other countries of CEE was quite different. Since 1990, the more "western" countries of CEE, such as Poland (Zatonski et al. 1998), Hungary, the Czech Republic (Bobak et al. 1997) and Slovakia have experienced rapid improvements in life expectancy while the more "eastern" ones, such as Romania and Bulgaria, only began to show improvement in the late 1990s. Since data for Slovenia became available, in the mid-1980s, life expectancy has exceeded that in its former communist neighbours, improving consistently since then (Figure 3.2).

Aggregate measures of mortality, such as life expectancy, have the advantage of simplicity but they obscure details of differences in death rates at different

Figure 3.2 Life expectancy at birth (in years) in selected central and eastern European countries and in the European Union

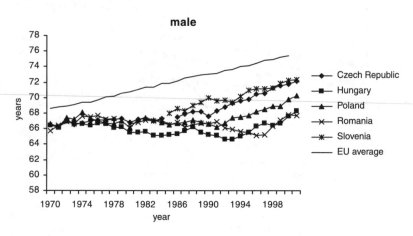

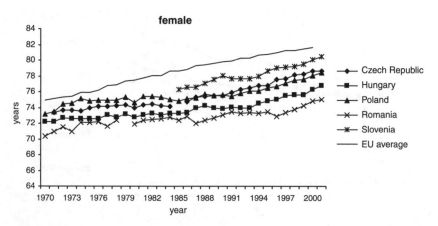

Source: WHO European Health for all database, 2003

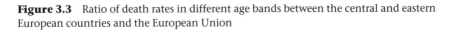

Figure 3.3   Ratio of death rates in different age bands between the central and eastern European countries and the European Union

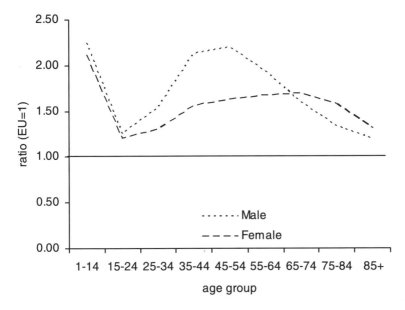

ages. Figure 3.3 shows the ratio of death rates in different age bands between the CEE countries and the EU. In childhood and among men in the 35–44 age group death rates are over twice as high as in the EU. The gap is narrowest in adolescence and old age.

This is, however, only a snapshot and for a fuller picture it is necessary to look at changes over time. Thus, although deaths in childhood are still much higher in CEE than in the EU, rates have fallen steadily throughout the 1970s and 1980s, a decline that has accelerated in the 1990s. There is one important exception. In Romania death rates among 5–9 year olds increased sharply, albeit from a low initial level, at the end of the 1990s as a consequence of the policy of inadvertently giving HIV-contaminated blood transfusions to many undernourished children who had been abandoned in "orphanages" in the late 1980s (Kozintez et al. 2000).

Figure 3.4 shows trends in death rates for men aged 35–44, an age group where the gap with the current EU was especially large. Again it highlights the diversity, with death rates increasing rapidly in the early 1990s, reaching over five times the level in the EU in Latvia, with similar, if slightly smaller, increases in the neighbouring Baltic republics and in Hungary, while there was a consistent, if gradual, decline in mortality throughout this period in the Czech Republic and Slovenia.

Ultimately, however, it is necessary to look at patterns of different causes of death. Here too there is considerable diversity, although again there are some sub-regional similarities. Thus, the countries of central Europe, such as Poland, the Czech Republic and Hungary, experienced short-lived increases in

Figure 3.4 Trends in death rates for men aged 35–44

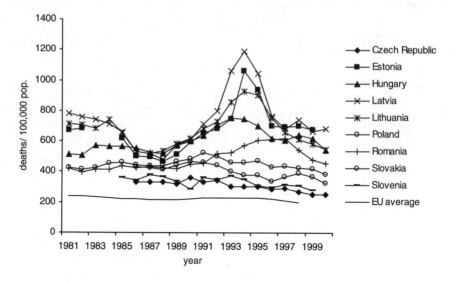

deaths at the time of transition, largely due to deaths from external causes, especially traffic accidents, which then declined steadily during the remaining years of the 1990s (Winston et al. 1999). Later sustained improvements in life expectancy, beginning at different times in the 1990s, have largely been due to falls in cardiovascular disease, in some cases such as Poland falling quite steeply. Similar falls in Romania and Bulgaria occurred in the final years of the 1990s.

Once again the situation in the Baltic republics has been quite different. The changes seen in these countries can only be understood with reference to events in 1985, when Mikhail Gorbachev implemented an initially highly effective and wide ranging anti-alcohol campaign (White 1996), leading to an immediate improvement in life expectancy. This was due largely to a decline in cardiovascular diseases and injuries with smaller contributions by other causes associated with alcohol, including acute alcohol poisoning and pneumonia. These causes of death subsequently increased, not only in the Baltic republics but also in the Russian Federation (and to some extent in Ukraine and Belarus), accelerating upwards in the early 1990s before falling once again after 1994 in all these by now independent countries. These phenomena have been studied most closely in the Russian Federation, where it is now clear that heavy alcohol consumption has been an important factor (McKee et al. 2001).

In summary, while levels of mortality overall are somewhat higher in the countries of CEE, with the gap especially large for adult men, the picture is extremely diverse. At the risk of simplification, three broad subgroupings can be ascertained. These are the three Baltic republics, the two countries of southeast Europe (Romania and Bulgaria), and the remaining countries of central Europe.

Looking beyond mortality

Mortality rates have many advantages as indicators of the health status of a population, as they can be tracked over many years and death is unambiguous, even if ascertainment of the precise cause may sometimes be difficult. Measures of morbidity are more problematic and traditionally focus on notifications of infectious diseases. As yet there are few examples of the diseases registries established in some western countries that would allow tracking of change, with the exception of cancer registries. Another measure of health for which there are comparable data available is the presence of long-standing illness, derived from the Eurobarometer surveys (Figure 3.5). The rates of reporting such illnesses are high in candidate countries, except in Cyprus and Malta, where they are similar to those seen in the current EU.

It is possible to combine data on ill health and premature death to generate a measure of health-adjusted life expectancy (HALE), a summary measure of the equivalent number of years in full health that a newborn can expect to live based on current rates of ill health and mortality. Thus, while life expectancy (representing the impact of mortality) within the transition countries ranges from 71.3 years in Romania to 75.2 years in the Czech Republic, levels of HALE in the transition countries are significantly lower, varying from 57.7 years in Latvia to 66.9 years in Slovenia (Figure 3.6).

Figure 3.5 Percentage of the population reporting a long-standing illness in European Union and candidate countries

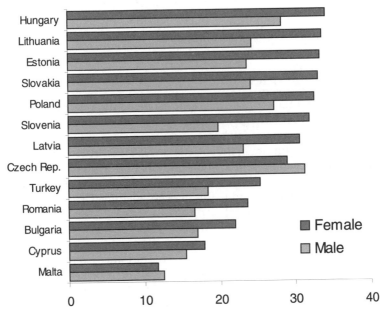

Source: Authors calculations from Eurobarometer 2002 data

Figure 3.6   Health adjusted life expectancy in European Union and candidate countries

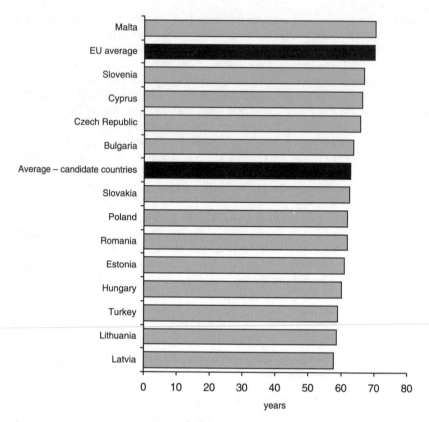

Source: WHO European Health for all database, 2003

The health of minorities

The Copenhagen Criteria contain an explicit statement about the importance of stable institutions that guarantee democracy, the rule of law, human rights, and respect for and protection of minorities. Subsequently, Agenda 2000 noted that the integration of minorities in the societies of CEE was, in general, satisfactory, "except for the situation of the Roma minority in a number of [applicant countries], which gives cause for concern". The Opinions on Readiness for Membership that stemmed from this process identified particular concerns about discrimination and social hardship in Bulgaria, the Czech Republic, Hungary, Poland, Romania and Slovakia.

The commitment by the EU to combat discrimination was enshrined in the new Article 13 of the Treaty of Amsterdam. This has since led to Directive 2000/43/EC implementing the principle of equal treatment of persons irrespective of racial or ethnic origin (European Commission 2000). As part of the *acquis*, candidate countries are required to implement this legislation prior to accession.

The Roma, or gypsy, population constitute sizeable minorities in many candidate countries in CEE. Obtaining accurate figures is problematic, for many reasons, but the estimates in Table 3.1 are the best available.

The Roma population share many common traditions but comprise diverse branches, characterized by differences in culture and language. Thus, the Romani language consists of up to 100 dialects, often with few shared words except for basic concepts related to food and family (Hancock 1999). While their position within society varies both between and within countries, in many places they suffer from marginalization and discrimination, which has worsened since the collapse of communist regimes (Paci 2002).

Originally from north eastern India, the Roma people began a slow westward migration about 1000 years ago. By the fifteenth century they were well established in the Balkans, with smaller groups throughout western Europe. At first they were welcomed, but the intolerance that accompanied the reformation and the rise of the nation state in the sixteenth century soon led to persecution. In the eighteenth century Austria-Hungary required Roma children over 5 to be taken from their parents and brought up in non-Roma families. In Romania, Roma people were kept as slaves until the 1860s (Fonseca 1995) and up to 500 000 were exterminated in Nazi camps. The post-war communist regimes conferred some degree of protection, albeit sometimes at the cost of forced assimilation. Since 1990 many Roma people have continued to be subject to widespread and often institutionalized racism, with an increase in attacks from the majority community, sometimes with semi-official approval.

Against this background, it is unsurprising that health policy-makers and researchers have paid little attention to the health needs of Roma people, even though their distinctive way of life suggests these needs may be different from those of the majority population (McKee 1997). Understanding these needs is inevitably complicated by the problem of defining the Roma population because of their reluctance to identify themselves and enforced assimilation. However, what evidence exists suggests that life expectancy is considerably lower (up to 10 years) than that of the majority population and infant mortality is up to four times higher (Braham 1993). Information on the causes of their high levels of premature death is subject to the uneven pattern of research,

Table 3.1   Estimates of the Roma population in candidate countries of CEE

Country	Estimated number of Roma people
Bulgaria	700 000–800 000
Czech Republic	250 000–300 000
Hungary	550 000–600 000
Latvia	8200
Poland	50 000–60 000
Romania	1 800 000–2 500 000
Slovakia	480 000–520 000
Slovenia	6500–10 000

Source: European Commission 2002

which has focused on genetic or infectious disorders (symbolizing the risk of contagion of the majority population) rather than non-communicable diseases (Hajioff and McKee 2000), the rates of which reflect the poverty, lack of education, overcrowding and unemployment from which they suffer (Koupilova et al. 2001).

As noted above, the EU has placed a high priority on the rights of the Roma people in the accession negotiations. It has also provided resources to empower them and to improve their living conditions through the Phare programme. However, there is still much to be achieved. In an insightful commentary on the impact of enlargement on the Roma population, Kovats emphasizes the importance of not developing structures that serve further to marginalize the Roma people through the creation of separate structures, and to recognize the need to treat Roma people within their individual national and local contexts (Kovats 2004).

Understanding the health divide in Europe

Earlier sections, looking at overall mortality rates, showed the existence of a health divide between the existing Member States and the candidate countries in CEE. This section will seek some explanations for this divide. There is rarely a single reason why an individual dies prematurely. Consequently, this chapter will look at the range of factors involved. At one level, taking a biomedical approach, it is possible to describe the differences in rates of specific diseases. On a second level it is possible to look at the biological risk factors, such as smoking or alcohol consumption, that underlie these differences in diseases. On a third level, it is possible to enquire about the underlying reasons why people are exposed to risk factors, asking questions about choice and empowerment. Finally, even if people acquire diseases, in many cases modern health care can prevent untimely death so a final level of analysis looks at the effectiveness of the health care response.

This analysis begins by looking at the specific diseases that contribute to the health divide and their major risk factors. Of necessity it will be selective. However, even a superficial examination of the data highlights the importance of a few specific conditions in explaining this divide, cardiovascular disease, injuries and violence, cancer, and some alcohol-related diseases such as cirrhosis. Each will be considered in turn.

The high levels of cardiovascular disease in CEE reflect high levels of many of the usual risk factors, such as fat consumption and smoking. Differences in access to and quality of health care for cardiovascular disease may also explain some part of the differences in mortality for this condition and it is also increasingly recognized that the traditionally very low levels of fruit and vegetables in diets in this region have also played a role (Bobak et al. 1998; Pomerleau et al. 2001). However, these mechanisms cannot explain all of the observed effects and it is likely that alcohol is playing an important role in all of northern Europe, but especially in the Baltic States where, as in the Russian Federation, alcohol such as vodka is typically drunk in bouts (Bobak et al. 1999), unlike the somewhat steadier consumption in southern and western Europe.

Figure 3.7 Death rates (per 100 000) from road traffic accidents in selected countries

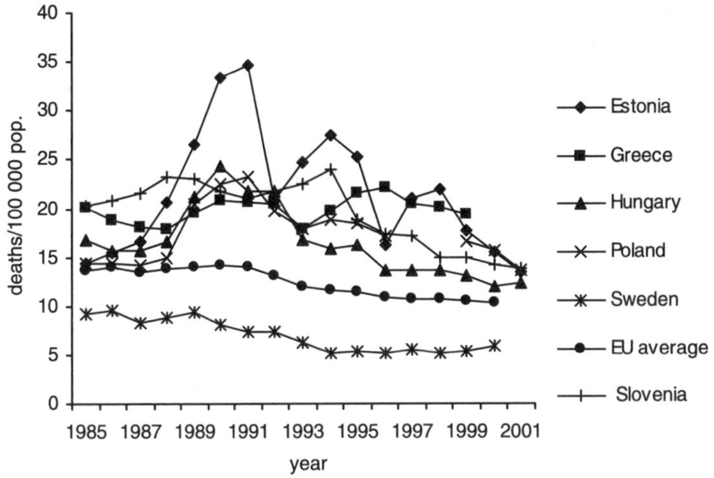

Source: WHO European Health for all database, 2003

All former communist countries experienced a short-lived, but important increase in deaths from injuries, especially those due to traffic (Figure 3.7). This was especially large in the Baltic states where, although death rates have returned towards their previous levels, they are still much higher than in many current Member States (although as the inclusion in the graph of the Member States with both the highest and lowest current rates shows, the distinction is not absolute). While all causes of injury are more common, the gap is particularly great for homicide and suicide (Figure 3.8), although again, rates in some Member States exceed those in some candidate countries, however, drowning and deaths in fires are, overall, very much more common than in the EU. Clearly many factors contribute to these deaths. In the case of road traffic injuries they include poor quality of roads and lax enforcement of speed limits, but it is also clear that alcohol plays an important role.

Death rates from unintentional injuries reflect many factors related to risk and its perception, and to the environment. Throughout the countries of CEE there have been few of the design features that enhance safety in the west, although this is now changing. In some cases effective health care could save lives but it is either unavailable or of poor quality, especially in rural areas suffering from poor communications and transport infrastructure.

Childhood injuries are an important contribution to the overall injury burden in both EU and candidate countries. From 1991 to 1995, had childhood injury death rates in the candidate countries been at the EU average level (UNICEF 2001), there would have been over 2000 fewer deaths per year among children aged 1–14 (this does not include Malta, Cyprus and Turkey).

Within this high burden of disease there is a large east-west gap in injury mortality rates. A study of figures of childhood injury mortality for 1991–1995 showed that all candidate countries (data not including Turkey, Malta and

Figure 3.8 Death rates (per 100 000) from suicide in selected countries

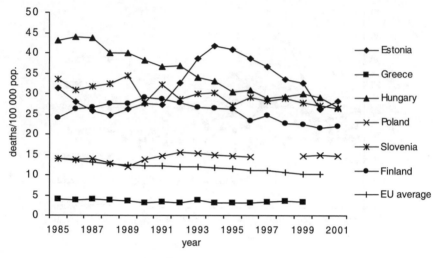

Source: WHO European Health for all database, 2003

Cyprus) had much higher injury mortality rates than in any current Member State with the exception of Portugal. At the lowest end of the spectrum, 5.2 children per 100 000 children aged 1–14 died of injuries in Sweden. At the opposite end, in Latvia the figure was 38.4 (a rate of one child in every 200 between his or her first and fifteenth birthdays).

The term "cancer" covers many disease processes, each with different risk factors. However, smoking is a major factor in cancers at many sites and has been extremely common among men in all of eastern Europe (Pudule et al. 1999). Consequently, death rates from lung cancer among men, which is almost entirely caused by smoking, are extremely high, in some cases reaching levels never previously observed anywhere in the world (Zatonski et al. 1996). In contrast, smoking has always been relatively uncommon among women. This is now changing, and female smoking rates, especially among young women in major cities, are increasing rapidly, encouraged by aggressive advertising by western tobacco companies (Figure 3.9) (Hurt 1995). Consequently, lung cancer rates among women will soon begin to rise (Bray et al. 2000).

The policy response to tobacco was initially weak but more recently several countries, in particular Poland (Fagerstrom et al. 2001), Hungary and the three Baltic states, have enacted anti-tobacco programmes that are stronger than those in many EU countries.

Cervical cancer is also relatively common, reflecting the high rates of sexually transmitted diseases and, until recently, the difficulty in obtaining barrier contraceptives (Levi et al. 2000). Unfortunately, the few effective cervical screening programmes are rare exceptions and screening is often opportunistic, with little quality control, and is thus generally ineffective.

Figure 3.9 Smoking rates in candidate countries, 2002

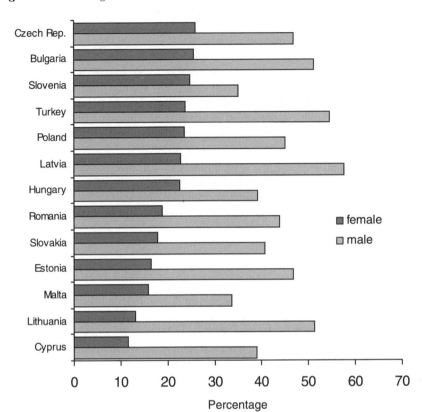

Source: Authors calculations from Eurobarometer 2002 data

In the space available it is not possible to go into detail about the other causes of cancer. However, it can be predicted that, in the future, deaths from some cancer sites, such as stomach cancer, will continue to decline while others, such as breast and prostate, will come closer to those in the west.

Infectious disease is no longer the threat that it once was, reflecting the commitment to disease control by the Soviet imposed public health system (Field 1957). The Soviet model was especially successful in reducing vaccine preventable diseases, in part because of its pervasive system of monitoring and use of compulsion. However, growing social inequalities, with increasing marginalization of certain groups, combined with a failure to adopt modern concepts of disease surveillance and a breakdown of earlier control systems following independence has allowed some diseases to re-emerge (Markina et al. 2000).

Some of the greatest concerns have been about rises in sexually transmitted diseases (STDs), HIV and tuberculosis. Recorded rates of STDs have since fallen although there are concerns as to whether this reflects a true reduction in incidence or a decline in notification, as treatment is increasingly being provided privately (Platt and McKee 2000). Rates of HIV infection are still low, in global terms, but are rising extremely quickly in many parts of CEE (Dobson 2001). At present, spread is primarily due to needle sharing among addicts but the epidemic is beginning to move into the wider population by means of sexual spread.

Rates of tuberculosis have also increased markedly in the 1990s in some countries. In particular, in the Baltic states, especially among prison populations, conditions are highly conducive to rapid spread and treatment is often inadequate (Stern 1999). A particular concern is the high rate of drug resistant disease (Farmer et al. 1999) and the co-existence of HIV and resistant tuberculosis have yet to elicit effective policy responses.

Finally, changes in land use and adoption of new agricultural practices are contributing to increases in some animal borne infections, such as leptospirosis in Bulgaria (Stoilova and Popivanova 1999) and in tick-borne encephalitis in the Baltic states (Randolph 2001).

The underlying factors

Lifestyle choices are heavily influenced by social circumstances and they can only be understood fully by considering the context in which they are made. The social forces driving trends in mortality in these countries are still inadequately understood, although some parts of the picture are clear.

In general the transition has had a beneficial effect on health, with considerable gains in some areas. The opening of markets has ensured market availability to fresh fruit and vegetables all year round and to healthier (by virtue of lower sugar or fat content) forms of common foods. Similarly, the emergence of an active consumer market has encouraged greater attention to safety and to routine maintenance, with a concomitant reduction in injuries. However, open borders cannot be selective, only admitting "goods" while excluding "bads". Thus, those promoting dangerous substances, such as tobacco and narcotics, have been able to create new markets for their products, whether among young women, in the case of the tobacco industry, or those on the margins of society, in the case of those trading in narcotics. Both have taken advantage of the turmoil in parts of the former Yugoslavia to increase the flow of smuggled goods into the rest of Europe, with the tobacco industry using this route as a means of circumventing sales taxes in many countries.

So not everyone has fared so well. In addition to the greater exposure to substances hazardous to health, income inequalities have widened and some groups have been left behind in the quest for modern market economies. It is now clear that the most vulnerable are those who have experienced the most rapid pace of transition (Walberg et al. 1998) and who are least able to draw support from social networks (Kennedy et al. 1998). The individuals most affected have been men, with low levels of education (Shkolnikov et al. 1998), low levels of social support (such as the unmarried) (Hajdu et al. 1995) and low levels of control over their lives (Bobak et al. 1998).

The role of health care

Increasing access to timely and effective health care interventions have done much to reduce mortality in western countries (Mackenbach et al. 1998). It has been estimated that, in 1988, about 25% of the mortality gap between east and west Europe between birth and age 75 could have been explained by failures of medical care (Velkova et al. 1997). A more recent analysis, comparing the Baltic states with the United Kingdom (selected as an example of a western European country) shows that the east-west gap in deaths from avoidable causes began to emerge about 1970. At that time many modern pharmaceuticals and innovative surgical techniques were being adopted in the west, but not to anything like the same extent in the east (Andreev et al. 2003).

While the specific impact of health care on measures of population health is often difficult to detect, there are several well-documented examples of where this has been identified (Becker and Boyle 1997; Nolte et al. 2002). Research on neonatal mortality has sought to separate the impact of health care from broader social determinants, with the former assessed by birth weight specific survival and the latter by the overall birth weight distribution. In the Czech Republic (Koupilová et al. 1998) there were considerable improvements in birth

Figure 3.10   Change in deaths from testicular cancer age 20–44: 1975–1979 to 1995–1999

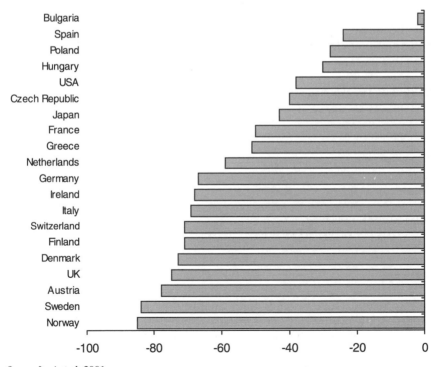

Source: Levi et al. 2001

weight specific mortality, and by implication, the quality of care. As a consequence, closing the remaining gap with the EU will require policies that address the social determinants of low birth weight.

Another area where the impact of health care can be identified is cancer survival. Research from the 1980s and early 1990s showed that cancer survival was somewhat lower in the countries of CEE than in the west, almost certainly reflecting the lack of access, at that time, to the then emerging expensive new chemotherapeutic drugs. However, in the 1990s, some countries have experienced considerable improvements, as can be seen from the case of testicular cancer (Levi et al. 2001) (Figure 3.10) although the degree of improvement is less than in western Europe.

Malta and Cyprus

The second group of candidate countries comprise the Mediterranean islands of Malta and Cyprus. In both, life expectancy at birth is now almost the same as the EU average (Table 3.2) and thus considerably higher than in the countries of CEE.

If Malta and Cyprus were already in the EU they would rank 2nd and 11th, respectively, (of 17) in terms of male life expectancy at birth and 13th and 14th, respectively, in terms of female life expectancy. Yet while Malta has relatively low death rates from many common causes of death, deaths from some diseases, such as ischaemic heart disease, are relatively high. Interestingly, given its geographical position, in the Mediterranean, and its cultural inheritance, bringing together different influences including many elements of a British diet, it has a pattern of mortality that resembles more closely that in the United Kingdom than that in its Mediterranean neighbours such as Italy.

Table 3.2   Life expectancy at birth in Malta and Cyprus compared with the EU and countries of CEE

Life expectancy at birth (years) in 1999	EU average	Countries of CEE	Cyprus	Malta
Male	75.11	68.74	75	75.12
Female	81.37	76.5	80	79.38

Data for latest available year.
Sources: WHO European and Eastern Mediterranean Regional Offices

Turkey

In this analysis Turkey stands alone among the candidate countries, largely because of the relative lack of comparable data on adult health, which prevents a detailed analysis of the health of the Turkish population. On the basis of mortality estimates, figures for life expectancy have been produced, but they should be interpreted with caution. They indicate that life expectancy at birth

Figure 3.11   Life expectancy in the EU, CEE and Turkey

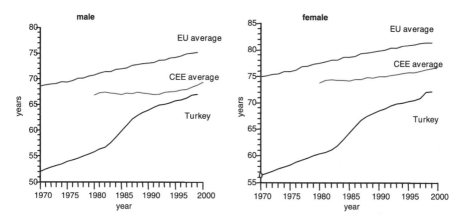

has been increasing relatively rapidly in the 1980s but still lags behind the CEE average and, especially, the EU average (Figure 3.11).

A recent review suggested that Turkey is experiencing high levels of cardio-vascular disease (Onat 2001). This is supported by a detailed analysis of available mortality data and studies on Turkish migrants in Germany that suggests that the available data substantially underestimate the true burden of cardiovascular disease in the Turkish population (Razum et al. 2000). Other research on Turkish migrants to Germany suggest that rates of cancer, where the lag period between exposure to risk factors and disease is often several decades, remain lower than in the German population (Zeeb et al. 2002). Turkey does, however, differ from many countries at a similar state of economic development in having imple-mented effective and wide-ranging tobacco control policies. This has been achieved in the face of efforts by the transnational tobacco industry to under-mine such activities. For example, there were attempts by the industry to stage Formula 1 events in the country that would have undermined the ban on tobacco sponsorship. Similarly there were efforts to provide grants to academic departments for "child smoking prevention" campaigns, campaigns now widely recognized as in fact resulting in increased child tobacco use. In the area of tobacco control, therefore, Turkey has taken a more principled position than some existing EU Member States (Gilmore et al. 2002). There is rather better information on the health of mothers and children, with one of the few nationally representative sources of health data in Turkey being the 1998 Demographic and Health Survey (DHS) (http://www.hips.hacettepe.edu.tr). The DHS, which is one of a series of surveys dating from the 1970s, documents a declining, but still relatively high rate of infant and childhood mortality, with marked regional variations. At present, therefore, in the absence of reliable or complete routine health data, it is only possible to say that it appears to be experiencing the double burden seen in many middle income countries outside Europe of a level of childhood mortality that, while falling, is still relatively high while traditionally low levels of non-communicable disease in adulthood are rising.

Summary

The candidate countries are as diverse in their health status as they are in other parameters. They can be divided, in broad terms, into three groups: Turkey, the two Mediterranean island countries, and the ex-communist countries of central and eastern Europe, however, especially within the last grouping, differences in health status, already substantial in 1990, have in many cases increased further.

Although the lack of data makes it difficult to assess the health of the Turkish population, it seems probable that their health needs are considerable, with a double burden of high mortality from traditional causes in childhood and growing rates of non-communicable diseases as seen in more developed countries. The strong stance taken by Turkey on tobacco control is, however, a very positive measure that will reduce levels of premature death in the future. In contrast, Malta and Cyprus have patterns of health that are similar to those in existing EU Member States.

Much more is known about patterns of health, and their causes, in the countries of CEE. While transition has brought about overall improvements in premature mortality, the picture remains uneven, with some groups doing better than others. Death rates from many non-communicable diseases remain much higher than in western Europe. This seems to reflect, to a considerable extent, traditionally high levels of smoking (among men) and poor dietary intake, with especially low levels of fresh fruit and vegetables. Death rates are also high from injuries and violence and, taken with the high rates of cirrhosis in some countries, this indicates the important role played by alcohol. However, it is important to look beyond the immediate risk factors to understand the role that social and economic transition has played, both positive and negative, in a process that has brought both winners and losers. Finally, it is clear that while great improvements in health care have been achieved, there is still much to be done.

References

Andreev, E.M., Nolte, E., Shkolnikov, V.M., Varavikova, E. and McKee, M. (2003) The evolving pattern of avoidable mortality in Russia, *International Journal of Epidemiology*, 32:437–46.

Becker, N. and Boyle, P. (1997) Decline in mortality from testicular cancer in West Germany after reunification, *Lancet*, 350:744.

Bobak, M., Brunner, E., Miller, N.J., Skodova, Z. and Marmot, M. (1998) Could antioxidants play a role in high rates of coronary heart disease in the Czech Republic?, *European Journal of Clinical Nutrition*, 522:632–6.

Bobak, M., McKee, M., Rose, R. and Marmot, M. (1999) Alcohol consumption in a national sample of the Russian population. *Addiction*, 94:857–66.

Bobak, M., Skodova, Z., Pisa, Z., Poledne, R. and Marmot, M. (1997) Political changes and trends in cardiovascular risk factor in the Czech Republic, 1985–92, *Journal of Epidemiology and Community Health*, 51:272–7.

Braham, M. (1993) *The untouchables: a survey of the Roma people of central and eastern Europe*. Geneva: UNHCR.

Bray, I., Brennan, P. and Boffetta, P. (2000) Projections of alcohol and tobacco-related cancer mortality in Central Europe, *International Journal of Cancer*, 87:122–8.

Dobson, R. (2001) AIDS-dramatic surge in ex-Soviet Union, no respite worldwide, new data show, *Bulletin of the World Health Organization*, 79:78.

European Commission (2000) Council Directive 2000/43/EC implementing the principle of equal treatment between persons irrespective of racial or ethnic origin. Official Journal of the European Communities 19.7.2000 L180/22.

European Commission (2002) DG Enlargement. EU support for Roma communities in central and eastern Europe. Brussels: European Commission.

Fagerstrom, K., Boyle, P., Kunze, M. and Zatonski, W. (2001) The anti-smoking climate in EU countries and Poland, *Lung Cancer*, 32:1–5.

Farmer, P.E., Kononets, A., Borisov, S.E., et al. (1999) Recrudescent tuberculosis in the Russian Federation, in P.E. Farmer, L.B. Reichman and M.D. Iseman (eds) *The global impact of drug resistant tuberculosis*. Boston, MA: Harvard Medical School/Open Society Institute.

Field, M.G. (1957) *Doctor and patient in Soviet Russia*. Cambridge, MA: Harvard University Press.

Fonseca, I. (1995) *Bury me standing: the gypsies and their journey*. London: Chatto & Windus.

Gilmore, A., Nolte, E., McKee, M. and Collin, J. (2002) Continuing influence of tobacco industry in Germany, *Lancet*, 360:1255.

Hajdu, P., McKee, M. and Bojan, F. (1995) Changes in premature mortality differentials by marital status in Hungary and in England and Wales, *European Journal of Public Health*, 5:259–64.

Hajioff, S. and McKee, M. (2000) The health of the Roma people: a review of the published literature, *Journal of Epidemiology and Community Health*, 54:864–9.

Hancock, I. (1999) Standardization and Ethnic Defence in Emergent Non-Literate Societies, in T. Acton and M. Dauphanis (eds) *Language, Blacks and Gypsies*. London: Whitting & Birch.

Hurt, R.D. (1995) Smoking in Russia: what do Stalin and Western tobacco companies have in common?, *Mayo Clinic Proceedings*, 70:1007–11.

Kennedy, B.P., Kawachi, I. and Brainerd, E. (1998) The role of social capital in the Russian mortality crisis. *World Development*. 26:2029–43.

Koupilova, I., Epstein, H., Holcik, J., Hajioff, S. and McKee, M. (2001) Health needs of the Roma population in the Czech and Slovak Republics, *Soc Sci Med*, 53:1191–204.

Koupilová, I., McKee, M. and Holcik, J. (1998) Neonatal mortality in the Czech Republic during the transition, *Health Policy*, 46:43–52.

Kovats, M. (2004) Roma health: problems and perception, in J. Healy and M. McKee (eds) *Accessing health care: responding to diversity*. Oxford: Oxford University Press.

Kozintez, C., Matusa, R. and Cazacu, A. (2000) The changing epidemic of pediatric HIV infection in Romania, *Annals of Epidemiology*, 10:474–5.

Levi, F., La Vecchia, C., Boyle, P., Lucchini, F. and Negri, E. (2001) Western and eastern European trends in testicular cancer mortality, *Lancet*, 357:1853–4.

Levi, F., Lucchini, F., Negri, E., Franceschi, S. and la Vecchia, C. (2000) Cervical cancer mortality in young women in Europe: patterns and trends, *European Journal of Cancer*, 36:2266–71.

Mackenbach, J.P., Looman, C.W.N., Kunst, A.E., Habbema, J.D.F. and van der Maas, P.J. (1998) Post-1950 mortality trends and medical care: gains in life expectancy due to declines in mortality from conditions amenable to medical intervention in The Netherlands. *Social Science & Medicine*, 27:888–9.

Markina, S.S., Maksimova, N.M., Vitek, C.R., Bogatyreva, E.Y. and Monisov, A.A. (2000) Diphtheria in the Russian Federation in the 1990s, *The Journal of Infectious Diseases*, 181(Suppl 1):S27–34.

McKee, M. (1997) The health of gypsies. Lack of understanding exemplifies wider disregard of the health of minorities in Europe, *British Medical Journal*, 315:1172–3.

McKee, M. and Britton, A. (1998) The positive relationship between alcohol and heart disease in eastern Europe: potential physiological mechanisms, *Journal of the Royal Society of Medicine*, 91:402–7.

McKee, M., Shkolnikov, V. and Leon, D.A. (2001) Alcohol is implicated in the fluctuations in cardiovascular disease in Russia since the 1980s, *Annals of Epidemiology*, 11:1–6.

Nolte, E., Scholz, R., Shkolnikov, V. and McKee, M. (2002) The contribution of medical care to changing life expectancy in Germany and Poland, *Social Science & Medicine*, 55:15–31.

Onat, A. (2001) Risk factors and cardiovascular disease in Turkey, *Atherosclerosis*, 156:1–10.

Paci, P. (2002) Gender and Equity in the ECA Region (unpublished report). Washington, DC: World Bank.

Platt, L. and McKee, M. (2000) Observations of the management of sexually transmitted diseases in the Russian Federation: a challenge of confidentiality, *International Journal of STD & AIDS*, 11:563–7.

Pomerleau, J., McKee, M., Robertson, A. et al. (2001) Macronutrient and food intake in the Baltic republics, *European Journal of Clinical Nutrition*, 55:200–7.

Pudule, I., Grinberga, D., Kazdiauskiene, K. et al. (1999) Patterns of smoking in the Baltic Republics, *Journal of Epidemiology and Community Health*, 53:277–82.

Randolph, S.E. (2001) The shifting landscape of tick-borne zoonoses: tick-borne encephalitis and Lyme borreliosis in Europe, *Philosophical Transactions of the Royal Society of London. Series B, Biological Sciences*, 356:1045–56.

Razum, O., Akgun, S. and Tezcan, S. (2000) Cardiovascular mortality patterns in Turkey: what is the evidence?, *Soz Praventivmed*, 45:46–51.

Shkolnikov, V.M., Leon, D., Adamets, S., Andreev, E. and Deev, A. (1998) Educational level and adult mortality in Russia: an analysis of routine data 1979 to 1994, *Social Science & Medicine*, 47:357–69.

Stern, V. (1999) *Sentenced to die: The problem of TB in prisons in Eastern Europe and central Asia*. London: International Centre for Prison Studies, King's College London.

Stoilova, N. and Popivanova, N. (1999) Epidemiologic studies of leptospiroses in the Plovdiv region of Bulgaria, *Folia Medica (Plovdiv)*, 41(4):73–9.

UNICEF (2001) A League Table of Child Deaths By Injury in Rich Nations. Innocenti Report Card. Issue No 2. Florence: UNICEF.

Velkova, A., Wolleswonkel-Van den Bosch, J. and Mackenbach, J.P. (1997) The East-West Life Expectancy Gap: Differences in Mortality Amenable to Medical Intervention, *International Journal of Epidemiology*, 26(1):75–84.

Walberg, P., McKee, M., Shkolnikov, V., Chenet, L. and Leon, D.A. (1998) Economic change, crime, and mortality crisis in Russia: regional analysis, *British Medical Journal*, 317:312–18.

White, S. (1996) *Russia Goes Dry*. Cambridge: Cambridge University Press.

Winston, F.K., Rineer, C., Menon, R. and Baker, S.P. (1999) The carnage wrought by major economic change: ecological study of traffic related mortality and the reunification of Germany, *British Medical Journal*, 318:1647–50.

Zatonski, W., McMichael, A.J. and Powles, J.W. (1998) Ecological study of reasons for sharp decline in mortality from ischaemic heart disease in Poland since 1991, *British Medical Journal*, 316:1047–105.

Zatonski, W., Smans, M., Tyczynski, J. and Boyle, P. (1996) Atlas of Cancer. Mortality in Central Europe. IARC Scientific Publications No. 134. Lyon, France: International Agency for Research on Cancer.

Zeeb, H., Razum, O., Blettner, M. and Stegmaier, C. (2002) Transition in cancer patterns among Turks residing in Germany, *European Journal of Cancer*, 38:705–11.

chapter four

Health and health care in the candidate countries to the European Union: Common challenges, different circumstances, diverse policies

Carl-Ardy Dubois and Martin McKee

Introduction

After successfully growing from six to fifteen members through four successive enlargements over the last half-century, the signature of the Accession Treaty in Athens has brought the EU to a turning point as it faces its fifth and greatest enlargement ever in terms of scope and diversity. Ten new Member States (Poland, Hungary, Czech Republic, Slovakia, Estonia, Latvia, Lithuania, Slovenia, Malta, Cyprus) will achieve membership on 1 May 2004, creating a substantial increase in its area, its population and its cultural and historic capital. But accession is more of a process than an event. Preparation for accession to the EU, which has also been initiated by Romania, Bulgaria and Turkey has created unprecedented pressures and opportunities for social, political, economic and institutional changes. The process of adopting the *acquis communautaire* and Copenhagen criteria has fundamentally altered institutions and policies in the candidate countries. To achieve membership, each state was required to show that it had stable democratic institutions, had made significant progress towards a functioning market economy, and had harmonized national regulations with the existing body of EU law, amounting to not less than 80 000 pages of legal text organized in 31 Chapters.

According to the European principle of subsidiarity, the organization, financing and delivery of health services is the responsibility of the Member States. Yet health care, which absorbs between 3% and 9% of Gross Domestic Product in the candidate countries, is far from immune from the requirements of the single European market. Health care has had a European dimension ever since the inception of the European Economic Community in 1957, in the Treaty of Rome. This is reflected in a range of health related legislation including, for instance, workplace safety, tobacco control and control of communicable diseases. However, the growth of European legislation in relation to the many components of health care, whether they be people (such as health professionals), goods (such as pharmaceuticals), or services (such as insurance providers) means that the health sector has not been spared the effects of the process of enlargement. The candidate countries have had to adapt their health systems to ensure conformity with a series of health related elements of the *acquis communautaire* scattered among many different chapters. Moreover, it is important to recognize that, for most candidate countries, the accession process coincided with the task of rebuilding or reforming their health care systems as part of the broader process of political transition and in response to changing health needs of their populations.

The purpose of this chapter is to summarize the main trends relating to the evolution of health and health care in the current candidate countries. Several questions are addressed. What factors are driving health care reform in candidate countries? Are there identifiable paths being followed with regard to governance and funding of health care? How do the accession process and EU imposed standards and regulations affect the development of health policies? Even though accession to the EU has been delayed to 2007 for Romania and Bulgaria and even longer for Turkey, the analysis will include all countries that have initiated the accession process: the two parts of former Czechoslovakia (the Czech Republic and Slovakia), three former Soviet states (Estonia, Latvia, Lithuania), four former independent socialist states of central Europe (Romania, Bulgaria, Poland, Hungary), one former part of Yugoslavia (Slovenia), and three Mediterranean countries (Cyprus, Malta and Turkey) As this list makes clear, these countries are very diverse in their historical inheritance and current status, yet they do, for the present purposes, have in common the imperative of adopting a wide range of EU legislative provisions.

The paper will proceed as follows. The next section outlines theoretical approaches that have been adopted to analyse the evolution of public policies within the context of European transition and integration. It highlights critical variables that must be taken into consideration to understand the transformation of health care in the candidate countries. A second section focuses on challenges faced by these countries in their transition process and reveals a series of broad commonalties that have implications for health care organization. A third section explores variations in health systems and demonstrates how differences in initial structural conditions and institutional developments are associated with differences in policy choices in various areas. It shows that, in spite of common imperatives related to accession, the re-engineering of health systems in the candidate countries is following quite diverse pathways. In conclusion, we synthesize the insights gained from this analysis. It is argued that institution-building in the candidate countries is shaped by and embedded in the accession process. But health care systems as socio-historic constructions are characterized by a considerable inertia. While reforming their health services, candidate countries have to take into consideration both EU requirements and their national traditions and preferences. Overlooking the political, economical and institutional forces that operate at national level to channel changes in particular directions risks fostering creation of shallow institutions driven by short-term tactical considerations and designed only to satisfy external expectations. Restricting integration of the current candidate countries within a top-down, one-way process creates the risk of overlooking the potential contribution of the new members to the Union and may result in reversal of successful policies introduced by some countries before their accession.

Theoretical approaches to analysis of transition and integration

After the dislocation of the Soviet Empire and the collapse of the communist regimes in central and eastern Europe, the post-communist transformation has become a major theme of social science studies. At the same time, the processes of integration and enlargement by the EU have generated a rapidly expanding academic and policy interest in both Member States and prospective entrants. Although there is no enlargement theory per se, a coherent research agenda is being developed, building essentially on comparative analysis of pathways and outcomes of social and economic policies in the Member States and prospective members (Marrée and Groenewegen 1997; Grabbe 2001; Buller et al. 2002; Busse 2002a).

Theoretical approaches to studying European integration, EU enlargement and the transition of central and eastern European countries from socialism can be usefully placed into two main categories arising from two rival hypotheses:

The hypothesis of convergence emphasizes the prospect of transition to a market economy. A key contention underlying this hypothesis is that in embracing the western models of market economy and democratic polity, post-socialist and other transition countries are bound to converge to the supposedly superior systems and organizational forms of the industrialized West (Nee 1989; Dallago et al. 1992; Nelson et al. 1997). This means that the countries involved in the accession process were embarking on the same, clearly marked, road to the same final destination. Stabilization, liberalization and privatization of the means of production are promoted, all on a "one way" track, and representing an effective means to ensure efficiency of production, promote division of labour to maximize comparative advantage, ensure allocation of resources in line with consumer preferences, and avoid problems with incentives (World Bank 1996). Similar assumptions are also put forward in European studies which suggest that the twin processes of enlargement and integration of the EU generate a set of circumstances likely to induce convergence of national policies (European Commission 1995; Agh 1999a; Agh 1999b; Knill and Lehmkuhl 1999; Grabbe 2001). From this perspective, the different components of preparation for accession (technical assistance from EU, common programmes, internalization of market standards, legislative harmonization, absorption of Phare funds, setting standards and monitoring applications over the course of accession) are all interpreted as mechanisms used instrumentally by the EU to ensure diffusion of western standards and drive prospective entrants towards greater convergence with policy models already adopted by the Member States. With regard to health systems, this means that a host of influences inherent in the accession process are likely to drive health services in candidate countries towards the standards of the West, in the expectation that this will make them more economically viable, responsive and compatible with a market economy. Comparisons with existing Member States, the influence of the EU and its conditionalities, and a willingness to overcome apparent shortcomings in health care delivery provided candidate countries with incentives to undertake major reforms of their health care systems and to come closer to western institutional and organizational configurations. In this respect, actions that have been taken in diverse areas such as health care financing, health care provision, human resource development, professional training and pharmaceuticals are often grouped under the label of modernization and interpreted as ways for the candidate countries to adapt their health care systems to a market economy environment and become more consistent with the Member States. Thus the accession process poses a set of common challenges for the candidate countries and makes them subject to many similar exogenous influences. The same criteria and procedures are applied by the EU to all current candidates. In parallel, at least in the former communist states, the transition process is forcing them to make the structural adjustments needed in order to regenerate their economies, modernize their health care systems, and take measures to improve the health status of their populations. Thus the overall contribution of this approach is to stress the impact of the European dimension and other exogenous pressures on the process of reshaping health systems in candidate countries. It notes similar strategies developed in these countries to cope with common challenges as well as imperatives created concurrently by the accession process and the need to reverse inherited shortcomings of their health care delivery systems.

The hypothesis of institutional diversity emphasizes the resilience of national policies and institutions to outside pressures and draws attention to the diversity of national circumstances. It puts forward the importance of path dependence, that is the ways in which cultural norms and inherited institutions combined with new ones leading to the emergence of hybrid institutional and organizational forms specific to each country (North 1990; Stark 1992; Magnin 1996; Nelson et al. 1997). Different transformation paths and different destinations are likely to be generated by different histories and different contexts. For the candidate countries, this means that their contrasting geography, social structure and cultural values, the different ways in which communism collapsed, and the diversity in initial conditions resulting from national historical events are all intervening variables that may explain different responses to similar pressures or imperatives. From this perspective, EU enlargement is defined as a complex systemic transformation process imprinted by the distinctiveness of national trajectories, and displaying general similarities and persisting national peculiarities. Because the EU candidate countries differ in terms of openness of their economies, available resources, institutional history and development of their service sectors, they are likely to pursue distinct paths in the process of reforming their health services, notwithstanding similar pressures relating to the accession process. Applying the hypothesis of institutional diversity to the analysis of health care systems in the transition countries also suggests that expectations that a universal model of health care compatible with the market economy could replace the former arrangements are simply unrealistic. Diversity in initial conditions of candidate countries' health care systems, differences in domestic needs and capabilities, and unique political, social and economic conditions in each country would instead be reflected in diverse models of health sector reform. Furthermore, institutional configurations in the Member States constitute targets that are both multiple and moving (Hollingsworth et al. 1994). European health care systems, which already had adopted diverse institutional forms, have been undergoing significant changes over the last decade. Emerging configurations in the candidate countries are then subject to a variety of institutional influences and inspirations from the EU. In sum, this approach draws attention to the inertia that characterizes social structures and policies. It makes it possible to account for intervening variables such as economic, institutional and policy environments, which may generate different responses to the same exogenous pressures relating to the twin processes of accession to the EU and transformation of social institutions in the candidate countries.

Taken together, these two perspectives provide a potentially powerful analytical framework within which to analyse the evolution of health care systems in the candidate countries. The hypothesis of convergence offers a useful point of departure to examine similar challenges and pressures faced by health policy-makers in these countries which mostly share a common history of a planned economy followed by a transition to a market economy. The systematic attempts to harmonize rules and regulations with the EU, the political importance attached to membership by the candidate countries and the EU's determination to ensure compliance of the candidate with the *acquis communautaire* prior to their entry make a strong case for a commonalty of imperatives and possible convergence of the reforms being implemented. Concurrently, the hypothesis of persisting institutional diversity suggests that the convergence of policies, mainly macroeconomics, designed for a single market will not necessarily result in uniform health systems or health policies. Against a common background, there is significant scope for variation in the transformation processes among candidate countries and this is likely to be reflected in varied patterns of health care systems. Comparative studies of public policies have shown that similar challenges often manifest divergent constellations of problems in different countries. Policy choices and policy outcomes vary even among countries with similar features (Börzel and Risse 2000; Cowles et al. 2001; Héritier et al. 2001). Each country's characteristics defines the repertoire of feasible policy options. Thus, the accession process is only one variable among others. A complete picture must also take into consideration a broad variety of institutional, political and economic factors that influence the transformation of the health care systems in the candidate countries.

Common challenges faced by the candidate countries

As noted throughout this book, the 13 candidate countries are a diverse grouping although it is possible, with caution, to identify two main groups: a group of ten countries in central and eastern Europe (CEE) that share a common background of past socialist governance followed by a transition towards democratic polity and economic liberalization; and a second group of three Mediterranean countries (Cyprus, Malta and Turkey) historically characterized by a lower level of economic development than most western European countries but a long-standing tradition of openness to western influences, in particular in the cases of Malta and Cyprus, which have long been subject to British influences. But this sharp divide must not overlook the common features shared by all the current candidate countries. First, as emphasized by Agh (2003) throughout their long history, the countries of CEE have also been closely integrated with western Europe both in terms of trade and culture and prior to the imposition of communist rule most had democratic governments. Second, although the changes required to achieve the requirements of accession may have been greater for the states of CEE due to 50 years of communist rule, it remains the case that all the current candidate countries (and as the examples in this book show, countries involved in earlier enlargements) had some distance to travel in order to achieve the objectives of reforming their systems of social protection and implementing the fundamental legal, economic and political changes required for accession to the EU. Common challenges and trends shared by the 13 candidate countries relate to the health context, the macroeconomic context, the political organization of the health system, and the micro-efficiency of the health services.

The health context

Patterns of health in the candidate countries are examined in detail in Chapter 2. For the present purposes, the most important points to note are that, despite recent improvements, the burden of disease in the CEE candidate countries is substantially higher than in existing Member States, with particularly high levels of non-communicable diseases. Looking ahead, they face ageing populations as fertility rates have fallen below replacement levels in most countries. Only Slovakia and Poland have experienced an increase in populations over the last decade. The total population of the candidate countries, estimated to be about 105 million in 2000, has fallen by nearly 2 million over the last 10 years whereas life expectancy has shown significant improvements during the same period (WHO Regional Office for Europe 2002). This means that the expected costs of caring for an older population and of delivering effective treatment of chronic disease and disease prevention are emerging as key issues to be addressed by all the candidate countries. This will require health care delivery systems to meet new types of demands requiring high cost, highly specialized, technologically driven and multidisciplinary care. In some countries the situation is complicated further by the re-emergence of pre-existing infectious diseases that were thought to have been under control, in particular tuberculosis and syphilis.

The macroeconomic context

Financing of health systems has become one of the most critical challenges facing governments across Europe, leading to continuing debate about reform. However, in many candidate countries these pressures have become even more acute, prompting often radical reforms as a consequence of a series of factors including the past legacy of under-capitalization of health care infrastructure (particularly in the post-communist countries but also to a certain extent in Turkey and Cyprus), the temporary collapse of economies in CEE candidate countries in the early 1990s, the exacerbation of tensions between competing priorities during the accession process, and the importance of an informal or "shadow" sector as integral part of the economy in many candidate countries. Common challenges faced by the candidate countries in this respect are as follows.

The availability of resources for healthcare

With the exception of Malta and Slovenia, which allocate a share of GDP close to the EU average to health care, the candidate countries are in general perpetuating a situation in which they spend a relatively modest proportion of their national income on health care. According to the most recent estimations, the share of GDP allocated to health care averaged 6.2% in the candidate countries in comparison with 8.5% in the Member States (WHO 2002). Even more significant is the fact that six countries (Hungary, Bulgaria, Slovakia, Slovenia, Estonia, Latvia) out of the 13 candidates experienced a fall in the share of national income dedicated to health care between 1995 and 2000. Although public health expenditures still account for the most important part of total health spending, ranging from 53.8% in Cyprus to 91.4% in the Czech Republic, the general trend is towards reducing these proportions and looking for additional sources of funding. Thus private expenditure through direct out-of-pocket payments and voluntary health insurance have tended to increase in most of the candidate countries over the last decade (WHO 2002).

The size of the shadow economy

In most candidate countries, the size of the shadow economy, accounting for up to 33% of the labour force (Estonia) and 36% of GDP (Bulgaria) creates serious impediments to reforming health care financing and optimizing the use of health care resources (Schneider 2002; European Commission 2003). Informal and under-the-table payments have emerged as a significant proportion of health care financing, particularly in Estonia, Bulgaria, Latvia, Slovakia and Turkey where low levels and, in some cases, decreases in health care resources have led to underpaid staff, lack of basic equipment in public facilities and access to some basic services becoming dependent on capacity to pay informal charges. According to some estimates, the frequency of informal payments for health services may reach 60% in Slovakia, 31% in Latvia and 21% in Bulgaria (Lewis 2002). This shadow economy in health care has at the very least two important implications. First, under-the-table payments are reducing the effectiveness of public policies since it is patient ability and willingness to pay that determines where resources flow into the system. Second, because a large shadow economy increases the risk of evading social contributions, it is incompatible with health insurance systems based on payrolls which have emerged as the predominant form of health care funding in the candidate countries, and which depend on high formal employment rates.

Adaptation of health care systems to the requirements of the single European market

A number of health related actions undertaken over the years by the EU to implement its single market policies have also altered the macroeconomic environment in which health care systems exist and have important implications for prospective entrants.

A first set of issues is raised by the opportunities offered to the health sectors in the candidate countries by elimination of barriers to free movement of goods. Manufacturers of medical devices and pharmaceuticals may be attracted to future Member States that have a competitive advantage due to less costly labour. But a prerequisite is the enforcement of international standards relating to intellectual property protection for such products. In addition, inherent tensions between the free movement of goods and diversity of pricing and reimbursement systems have led to the development of parallel trade. As shown by the experience of Spain's accession, medicines sold in acceding countries might be diverted to more lucrative western European markets, so reducing access to them in their original destinations (Lobato 2002). Joining the single market for health products also requires that most candidate countries close the gap with the EU in terms of quality, safety and efficacy standards and ensure that products produced under their jurisdictions meet the necessary international standards (Kanavos 2002). These issues are considered in more detail in Chapters 15 and 16.

A second set of issues is raised by the free movement of patients, especially since the Kohll and Decker judgements by the European Court of Justice. These, and subsequent rulings, have extended the right of patients to seek treatment abroad and clarified that health care provision is, in certain circumstances, considered as a service under European law and so subject to rules on the internal market. This gives candidate countries an opportunity to attract patients, and thus resources, from other Member States by providing cheaper services, while at the same time facing incentives to improve the quality of their services (Busse 2002b). However, the prospect of significant numbers of their own citizens seeking treatment abroad may pose a threat to the finances of their health care systems as the costs of care in current Member States are likely to remain higher for some time. These issues are addressed in more detail in Chapter 11.

A third set of issues is raised by the rules on free movement of professionals within the European single market. These have required candidate countries to update their legislation on professions and, in some cases, restructure training programmes (Cachia 2002; Zajac 2002). These developments have, however, been seen by some as threatening the possibility that a significant number of highly qualified health workers in some candidate countries taking advantage of the single market to emigrate towards the more wealthy Member States. These issues are dealt with in more detail in Chapters 7–10.

The political organization of the health care systems

Countries across Europe face a common challenge of dividing competencies and powers between different administrative and political levels. At an EU level, the Treaty on European Union has confirmed the principle of subsidiarity, in which governance functions should be discharged at the lowest possible level of government. In the health sector, decentralization has emerged as a major thrust of health reform initiatives. Although facing increasing questioning about the appropriate balance between centre and periphery, it has been seen as an effective means of achieving a number of objectives such as to deliver services more responsive to local needs, improve democratic accountability, and create incentives for efficiency. The candidate countries have clearly followed this trend and the accession process has coincided with convergent efforts made in each state to transform the health sector in a less hierarchical and more decentralized system. In Malta, Cyprus and Turkey, decentralization is still an important component of the health reform agenda even though the changes have so far been relatively modest and have mainly involved a shift to a more pluralistic provision of health services (Aktulay 1996; Muscat 1999; European Commission 2003). In the ten countries of CEE, decentralization has been part of the systematic rejection of the communist model of health care governance, which was characterized by a strictly hierarchical structure and a centrally organized budget system, leaving no room for popular choice or local initiative (Afford 2001). A general pattern in health care reforms in CEE has been to devolve to local and/or regional authorities an increased role in provision and, in some cases, financing of health services. Other measures such as the creation of semi-autonomous health insurance agencies and limited privatization of ownership of health care facilities have confirmed the move from the previous centralized structures towards a more pluralistic system. However, while designing these new structures, the candidate countries have also been faced with a common set of emerging policy issues such as defining clearly the distribution of power and competencies among the newly created entities (central versus regional and local; owners versus founders; purchaser versus provider; public versus private), as well as containing costs, preventing irrational duplication, and minimizing disparities between regions (Belli 2001).

The microeconomic efficiency of health services

Microeconomic efficiency refers to both allocative and technical efficiency in the various parts of the health sector. The goal is to achieve a combination of services that minimizes cost while maximizing health outcomes within the resources available for health services. It requires a search for technological innovations, organizational reconfigurations, and combinations of inputs that can most increase efficiency. In this respect, the candidate countries face the challenge not only of providing sufficient resources for health care but also to optimize the funding methods used and develop the most efficient arrangements for the provision of health services. The CEE countries inherited health care delivery systems characterized by labour rather than capital intensive provision and characterized by major shortcomings such as overprovision of poorly equipped hospitals, an emphasis on specialization, a vertical and segmented approach to disease management, underpaid staff with low status, and a lack of incentives to efficiency. To some extent the three Mediterranean countries face similar problems. For instance, institutional fragmentation in Turkey has led to considerable duplication of facilities with under use of staff and resources (European Commission 2002a). In Cyprus it is reported that outdated and inefficient management of the public health system has created opportunities for the private health sector to expand, with implications for equity (European Commission 2002b). Weakness in the mechanisms to refer patients between levels of care remains an important issue in Malta, Turkey and Cyprus. Clearly there is still quite a large potential for improving the microeconomic efficiency of health care delivery in some candidate countries so as to ensure that the limited resources available are used more effectively. A series of convergent measures are part of efforts that have already been made towards this goal, including the following: reductions in hospital capacity, strengthening of primary care, and financing reform.

In summary, candidate countries that are engaged in the twin processes of transition to a market economy and accession to the EU face a number of similar challenges related to:

- the health conditions of their populations;
- a macroeconomic environment characterized by strong fiscal pressures, competing priorities and imperatives of adjusting to a single market;
- many pressing demands for democratizing the governance of health care and designing structures that are more responsive to local needs and expectations;
- deficiencies in the organization of health care at micro-level, leading in some places to a need to reform outdated management structures and create incentives for efficiency.

Some common trends have emerged in the responses to these challenges. They include strengthening of public health capacity, creation of new health care funding bodies with varying degrees of autonomy, diversification of sources of funding (not always by design), creation of a more pluralist model of health care provision, strengthening of health care governance, and changes in methods of paying providers.

But also diversity in trajectories followed by health care systems

The identification of common challenges and evidence of similar policy responses do not mean that health care systems in candidate countries form a homogenous group or are converging towards a single model. A full analysis must also explore the differences between them. This section focuses on the diverse historical, political and economic journeys travelled to reach the stage of accession and highlights a variety of institutional forms which have emerged in the course of the health care reforms.

First, it is apparent that the histories of the candidate countries are diverse. Even in central and eastern Europe, where there was a shared history of communist rule, the legacy from the socialist era differs between countries. The Baltic states were part of the USSR, thus, unlike the other countries that began the process of transition with the governmental machinery of independent states, they faced the need to create anew the basic state institutions. Four of the thirteen candidate countries (the Czech Republic, Slovakia, Hungary, Slovenia) were once part of the former Austro-Hungarian empire and inherited its institutional tradition of work-related social security systems. Malta and Cyprus, which were part of the British Empire until the 1960s, and remain in the British Commonwealth, have inherited the models of health care provision introduced by the British colonial administration. Following the split of Czechoslovakia, the evolution of social and economic policies in the two newly created countries has reflected distinct collective memories of the communist era. While in the Slovak lands the communist regime brought a relative affluence that had never before existed, the Czech lands experienced a relative deceleration or even deterioration in conditions that contrasted with the liberalization, political freedom and relative affluence experienced during the inter-war period (Radicová and Potucek 1997).

Geography also matters. The geographical location of the Baltic countries has created a natural orientation towards the Scandinavian states, strengthened in the case of Estonia by a shared linguistic heritage with Finland. Poland, which shares borders with Germany, has been subject to its influence in designing its social policies. In particular, the German Bismarckian health care model had been introduced in Poland prior to the Second World War, so that its reintroduction after the collapse of the communist bloc created a link with an earlier independent Poland, facilitating the role played by German policy advisers who were active in the reform process (Mihalyi 2000).

On the political level, although the candidate countries, as are the current Member States, are adhering to a model based on Europe of the regions, the organization of public services and the share of responsibilities and powers between central, regional and local authorities differ from one country to another and result in major differences in health care governance. In some countries, such as Estonia and Lithuania, municipalities with elected councils are granted exclusive competencies in regard to the governance of public services and can levy their own taxes. Other countries have developed an intermediate tier (provinces, autonomous counties, districts) with varying responsibilities and powers. Other countries still retain the bulk of powers at the centre while deconcentrating some limited responsibilities (Green 1998). Demographic and geographic factors associated with the size of different countries, their population density, and whether they are predominantly urban or rural, matter in many ways, influencing relations between citizens and public health authorities and public participation in the health care decision-making process. It is also important to recall that most countries have experienced boundary changes more than once in the twentieth century, changes that in some cases have persisting consequences.

On the economic level, there are considerable disparities between the candidate countries and these variations are of utmost importance in understanding the levels of resources allocated to health care and the capacity to implement health care reforms. At the onset of the transition in the early 1990s, a collapse in GDP has been experienced to varying extents in all countries of CEE, resulting in cuts in expenditure on health. Poland had a short, relatively mild recession (6% drop in production over two years) whereas the Baltic countries experienced a long and deep recession (35–51% over five to six years) (World Bank 2002). In 1998, Poland, the Czech Republic, Hungary, Slovakia and Slovenia have either recovered their 1989 level of GDP or came very close to it, in contrast with the Baltic states, Romania and Bulgaria which, at the same date, had recovered less than three-quarters of the 1989 level (EBRD 1999).

Collective memory and pathways to reform are also important variables. During the decades preceding accession, Cyprus, Malta and to a lesser extent Turkey have had very close economic relations with western Europe whereas trade relations in CEE were dominated by Comecon. Some communist states, notably Hungary, and Poland (as well as Slovenia, whose position was different as part of Yugoslavia) introduced elements of market-based reforms and were exposed to western markets even before the collapse of the Soviet Union. This is reflected in a higher score on a liberalization index measured at the onset of transition in 1990 (de Melo and Gelb 1996; EBRD 2000). Poland and the countries of the former Austro-Hungarian empire (Hungary, Czech Republic, Slovakia and Slovenia), which are often considered as the fastest reformers among the post-communist countries, rank with Cyprus and Malta among the seven wealthiest candidate countries. Each had the opportunity to draw on previous market experiences to design institutional frameworks supporting economic transition. Variations also exist in the pace of market liberalization and privatization. Some countries, such as Poland and the Czech Republic, opted for a radical shock therapy resulting in rapid establishment of markets and major adjustments of most economic sectors. Other countries adopted a more gradualist approach which gave primacy to establishing the new institutions needed to support the desired changes.

Thus, the 13 candidate countries began the process of accession with different initial conditions, which go some way to explaining current variations in both economic outcomes and success in transforming the various sectors of their economies, including health care. Health systems are socio-historic constructions that reflect various historical, political and economic influences. In the light of the diverse circumstances described, it is difficult to envisage a single health care model for candidate countries or to expect a single pathway of health system transformation. While it is apparent that the transition and accession processes both give rise to a common set of challenges and imperatives that may explain some similar trends in the development of the health systems, there remain considerable differences between countries. Health care reforms are planned and implemented at national level, within the institutional framework of each country, according to the specific circumstances and value structures of each society. Both exogenous and endogenous factors are driving health system reform in the candidate countries, leading them in diverse directions, reflected in diverse institutional forms. This diversity can be seen in several key areas of health care reform, including funding, governance and entitlements.

Collection and pooling of funds

The Semashko model, which prevailed within the former communist countries of CEE and the tax-funded model, adopted to varying extents by Malta, Cyprus and Turkey have both, in their different ways, resulted in health care systems mainly funded from the state budget. Reforms of health care funding in the candidate countries from the early 1990s were driven by the same principles of liberalization of social welfare and were intended to increase the financial resources available for health care, with a shift away from the centralized state model, and as a means of enforcing accountability of both providers and users of health care resources. To achieve these objectives two main strategies have been envisioned and are being implemented: creation of social insurance funds and increases in private financing of health expenditures. Although these common strategies might suggest convergence of funding policies, the financial and institutional arrangements for the new schemes differ in many ways.

One is the mix of sources of funding. Despite the evident shift to social insurance contributions, funding of health care in most countries still relies on a mix of sources including general taxation, social insurance contributions, voluntary insurance premiums and user charges. Analysis of the financing pattern in the candidate countries shows three distinct clusters:

In Slovakia, the Czech Republic, Hungary, Slovenia, Estonia, Romania, Poland and Lithuania, earmarked funds collected under the social insurance scheme comprise the greatest part of health spending and cover up to 95% of health expenditures. It should be noted that the first four countries of this group were formerly part of the Austro-Hungarian empire, which had adopted the Bismarck model of health insurance. Latvia and Bulgaria are moving towards a health insurance system.

In Cyprus, Malta and Turkey, general taxation provides the main source of health care funding but it amounts to less than 50% of health expenditures and the general trend until recently has been towards increasing the private share under the form of voluntary premiums or user charges. In this group of countries, out-of-pocket payments constitute the second most important source funding for health care. Three health insurance funds are operating in Turkey but have a limited scope and they provide coverage of only specific groups. Initiatives to implement a national system of social insurance in Malta and Cyprus are still in a very early phase of their development.

The second is the degree of concentration of the health insurance sector. It is too early to form a definitive assessment of the orientation of the health insurance market in the candidate countries, but it already appears that there are different trends in respect of the structure of the health insurance market (Busse 2002a). At least two clusters may be identified.

Some systems, such as those implemented in Slovakia, the Czech Republic,

Latvia, Poland and Romania, are relatively fragmented, thus reproducing a main characteristic of the German archetypal model. In the mid-1990s there were as many as 27 competing health insurance funds in the Czech Republic, 12 in Slovakia and 32 territorial sickness funds in Latvia. Their numbers have since been reduced but the principle of plurality has been safeguarded with nine health insurance funds in the Czech Republic, five in Slovakia and eight in Latvia. In Poland and Romania, regional health fund monopolies, with considerable autonomy, divide up the administrative territories, coexisting with a limited number of additional countrywide funds.

Other systems, such as those implemented in Hungary, Estonia, Lithuania, Slovenia and Bulgaria appear to reproduce a characteristic of the French health insurance model, with its trend towards a more concentrated, less fragmented health insurance market. The providers of health insurance in this group of countries are limited to single national funds. Regional funds, when they exist, are directly subordinated to the central funds.

The third is the degree to which the social insurance sector is steered. When implementing reforms of health care funding, policy-makers in the candidate countries were faced with the challenge of finding the right balance between, on the one hand, the will to create independent public institutions to manage the funds and, on the other hand, the risk that the governments might lose control of decision-making and thus of significant financial resources. In Hungary, it turned out that the extensive financial and political independence of the National Health Insurance Funds induced moral hazard, resulting in recurrent deficits which were automatically refinanced by the government at the expense of other sectors. Since 1998, the Hungarian Government reversed the situation in appropriating direct responsibility for the health insurance funds (Mihalyi and Petru 1999). A similar trend has been followed in the Czech Republic, Estonia and Turkey where the management of the health insurance funds is primarily a state responsibility. In contrast, Slovakia, Slovenia, Bulgaria and Lithuania have implemented a structure of governance in which power is shared between representatives of the government, employers and the insured. In Poland and Latvia, the governance of the health insurance funds falls under the jurisdictions of local governments (regional councils in the first case and municipalities in the other).

The fourth is the nature of risk equalization schemes or pooling systems. Where there are multiple social health insurance funds (Poland, the Czech Republic, Slovakia, Latvia, Romania), a risk equalization mechanism is needed to maintain the objective of solidarity and consequently prevent risk selection (cream skimming), reduce existing differences in the risk structure between the insurance companies and prevent fiscal insolvency of health insurance funds with adverse risk structures. The risk equalization schemes in the current candidate countries are still largely embryonic, but again it is clear that there is no uniformity in the initiatives that have been taken. In Poland and Slovakia, the overall revenue of the health insurance funds is subject to the equalization process (Mihalyi and Petru 1999; Hlavacka and Sckackova 2000). Romania and the Czech Republic use a formula that reallocates only a part of the revenue, respectively 25% and 60% (Busse 2000; Vladescu et al. 2000). In Latvia, the funds are de facto redistributed because the territorial sickness funds remain largely funded by a tax-financed system (Karaskevica and Tragakes 2001).

Governance of health services

Beyond the broad pattern of increasing transfer of responsibilities to local levels and delegation of financing to health insurance funds, a variety of paths are being followed by the candidate countries in the process of redesigning governance structures for health care. Variations observed fall into two main categories, corresponding to two main targets of current reforms:

Governance of primary and secondary care

The process of decentralizing the governance of primary and secondary care in the candidate countries exhibits four distinctive patterns. Estonia, Lithuania and Bulgaria have adopted a model with features similar to that in Finland, creating the most advanced form of decentralization among the candidate countries. Municipalities with elected local governments are granted a high degree of political control over the organization and provision of primary and secondary care. Local self-governments decide on municipal budgets for health care and hold authority to privatize some services. Municipalities as owners are responsible for the maintenance and capital costs of their health care facilities, including local hospitals and polyclinics. General practitioners, as independent providers, contract with the sickness funds and operate in polyclinics and other ambulatory facilities owned by the municipalities and increasingly by private providers. In Bulgaria and Estonia, partial responsibility for financing was transferred to municipalities (Hinkov et al. 1999; Jesse 2000). For instance, elected municipalities in Estonia spend up to 58% of total income tax and can raise additional taxes for expenditures on local services.

Hungary and Latvia have adopted arrangements which are similar to those developed in Sweden, Norway and Denmark. Two tiers of elected local self-governments, autonomous counties at the intermediate level and municipalities at the basic level, divide up responsibilities for organization and provision of primary and secondary health services while tertiary care remains a state responsibility (Green 1998). Counties are responsible for providing secondary care in district general hospitals. Hospital personnel are mainly salaried employees accountable to the county councils through an executive structure. Municipalities are legally responsible for planning and ensuring the provision of primary care. They employ salaried health care teams or contract with independent general practitioners to provide services (Gaal et al. 1999; Karaskevica and Tragakes 2001). The ownership of the bulk of primary care facilities, polyclinics and hospitals has been transferred to local governments (counties and municipalities)

In Poland, the Czech Republic and Romania, the provincial authorities at the intermediate level dominate the planning and the provision of health services. But there is a trend towards bringing the management of some hospitals and primary care facilities under the control of a few larger municipalities. The provincial structure is characterized by a system of dual subordination combining an Assembly indirectly elected by representatives of municipalities with an executive headed by a centrally appointed governor (Green 1998). The implication is that primary and secondary care are primarily planned and directed by the Ministry of Health through provincial health boards in which representatives of the municipalities can participate. Recent changes in the Czech Republic and Poland have confirmed a trend towards increasing influence of municipalities, with a greater role for the private sector. In Poland, the control of integrated health care organizations delivering primary care has been transferred to larger municipalities (Karski and Koronkiewicz 2000). In the Czech Republic, primary care is increasingly provided by independent general practitioners who operate private practices within health centres and polyclinics owned by municipalities (Busse 2000).

In Malta, Cyprus, Slovenia, Slovakia and Turkey, notwithstanding recent attempts to introduce a decentralized governance of health services, the balance of powers within the health care system is still tilted towards the centre. The systems in Malta, Slovenia and Cyprus are characterized by highly centralized structures (Muscat 1999; Albreht et al. 2002; European Commission 2002b). Central governments have the overall responsibility for planning, funding, administering and delivering primary and secondary care. Moreover, the small size of these countries mitigates against creating regional level health authorities. In these three countries, privatization has featured as the most favoured option for decentralization, notably in the primary care sector where there has been a move towards having independent practitioners contracted with the health funds to provide health services. In Turkey and Slovakia, the thrust for decentralization set out in the health sector reform has many features of deconcentration. The provincial health administration in Turkey and the district offices in Slovakia, which provide primary and secondary care, are primarily subordinate units of the Ministry of Health and administrative arms of the central government (Aktulay 1996; Hlavacka and Sckackova 2000).

Governance of public health

Two distinct paths in the governance of public have emerged from recent transformations of health systems in the candidate countries. National governments in seven states of CEE (Slovakia, Slovenia, Hungary, Bulgaria, Estonia, Latvia and Lithuania) as well as Cyprus and Malta have taken direct responsibility for public health services through the creation of a national agency for public and environmental health. In most cases, responsibilities are shared with deconcentrated units which operate at district level, in parallel and not as an integral part of local self-governments (Green 1998). It is expected that these national health agencies will make it possible to address more effectively important public health concerns because they have more capacity than local units to provide specific and complex services and because they often have the scope to raise extra funding for additional activities.

In three states of CEE (Czech Republic, Poland and Romania) as well as Turkey, public health responsibilities are primarily devolved to provincial governments. For the three former communist states in this group, this means that they are still operating the inherited infrastructure of sanitary-epidemiological stations in which the combined functions of preventive public health and environmental health protection were run within a framework determined by the Ministry of Health.

Entitlements, benefits, coverage, users' choice and sharing of costs

Although governments in all the candidate countries have subscribed to the principles of solidarity and universality of care, the range of services covered, their accessibility, the scope of users' choice, the sharing of costs and the mechanisms of reimbursements vary from one country to another. In some states such as Malta, Slovenia, Slovakia and Czech Republic, the public health care system ensures coverage of all citizens and/or permanent residents whereas in Bulgaria, Hungary, Lithuania, Poland and Romania entitlement is based on contributions to the health insurance plan, creating threats to the equity of the health system (European Commission 2003). In Cyprus, the public sector restricts the free provision of health services only to government employees, families with four or more children, certain categories of chronically ill persons and individuals and households with low incomes. The higher income groups must pay user charges to access public health services (European Commission 2002b).

Defining a systematic basic benefit package remains an ongoing issue in many candidate countries and again the policies vary considerably. Slovakia exemplifies a state where health care benefits are very comprehensive with a wide range of services covered. Services such as rehabilitation, spa treatment, spectacles and most basic dental procedures are provided (European Commission 2002c). Other countries such as Latvia have shown a trend towards reducing the "Basic Care programme" which is reviewed annually (European Commission 2002d). In Cyprus and to a lesser extent in Malta, due to the small size of the health market, the production of some highly specialized services is not financially viable. Consequently, the Maltese and Cypriot Governments fund overseas treatment for conditions necessitating such highly specialized care.

As a means of controlling demand, co-payment is a common option used by all the candidate countries, but in diverse ways. While most countries restrict co-payments for basic benefits to drugs and specific services such as dental care, a few countries such as Cyprus and Estonia require co-payments even for outpatient visits. Freedom of choice for users of health services is a further issue. Users' choices in the candidate countries are restricted to varying degrees while each country is choosing among different options or combining several policy tools to foster appropriate use of services: gatekeeping function, choice restricted within a specific pool of providers or a territorial unit, rules of reimbursements, and co-payments.

Thus, on many key areas of health care reforms in the candidate countries, there is a strong case against the assumption that there is a single health policy track. Although the changes relating to health care funding, governance of health services, and organization of health care are still in process and in some cases operating at a rapid pace, the evidence to date suggests that multiple paths are being followed by the different countries involved in the accession process.

Conclusion

The 13 candidate countries are all implementing major changes to their health systems, although these are largely independent of the process of EU accession. Many of the candidate countries face a similar set of challenges, reflecting the health of their populations and organization of their health care systems. Common problems arise from inadequate infrastructure, scarcity of resources and out-of-date management systems. Current reforms show many similar trends, including a shift towards health insurance, plurality in the provision of health services and increased devolution to lower tiers of governments. Yet the evidence reviewed in this analysis warns against the simplistic assumption that there is an ineluctable process of convergence. First the unique characteristics of the candidate countries, the diversity in their institutional histories, and the variations in their starting conditions during the process of transition mean that their institutional changes are likely to follow diverse paths. It has been shown that the candidate countries use various policy options to implement similar objectives, consistent with the distinct endogenous conditions shaping options and choices in each country. Second the accession process and the transition of the post-communist countries has occurred in a context of growing uncertainty as to which health care structure is most appropriate to deal with common challenges, also faced by western European systems, such as cost containment, control of technologies, shifting relationships between the different levels of care and the need for better management of both demand and provision. Within the EU, several competing models suggest different policy alternatives to deal with common challenges. For many of these issues, solutions are often tailored to the unique characteristics and traditions of each country.

The diversity of contexts, the emphasis on subsidiarity in European health policy, and the fragmentation of issues impacting on health care within the *acquis communautaire* mean that there is no single EU approach to health care that can be aimed at. Yet it is also true that purported EU requirements are used as a justification for actions driven by domestic agendas and, at the same time, true EU requirements have simply led to the creation of institutional facades designed to satisfy external expectations and demands while parallel institutions and practices that reflect domestic preferences persist (Verheijen 1999; Dimitrova 2002).

While further rounds of enlargement seem inevitable and because the current acceding countries will have to complete the process of integration after gaining full membership, EU accession and subsequent integration of the new members is a two-sided process, which must take into consideration the unique circumstances of each acceding country, drawing on knowledge of successful existing practices and recognizing the potential contribution of each new member to the broad spectrum of experience that already exists within the EU.

References

Afford, C.W. (2001) Failing health systems: failing health workers in Eastern Europe. Report on the Basic Security Survey for the International Labour Office and Public Services International Affiliates in the Health Sector in Central and Eastern Europe. Geneva: International Labour Office.

Agh, A. (1999a) Europeanization of policy making in East Central Europe: the Hungarian approach to European Union accession, *Journal of European Public Policy*, 6(5):839–54.

Agh, A. (1999b) Processes of democratization in the Central European and Balkan States: sovereignty-related conflicts in the context of Europeanization, *Communist and Post-Communist Studies*, 32(3):263–79.

Agh, A. (2003) Public administration in Central and Eastern Europe, in B.G. Peter and J. Pierre (eds) *Handbook of Public Administration*. London: Sage.

Aktulay, G. (1996) *Health Care systems in Transition: Turkey*. Copenhagen: WHO Regional Office for Europe.

Albreht, T., Cesen, M., Hindle, D. et al. (2002) *Health Care Systems in Transition: Slovenia*. Copenhagen: European Observatory on Health Care Systems.

Belli, P. (2001) *Ten years of health reforms in the ECA region. Lessons learned and option for the future*. Harvard, MA: Harvard School of Public Health: Harvard Center for Population and Development Studies.

Börzel, T.A. and Risse, T. (2000) When Europe hits home: Europeanization and domestic change. European Integration online Papers (EIoP), 4, 15, http://eiop.or.at/eiop/texte/2000-015a.htm.

Buller, J., Evans, M. and James, O. (2002) Understanding the Europeanisation of public policy, *Public Policy and Administration*, 17(Special issue):2.

Busse, R. (2000) *Health Care Systems in Transition: Czech Republic*. Copenhagen: European Observatory on Health Care Systems.

Busse, R. (2002a) Health care systems in European Union pre-accession countries and European Integration, *Arbeit und Sozialpolitik*, 41–50.

Busse, R. (2002b) Border-crossing patients in the EU, *Eurohealth*, 8(4):19–21.

Cachia, J. (2002) Human resources in Maltese healthcare. Solutions for common needs, *Eurohealth*, 8(4):17–18.

Cowles, M.G., Caporaso, J.A. and Risse, T. (2001) *Europeanization and domestic change*. Ithaca: Cornell University Press.

Dallago, B., Horst, B. and Wladimir, A. (1992) *Convergence and system change. The convergence hypothesis in the light of transition in Eastern Europe*. Aldershot: Dartmouth.

de Melo, M. and Gelb, A. (1996) A comparative analysis of twenty transition economies in Europe and Asia, *Post-Soviet Geography and Economics*, 37(5):265–85.

Dimitrova, A. (2002) Enlargement, institution-building and the European Union's administrative capacity requirement, *West European Politics*, 25(4, supplement):171–90.

EBRD (1999) *Transition Report 1999: Ten Years of Transition*. London: European Bank for Reconstruction and Development.

EBRD (2000) *Transition Report 2000*. London: European Bank for Reconstruction and Development.

European Commission (1995) White paper on the preparation of the associated countries of Central and Eastern Europe for integration into the internal market of the union. Brussels: European Commission.

European Commission (2002a) Study on the social protection systems in the 13 applicant countries. Turkey. Country Report. Brussels: European Commission, Employment and Social Affairs.

European Commission (2002b) Study on the social protection systems in the 13 applicant countries. Cyprus. Country Report. Brussels: European Commission, Employment and Social Affairs.

European Commission (2002c) Study on the social protection systems in the 13 applicant countries. Slovakia. Country Report. Brussels: European Commission, Employment and Social Affairs.

European Commission (2002d) Study on the social protection systems in the 13 applicant countries. Latvia. Country Report. Brussels: European Commission, Employment and Social Affairs.

European Commission (2003) The social protection systems in the 13 candidate countries (25/3/2003). Studies carried out for the Commission by GVG – Gesellschaft für Versicherungswissenschaft und -gestaltung e.V. Final report. Brussels: European Commission. Directorate-General for Employment and Social Affairs.

Gaal, P., Rekassy, B. and Healy, J. (1999) *Health Care Systems in Transition: Hungary.* Copenhagen: WHO Regional Office for Europe.

Grabbe, H. (2001) How does Europeanisation affect CEE governance? Conditionality, diffusion and diversity, *Journal of European Public Policy*, 8(6):1013–31.

Green, G. (1998) Health and governance in European cities. A compendium of trends and responsibilities for public health in 46 Member States of the WHO European Region London: European Hospital Management Journal Limited.

Héritier, A., Kerwer, D., Knill, C., et al. (2001) *Differential Europe. The European Union impact on national policymaking.* Oxford: Powman & Littlefield Publishers, Inc.

Hinkov, H., Koulaksuzov, S., Semerdjiev, I. and Healy, J. (1999) *Health Care Systems in Transition. Bulgaria.* Copenhagen: European Observatory on Health Care Systems.

Hlavacka, S. and Sckackova, D. (2000) *Health Care Systems in Transition: Slovakia.* Copenhagen: European Observatory on Health Care Systems.

Hollingsworth, J., Schmitter, P. and Streeck, W. (1994) *Governing capitalist economies: performance and control of economic sectors.* Oxford: Oxford University Press.

Jesse, M. (2000) *Health Care Systems in Transition. Estonia.* Copenhagen: European Observatory on Health Care Systems.

Kanavos, P. (2002) European Union pharmaceutical policy: The challenges and opportunities of enlargement, *Eurohealth*, 8(4):24–6.

Karaskevica, J. and Tragakes, E. (2001) *Health care systems in transition: Latvia.* Copenhagen: European Observatory on Health Care Systems.

Karski, B. and Koronkiewicz, A. (2000) *Health care systems in transition: Poland.* Copenhagen: European Observatory on Health Care Systems.

Knill, C. and Lehmkuhl, D. (1999) How Europe matters: different mechanisms of Europeanization, *European Integration online Papers (EIoP)*, 3:7.

Lewis, M. (2002) Informal health payments in central and eastern Europe and the former Soviet Union: issues, trends and policy implications, in E. Mossialos, A. Dixon, J. Figueras and J. Kutzin, *Funding health care: options for Europe.* Buckingham: Open University Press.

Lobato, M. (2002) Pharmaceutical policy Lessons from Spanish accession, *Eurohealth*, 8(4):27–8.

Magnin, E. (1996) Complexité et trajectoire tchèque de transformation économique post-socialiste, *Revue d'Etudes Comparatives Est-Ouest*, 27:1.

Marrée, J. and Groenewegen, P.P. (1997) *Back to Bismarck: Eastern European health care systems in transition.* Aldershot: Avebury.

Mihalyi, J. (2000) Post-socialist health systems in transition: Czech Republic, Hungary and Poland. Working Paper WP4/2000, Department of Economics, Central European University.

Mihalyi, P. and Petru, R. (1999) Health care in the Czech Republic, Hungary and Poland – the medium-term fiscal aspects. Warsaw: Center for Social and Economic Research.

Muscat, N.A. (1999) *Health Care Systems in Transition: Malta*. Copenhagen: European Observatory on Health Care Systems.

Nee, V. (1989) A theory of market transition: from redistribution to markets in state socialism, *American Sociological Review*, 54:663–81.

Nelson, J.M., Tilly, C. and Walker, L. (1997) *Transforming post-Communist political economies. Task Force on Economies in transition, Commission on Behavioural and Social Sciences and Education, National Research Council*. Washington, DC: National Academy Press.

North, D.C. (1990) *Institutions, institutional change and economic performance*. Cambridge: Cambridge University Press.

Radicová, I. and Potucek, M. (1997) *Two Social Policies from One: The Czech and Slovak Example. Social Consequences of Economic Transformation in East-Central Europe*. Vienna: (SOCO) program of the Institute for Human Sciences.

Schneider, F. (2002) *The size and development of the shadow economies of the 22 Transition and 21 OECD countries*. Bonn: IZA.

Stark, D. (1992) Path dependence and privatization strategies in East Central Europe, *East European Politics and Societies*, 6(1):17–54.

Verheijen, T. (1999) *Civil services systems in Central and Eastern Europe*. Cheltenham: Edward Elgar.

Vladescu, C., Radulescu, S. and Olsavsky, V. (2000) *Health Care Systems in Transition: Romania*. Copenhagen: European Observatory on Health Care Systems.

WHO (2002) *The World Health Report 2002, Reducing risks, promoting healthy life*. Geneva: World Health Organization.

WHO Regional Office for Europe (2002) *Health status overview for countries of Central and Eastern Europe that are candidate for accession to the European Union*. European Communities and World Health Organization. Copenhagen: WHO Regional Office for Europe.

World Bank (1996) *From plan to market: World Development Report 1996*. Washington, DC: World Bank.

World Bank (2002) *Transition – The First Ten Years – Analysis and lessons for Eastern Europe and the Former Soviet Union*. Washington DC: World Bank.

Zajac, M. (2002) EU accession: Implications for Poland's health care personnel, *Eurohealth*, 8(4):13–14.

chapter five

Investing in health for accession

Nicholas Jennett[1]

Introduction

There is one factor above all others that makes the forthcoming accession of countries to the EU unlike any other. This is the issue of the economic perform- ance of the new members. There is still a wide gap between the incomes of the current 15 Member States (EU 15) and the acceding and candidate countries. The ten central and eastern European (CEE)[2] candidates' gross domestic product (GDP) per head as a percentage of the EU average, measured in purchasing power parities, went up from 38% in 1999 to 39% in 2000. If all 13 candidate countries (including Turkey) are included, it stood unchanged at the previous year's level of 35%. It is arguable that this gap is the biggest single challenge to the accession process.

It is true, of course, that the EU has experience of accession by relatively poor countries. In this context, the accessions of Ireland (1973), Greece (1981), Spain (1986) and Portugal (1986) are the most relevant examples. Ireland is often quoted as Europe's most stunning success story: on accession, Ireland's income per head was 54% of the EU average. But over the last decade the country has achieved a real growth rate of around 6.5% per annum. Eurostat estimates that in terms of GDP per head in purchasing power parity (PPP) terms, Ireland will reach over 120% of the EU average in 2002. Greece, Spain and Portugal have also achieved significant economic progress from low levels of income per head on accession (62% of the EU average in the case of Greece, 71% for Spain and 55% for Portugal) (European Commission 2001a).

The economic achievements of these entrants have been impressive. How- ever, it is also clear that accession per se is not a "quick fix". Greece, for example, achieved no catch up in its first post-accession decade – indeed, relative income levels fell. Ireland's growth rate only accelerated in the years well after accession.

But even putting these issues aside, there are a number of important differences between accession then and accession now. First, and as indicated above, the accessions of Ireland, Spain, Greece and Portugal were from an economic "starting base" significantly above the average levels of the current candidates. Second, the scale of the previous accessions was smaller and so the economic impact on the EU as a whole was less marked. In contrast, were all 13 accession and candidate countries[3] to accede today, EU average GDP per head (in PPP) would fall by more than 20%. Finally, the "rules of game" are different in this accession round. As the Commission has put it:

> Previous rounds of EU enlargement are only to a limited degree comparable to the present round. The economic structures of the countries and the rules and implications of EU membership were then very different. (European Commission 2001a)

It is clear that the Commission was referring *inter alia* to economic issues of great relevance to the candidates associated with regional and agricultural policy.

Although the acceding and candidate states are forecast to grow more quickly than the EU15 between 2001 and 2004, in many cases this growth is insufficient to make a significant impact on catching up. This is illustrated in Table 5.1.

At these rates of growth, only five of the acceding countries (Cyprus, Czech Republic, Estonia, Hungary and Slovenia) will have achieved 75% of EU average income by 2027. Bulgaria, Lithuania, Malta, Poland, Romania and Turkey will each take in excess of 30 years to achieve a GDP per head of 75% of the EU mean (European Commission 2001a). Catching up to the EU mean would take three decades or longer for virtually all candidate countries. These figures are a matter of very considerable concern; to quote the Commission again: "The

Table 5.1 Economic performance of candidate countries in relation to EU15

	Real growth forecast 2001–2004	GDP per head in PPP (% of EU average)		
		1995	2000	2004
Acceding States				
Cyprus	4.5	79.4	82.6	90.0
Czech Republic	3.8	62.2	60.1	63.8
Estonia	5.8	32.0	38.0	43.6
Hungary	5.3	46.1	52.8	59.4
Latvia	5.7	24.3	29.2	33.3
Lithuania	4.8	27.5	29.5	32.5
Malta	3.3	49.3	53.2	55.5
Poland	3.1	33.9	38.9	40.1
Slovakia	3.9	43.9	48.1	51.2
Slovenia	4.5	64.3	71.6	78.0
Candidate States				
Bulgaria	5.9	27.7	24.1	27.7
Romania	5.1	31.9	26.9	30.0
EU	2.3	100.0	100.0	100.0

challenge is how to design a more ambitious reform programme that would allow for higher, but still sustainable, growth" (European Commission Directorate General for Economic and Financial Affairs 2002).

This chapter argues that investment in health has an important, but so far neglected, part to play in such a new, ambitious programme for the candidate countries. This could take place through direct investment in health care or through paying stronger attention to the impact on health of other policies in the accession process. The next section in this chapter looks at the issue of health status in candidate countries (a more detailed discussion can be found in Chapter 3). It argues that the CEE candidate countries have an important *comparative advantage* in investing in health. Subsequent sections then look at the theoretical arguments for such investment and, in contrast, the neglect of health considerations during the accession process. The chapter concludes by examining what the EU and accession countries could do to improve this situation.

Health and the acceding and candidate countries

As shown in Chapter 3, the gap between the accession countries and Member States in terms of their health status is wide and well documented. Furthermore, there is little evidence that this gap is narrowing. Why does this matter? At one level, inequality itself is a strong argument for action. There is a real issue about the extent to which existing Member States and the new members can be regarded as participants in a single community while such inequalities persist.

Second, there is the (essentially self-interested) argument that existing Member States should be concerned about the state of health among their new partners because of the risks of some "export" of health problems (particularly those relating to infectious diseases) as movement of individuals becomes easier following accession.

But there is a third argument – that there may be a link between health and economic performance. This suggests that action to improve health may be important – perhaps even necessary – to address the problems of economic "catch up" referred to above. This argument justifies a close examination of the link between health status and economic performance. Data from a large number of countries shows that there is a strong positive statistical correlation between income per head (economic performance) and a range of indicators of health status. But a close look at this relationship reveals an interesting and important finding for the CEE acceding and candidate countries. It has been argued (Hager and Suhrcke 2001; UNICEF 2001) that these countries' performance in terms of health status is better than would be "suggested" by their level of economic development. This is illustrated in Figure 5.1 which analyses the relationship between infant mortality and income (measured by GNP) per head for a range of countries. The figure shows that all of the CEE acceding countries (Latvia, Lithuania, Poland, Hungary, Estonia, Slovakia, the Czech Republic and Slovenia) lie below the line of "best fit", suggesting that for their level of income, they have a lower than expected level of infant mortality. Infant mortality

Figure 5.1   Infant mortality in middle income developing countries, 1998

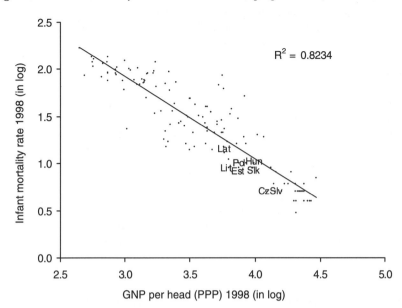

Source: World Bank (2000), World Development Indicators 2000, Washington, DC.

represents only one indicator of health status but similar conclusions would be drawn from an analysis of income and life expectancy.

This suggests that although health status is poor compared to existing Member States, the CEE countries enjoy relatively good health status compared to other countries at a similar level of economic development. This good health status *relative to their level of income* represents an important "head start" or comparative advantage in the growth stakes. Many candidate countries enjoy a similar comparative advantage in relation to their educational performance. In relation to both health and education, this is a consequence of a relatively strong legacy from pre-transition times. It is important that these advantages are not lost.

Health, human capital and growth – some theory and evidence

Why is this "head start" important? There is strong evidence that in parallel to investment in infrastructure and industry, economic growth requires societies to invest in human capital. A major World Bank study (Thomas et al. 2000) has recently concluded that no country has ever achieved sustained development without substantial investment in the education and health of its people. For example, there is a great deal of evidence (de la Fuenta and Ciccone 2002) for the role that *education* can play in promoting growth; a recent study of the spectacular growth record of the Irish economy confirms the importance of this form of human capital investment for the accession economies (Ferreira and

Vanhoudt 2002/01). The idea of investment in *health* also has a long academic tradition (Grossman 1972) and in the least developed countries, the work of the Commission on Macroeconomics and Health (2001) has made a powerful case for the importance of investment in health as a driver of economic development. An important Working Paper for the Commission (Bloom et al. 2001) found in a study of more than 100 countries that improvements in health have a significant positive effect on aggregate output.

The measure of "health" used in this study was life expectancy, and within the least developed countries these arguments are clearly understandable. For example, the AIDS pandemic in Africa will cause a decline in life expectancy in 51 countries in the next two decades, a demographic effect essentially without precedent in modern times. Seven countries in sub-Saharan Africa now have life expectancies of less than 40 years. In Botswana, life expectancy is now 39 years, instead of the 72 it would have been without the emergence of AIDS. By the end of this decade, 11 countries in the region will have life expectancies close to the age of 30. But the argument that investment in human capital through health care and other factors that improve health increases economic growth in more developed economies may seem less convincing. Could similar arguments relating health to economic performance apply in "developed" and in transition economies?

As noted above, there is clear evidence of a correlation between health and economic performance. The issue for middle income countries is whether good health causes good economic performance – or good economic performance causes good health. In practice, both are probably true. A number of academic studies on the causes of growth have now indicated that health and health care can play an important causal role in improving economic performance (Hager and Suhrcke 2001).

Why should investment in health have this effect? Most obviously, spending on health care per se is a valuable contribution to national output. Just like any other valuable service (including those of bankers, teachers and restaurant owners), activity in the sector adds directly to the sum of output and incomes in society. Across the EU as a whole, approximately 8.5% of national output is provided by the health care sector. The equivalent figure for CEE countries is around 5.8% (WHO 2002).

But there are other important arguments beyond the direct expenditure effect. First, whether through investment in health care (McKee 1999), public health interventions or initiatives to reflect the impact of health in other policies, better population health can lead to important induced growth effects. Some individuals will choose to devote their additional health capital (additional healthy life years) to market activities (working longer, more productively or with lower levels of absenteeism) which have a direct impact on GDP. In this context, although many health services and interventions are focused on people who are above the age at which they produce marketed outputs (even though most will continue to produce non-marketed outputs) by no means all are.

Second, regions or countries that have poor health status, and often poor health care facilities, may find it harder to attract or retain productive enterprises or individuals. This will also have an induced effect on income and growth levels. Third, investment in efficient health services will ensure that the long-term budgetary cost of care of a given quality is lower than it would otherwise have been. The improved output of these services (better health) should also reduce the costs of future social interventions (in health itself, disability, unemployment and so on). Finally, there are also some intriguing insights from a "new" perspective on the determinants of growth that has received much attention in recent years. This is the notion that alongside physical and human capital, the level of growth and development within a country or region is also dependent on its level of *social capital*.[4]

Social capital refers to the institutions, trust relationships and norms that shape the quality and quantity of a society's social interactions. Social capital is not just the sum of the institutions that make up society – it is the "glue" that holds them together. The core of the social capital argument is that economic and social development thrives when representatives of the state, the corporate sector and civil society create means through which they can identify and pursue common goals and where relationships between individuals (and between individuals and institutions) are characterized by trust (including the absence of corruption and "fair" treatment of individuals by public authorities).

Empirical studies of the impact of social capital are limited, but there is now some evidence that shows that social cohesion and trust are critical elements if societies are to prosper economically and if development is to be sustainable (Puttnam 2002). It is arguable that investment in the health sector has an important role to play in the development of social capital. In the first place, the "social solidarity" aspects of public health care can make a significant contribution to cohesion and trust. This underpins, for example, the importance of eliminating corruption in health services and the key issue of social solidarity in health care financing. Greater responsiveness of health services to individual and collective aspirations could also have a role in play in building social capital. To take an example, if individuals believe that health services will be "there when they (or their family) need them" they may prove to be more geographically mobile in search of employment. This is in the knowledge that decent services will be available for those family members who move to a new location, as well as for more dependent members of the family left behind. Finally, health is an important focus for activities of interest and voluntary groups in civil society, another important area for the development of social capital.

Overall, therefore, there are some strong arguments for the proposition that investment in improvements in health could be important in promoting economic growth within the candidate countries. In this context, it is important to build on the "head start" (or comparative advantage) that these candidates have in relation to their health performance.

What priority for investment in health in the process of accession?

Against this background, it might be expected that the priority attached to investment in health during the accession process would be high. In fact the opposite is true. Within the CEE candidate countries, investment in health continues to take low priority for two main reasons.

First, the importance of human and social capital investment compared to physical capital investment is still not appreciated in finance ministries. Resources for health are still often regarded as a form of consumption rather than investment expenditure. Given that the policy objective of many candidate countries is to reduce public sector deficits and contain public spending, health is often seen as a drain on national resources rather than as a means of adding to them. Slow progress in the reform of health care is often also cited as a constraint on additional investment in the sector.

Second, there has been an overemphasis on the narrow *acquis* issues in much of the enlargement debate. The fact that health care services are matter of national competence within the EU (that is, subject to subsidiarity) has tended to discourage consideration of the role that more effective services could play in boosting health and economic potential. More generally, and as referred to elsewhere in the book (see Chapter 14) the impact of *acquis* issues on wider health considerations has tended to be ignored during the accession negotiations. This represents a missed opportunity both for candidate countries and for existing Member States. The lack of concern over health within the candidate countries is neither economically, nor legally, justified.

What more is needed?

What could be done by Members States and candidate countries to address this missed opportunity? First, and in relation to direct investment, a proportion of EU pre- and post-accession funding for acceding countries could be reoriented towards investment for health improvement. In 2000–2006, the Phare programme (originally the Poland and Hungary Action for the Restructuring of the Economy programme) is providing some €1560 million per annum for institution building support through "twinning", technical assistance and investment to help applicant countries in their efforts to promote economic and social cohesion (European Commission 2001b). Over the period 1990 to 1998, around €9 billion was committed – but for reasons explained by Magda Rosenmöller (Rosenmöller 2002), only 1.2% of this was allocated to public health. In contrast, 24% was committed to traditional infrastructure (energy, transport and telecoms) (Phare 1998).

In terms of capital investment funding, the EU could extend the coverage of the Instrument for Structural Policies for Pre-Accession (ISPA) grant programme, which has an annual budget of €1040 million (at 1999 prices) (http://europa.eu. int/comm/enlargement/pas/ispa.htm). The programme, which comes under the responsibility of the Regional Policy Directorate General, finances major environmental and transport infrastructure projects. Transferring 10% of this amount to health investment would yield some €500 million over the period (Hager and Jennett 2002). Although it is late in the day for reorientation of these *pre*-accession programmes for some countries, the opportunity should be urgently taken to reflect health considerations in the programming of Structural and Cohesion Funds for the newly acceding countries.[5]

Second, a greater orientation on the health consequences of other policies, including those implicit in the accession process, is required. Many of the policies required to implement successfully the *acquis* have consequences for health – and some of these are negative. There is a clear danger that the economic advantages of accession could be undermined by unintended and disadvantageous consequences for health. As this chapter has argued, this will act to frustrate, rather than support, the economic convergence that candidates and Member States alike seek from accession.

As Karen Lock argues in Chapter 15, Health Impact Assessment (HIA) provides an operational methodology for the systematic analysis of the impact of wider policies on health. There are strong economic reasons for an enlarged EU to accord at least as much importance to HIA as it currently accords to Environmental Impact Assessment. Indeed, the importance of HIA is probably greater.

Conclusion

Investment in health – in human capital – is a clear prerequisite for the candidate countries and the EU to meet aspirations for accession. The EU has the means and mechanisms to simultaneously make a major impact on the quality of human capital formation within the candidate countries and protect the interests of the Union's existing citizens. The key constraints appear to be the willingness of the acceding countries to regard resources committed to health as investment in the future of their people and the willingness of the EU to accord the same significance to the protection of human health in other policies as it accords to the protection of the environment.

Notes

1 This paper represents the personal views of the author. The views expressed are not necessarily those of the European Investment Bank.
2 Including Bulgaria and Romania whose negotiations for accession are still ongoing.
3 That is, the ten acceding states plus Bulgaria, Romania and Turkey.
4 The World Bank has established a website entirely devoted to "social capital" – see www.worldbank.org/poverty/scapital/index.htm.
5 Poland, which will be the largest recipient of Structural Funds and of the Cohesion Fund among the new Member States, has commenced discussions with the Commission on a programme worth around €8.3 billion (Structural Funds) and €4.2 billion (Cohesion Fund) for the period 2004–2006. This will represent approximately 1.8% of the Polish GDP for the period. There is no health component within the programme proposed by the Polish Government.

References

Bloom, E., Canning, D. and and Sevilla, J. (2001) Health, Human Capital and Economic Growth. Commission on Macroeconomics and Health, Working Paper WG1:8 (available at www.cmhealth.org/docs/wg1_paper8.pdf).
Commission on Macroeconomics and Health (2001) Investing in Health for Economic Development (Jeffrey D Sachs, Chair) (available at www.cid.harvard.edu/cidcmh/CMHReport.pdf).

de la Fuenta, A. and Ciccone, A. (2002) Human Capital in a Global and Knowledge Based Economy, Final Report, May. Brussels: European Commission, DG Employment and Social Affairs.

European Commission (2001a) DG Economic and Financial Affairs Real Convergence in Candidate Countries – Past Performance and Scenarios in the Pre-Accession Programmes, ECFIN/708/01, November. Brussels: European Commission.

European Commission (2001b) Enlargement of the European Union – An historic opportunity. Brussels: European Commission.

European Commission Directorate General for Economic and Financial Affairs (2002) Enlargement Papers No. 7; Evaluation of the 2001 pre-accession economic programmes of candidate countries January. Brussels: European Commission.

Ferreira, L. and Vanhoudt, P. (2002/01) Catching the Celtic Tiger by its Tail. Economic and Financial Reports (available at www.eib.org/efs/reports/efr02n01.pdf). European Investment Bank.

Grossman, M. (1972) On the Concept of Health Capital and the Demand for Health, *Journal of Political Economy*, 80(2):223–55.

Hager, W. and Jennett, N. (2002) Human Capital for Accession, *Eurohealth*, 8(2).

Hager, W. and Suhrcke, M.A. (2001) European Bargain: Investing in CEEC Health. Brussels: Centre for European Policy Studies.

McKee, M. (1999) For debate – does health care save lives?, *Croatian Medical Journal*, 40(2):123–8.

Phare (1998) *Annual report 1998*. www.europa.eu.int/comm/enlargement/ pas/phare/ar98/index_ar98.htm – 21k. Phare.

Puttnam, R. (2002) *The Role of Social Capital in Development: An Empirical Assessment*. Cambridge: Cambridge University Press.

Rosenmöller, M. (2002) Health and support for EU accession: Phare and other initiatives. *Eurohealth*, Special Issue Autumn 8(8):36–8.

Thomas et al. (2000) *The Quality of Growth*. Oxford: Oxford University Press.

UNICEF (2001) *A Decade of Transition*, Regional Monitoring Report No. 8. Florence: UNICEF, Innocenti Research Centre.

WHO (2002) *European Health for all Database*. WHO Regional Office for Europe.

chapter six

Integration of East Germany into the EU: Investment and health outcomes

Ellen Nolte

On October 3, 1990, the German Democratic Republic dissolved into West Germany accompanied by formal ceremony and joyous celebration. In the same moment, the new territories joined the European Community, an event that passed with little fanfare or controversy even though something extraordinary had taken place. (Jeffrey Anderson, 1999)

The experience of the people of the former German Democratic Republic (GDR) following the fall of the Berlin Wall in November 1989 was indeed unique. Unlike its eastern neighbours, it became a fully fledged market economy within a few months. Its integration into the EU was a crucial step in the process of EU enlargement as it was the first former communist state, although a rather unusual one, to join (Blacksell 1995). These developments made East Germany's prospects different from all other former communist countries, especially as this new 16 million population market, with its sizeable future demands for imports, was financially largely guaranteed by West German backing.

This chapter revisits the process of how East Germany was integrated into the EU and how its health care system was transformed in the course of the political transition. It will specifically look at the context within which this process took place and reflect on reasons for the policy decision to adopt the West German model of health care. It will then explore mechanisms that were adopted to minimize the adverse effects of transition with regard to health care and finally examine briefly the possible impact of these changes on the population's health in East Germany.

German unification and European integration

The transition in East Germany was qualitatively different from its eastern neighbours. Other countries were engaged in a major process of state building, enacting new constitutions and establishing new institutions and laws on health and safety, while these already existed in the Federal Republic and were simply extended to the territory of the former GDR that became the new Länder. This also meant that from the date of German unification European Community law would be fully applicable to this territory as stipulated by Article 10 of the Unification Treaty (Presse- und Informationsamt der Bundesregierung 1990).

Importantly, simultaneously with German-German negotiations leading, eventually, to unification, the European Commission worked on strategies to integrate the former GDR into the European Community (Commission of the European Communities 1990). The way in which the GDR was to be incorporated was, however, not clear in the early stages of this discussion. It was, for example, conceivable that the GDR would independently accede to the EC before its unification with West Germany (Lippert 1993). This possibility was, however, largely precluded by the tremendous speed with which events unfolded following the fall of the Berlin Wall, which determined both the timing and mode of integration (Kohler-Koch 1991).

In April 1990, a special European Council in Dublin, Ireland, eventually agreed on a common approach on German unification and on Community relations with central and eastern European countries. The member governments decided "to handle the incorporation of East Germany into the EC as a de facto but not de jure enlargement of the Community" (Anderson 1999). The integration of the GDR thus did not follow the formal procedures for accession to the EC according to Article 237 of the EEC Treaty (Commission of the European Communities 1990). However, acknowledging that despite differing from "normal" accession, the incorporation of East Germany would pose several problems similar to the most recent enlargements of the Community, the Commission proposed a step-wise process of integration with transitional arrangements to ease convergence to the *acquis communautaire* (Anderson 1999). Following this line of reasoning it reached an exceptional decision to introduce transitory measures relating to the unification of Germany (Commission Decision 1990). This authorized Germany provisionally to maintain in force in the former GDR legislation that did not comply with certain specified Community Acts. These included legislation related to workers' health and safety (Council Directive 90/659/EEC); the harmonization of technical rules (Council Directive 90/657/EEC) (Box 6.1); and environmental protection (Council Directive 90/656/EEC; Council Directive 90/660/EEC) (Box 6.2). The transitional measures were subsequently converted into national law. However, almost 80% of Community law came into force in the former GDR immediately after unification; the remainder was to be incorporated by the end of 1992 or 1995 (Bundesregierung 1991).

Box 6.1 "All necessary measures"

Directive 90/657/EEC represented a particularly interesting set of transitional measures that affected a wide range of products manufactured in the former GDR, such as pharmaceuticals, chemical products, foodstuffs, cosmetic products and tobacco. It required the Federal Republic to take "all measures necessary to ensure that products not complying with [specified Directives] are not placed on the market in the territory of the Community other than the territory of the former [GDR]". Directives thus specified included those on labelling of tobacco products and maximum tar yield of cigarettes (89/622/EEC and 90/239/EEC) as well as Directive 75/319/EEC on proprietary medicinal products. While these measures would give manufacturers in the former GDR at least a two year transition period to conform with EC regulations, they were not allowed to market their products anywhere within the EC except the territory of the former GDR. In case of pharmaceuticals, transitional periods largely affected manufacturing licences, good manufacturing practices and inspection as well as marketing of pharmaceutical products that had been approved before unification.

Box 6.2 Cleaning up the environment

In their assessment of the consequences of German unification for the European Community, based on an environmental report by the GDR Ministry in June 1990, the Commission noted that "the environment in the GDR is in a catastrophic state". For example, air pollution was estimated as being four times the EC average and about half of water resources unusable for drinking water production; the environmental situation in the GDR was perceived as "seriously affecting human health. Even now the population [. . .] is obliged to live and work in unhealthy and inhuman conditions."

Consequently a series of transitional measures had to be adopted that, because of the severity of pollution and the initial lack of adequate technical equipment and facilities to reduce pollution, necessitated prolonged transition periods, in some cases up to 1996. In those cases, the German government was required to prepare and submit improvement plans to the Commission within one to two years (Toepel and Weise 2000).

Unifying health care

The strong dynamics of the process of political unification of the two German states also largely determined the transformation of the East German health care system, ultimately resulting in the replacement of its Soviet style system by a pluralist insurance-based system of medical care of high technological standard (Table 6.1) (OECD 1992; Wasem 1997a).

The process of reforming health care in East Germany has been described in detail elsewhere (Manow 1994; Robischon et al. 1994; Wasem 1997b). In brief, in both East and West Germany there was consensus among actors in the field

Table 6.1 Main components of the health care system in East and West Germany pre-1990

	East Germany	West Germany
Sources of financing	Combination of payroll taxes and general taxes; services free of user charges	Mainly insurance-based, contributory financing with some 14% financed by tax revenues; user charges
Structure of health insurance	Integral part of a "uniform social insurance" run by the Free German Trade Union Association (FDGB)	Independent part of a social insurance system, based on pluralist structure of mainly mandatory health insurance funds
Governance of the health care sector	Strictly hierarchical planning and steering structure controlled by the Ministry of Health	Neo-corporatist arrangements between (federal/state) governments and associations of providers/sickness funds
Health care provision	State-owned health care centres (polyclinics) with salaried staff; intended to integrate inpatient and ambulatory care	Private, office-based physicians and dentists; separation of inpatient and ambulatory care

Adopted from Wasem 1997a

of social and health policy that the social insurance system of the former GDR was in need of reform although the structure and content of this reform, especially in relation to health care, were less clear. In fact, there was much controversy among (West) German governmental and non-governmental actors, interest groups and even the administration itself. However, the speed with which the unification of the two states was driven required pragmatic solutions (Stone 1991) with virtually no space for innovative or experimental steps in reforming East Germany's health care sector.

The main areas of conflict concerned the structure of the health insurance system, funding mechanisms and the survival of the outpatient polyclinic system (Wasem 1997a). Importantly, however, although the proposed reorganization was of the East German health care system, those shaping the reform were exclusively West German (Manow 1994; Robischon et al. 1994). East German actors were only of secondary importance. Their rather weak negotiating role, a disadvantage seen not only in the health policy field, was due to a combination of factors relating to the continuing disintegration of political authority, growing administrative disorder and increasing mistrust in administrative bodies in the east, resulting in considerable inequality in bargaining resources, competence, expertise and power between east and west (Lehmbruch 1994).

This is illustrated by the observation that, in their coalition agreement, the first democratic government of the GDR, elected in spring 1990, planned to preserve some basic features of East Germany's health care sector, namely some form of unified health insurance and the polyclinic system as the main institutional setting for providing outpatient care. This proposal was mainly the result of successful lobbying of the West German Social Democratic Party in conjunction with the Federal Association of Local Sickness Funds (AOK Bundesverband) (Robischon et al. 1994). It faced, however, strong opposition from a number of actors including the associations of substitute funds who pressed for a transfer of the highly fragmented West German health insurance system to East Germany, an effort supported by the chambers of physicians and, eventually, by the governing coalition party itself, in particular by the Federal Republic's Chancellor Helmut Kohl, who then had strong negotiating power (Manow 1994; Wasem 1997a).

As a result of the negotiations on the Unification Treaty, the East German health care system was to be put on the same financial and organizational basis as that of the West German health care system by early 1991 (Presse- und Informationsamt der Bundesregierung 1990). Thus, with the exception of a five-year period of grace for the maintenance of polyclinics and related facilities, East Germany's health care reform was an almost unmodified transfer of West Germany's institutional structure (Robischon et al. 1994).

Rebuilding the system

To minimize the adverse effects of transition, the Fonds Deutsche Einheit (German Unity Fund) was set up by the federal government and the western Länder in mid-1990. It provided a total of DM 115 billion (€59 billion) over a period of five years to be invested in East Germany (Singer 1992). It was supplemented by the programme Aufschwung Ost ("Upswing-East") making available a further DM 24 billion (€12.3 billion) for the years 1991 and 1992 that was predominantly assigned to local investments in infrastructure, job-creation schemes as well as environmental improvement schemes (Sinn and Sinn 1992). The overall amount of public funds allocated to the new Länder from 1991 to 1999 was estimated at almost DM 1200 billion (€615 billion) (Bach and Vesper 2000). This represents a reallocation of an annual 7% of the West German GDP to the eastern Länder (Bach et al. 1998). Because of the sustained structural weaknesses and the degree of economic stagnation in the new Länder further financial transfers from the west to east are expected to be required.

These programmes also provided limited funds to support hospital investments. However, restructuring the health care sector in East Germany required substantial additional financial investments and a number of specific programmes were set up to support this process (Bundesministerium für Gesundheit 1998; Bundesministerium für Gesundheit 2000). These included a Soforthilfeprogramm (Immediate Aid Programme) of DM 520 million (€266 million) that was launched in 1990 to begin the process of upgrading East Germany's failing health care infrastructure, focusing on modernizing technical equipment. The same year also saw the provision of start-up financing of DM 3 billion (€1.53 billion) to enable establishment of social health insurance in the new Länder. In 1991, the Federal Government made available another DM 2 billion (€1.02 billion) as special loans to facilitate the setting up of private practice by the medical profession. Reforming the health care sector was further supported by separate federal funds aimed at assisting hospital (re)organization, mainly consultancies to individual hospitals on implementing the new legal and organizational framework, restructuring of polyclinics, and (re)training of selected health personnel (DM 14.9 million (€7.6 million) between 1991 and 1996) In addition, a number of grants were made available for time-limited local/regional projects, for example DM 87 million (€44.4 million) between 1991 and 1996 for the establishment of cancer centres. However, despite this substantial initial investment it was soon realized that the hospital sector in particular would need further sustained funding for rebuilding its infrastructure and modernizing facilities and equipment. Therefore the Krankenhausinvestitionsprogramm (Hospital Investment Programme) was introduced in 1992, providing another DM 21 billion (€10.5 billion) for the period 1995–2004 (subsequently slightly modified).

This financial investment was accompanied by a number of non-monetary measures to assist adaptation to the West German administrative and organizational structure. Federal and Länder governments set up a scheme of consultancies, with direct personnel support as well as advanced and continuing training for health personnel including public health officers (Amtsarzt), other staff of local/regional public health administrations, pharmacists and vets (Bundesministerium für Gesundheit 1998). This process was actively supported by the corporatist actors in the field of health policy. For instance, the West German Association of Sickness Funds Physicians soon began to train their colleagues in East Germany in setting up private practices and in establishing professional associations (Stone 1991). Local and substitute sickness funds expended much effort on training staff and offering ongoing technical support for their "adopted" area in the east (Freudenstein and Borgwardt 1992). As a result, local as well as substitute sickness funds soon established offices in the east and were able to start work by January 1991 (Spree 1994). While these arrangements certainly helped to establish the health insurance system and the system of ambulatory care in a relatively short period of time, their efforts were, however, not altogether altruistic but further served the aim of many professional and governmental actors to transfer the West German model of health care to the east (Stone 1991; Freudenstein and Borgwardt 1992; Robischon et al. 1994).

The changing pattern of population health

Considering the substantial transformation of the East German health care system since unification, one might expect some impact on changing mortality in the former GDR. Elsewhere we have shown that a brief increase in mortality immediately after the fall of the Berlin Wall was followed by sustained improvement in health in East Germany that exceeded even the most optimistic predictions. Between 1992 and 1997, life expectancy at birth increased by 2.3 years in men and by 2.4 years in women, substantially more than in West Germany, at 1.2 and 0.9 years, respectively (Nolte et al. 2000b). Subsequent analyses have demonstrated that these improvements were, at least in part, attributable to changes in medical care. For example, using the concept of "unnecessary untimely deaths" we showed that, in East Germany, mortality improvements attributable to medical care in the 1980s were due, largely, to declining infant mortality (Nolte et al. 2002). In the 1990s, they also benefited adults, specifically those aged 55 and over. We estimated that of an increase in life expectancy between birth and age 75 of 1.4 years in men and 0.9 years in women between 1992 and 1997 (West Germany: 0.6 and 0.3 years) 14–23% was accounted for by declining mortality from conditions amenable to medical intervention. Falling death rates from hypertension and cerebrovascular diseases and, among women, from cervical cancer and breast cancer have been important contributors. Similar trends were seen in Poland, although on a smaller scale. These findings thus suggest that the transformation of the East German health care system brought tangible improvements in mortality that were greater than in West Germany, where the existing system continued in place, or in Poland, where reform has been much slower. This conclusion is supported by other evidence of improved medical care in East Germany. Thus Nolte et al. reported that, since unification, there was a substantial decline in neonatal mortality, of over 30% between 1990 and 1997 (Nolte et al. 2000a). This was shown to be attributable, largely, to an improvement in survival at all birthweights but in particular among infants with low and very low birthweight. Differences in survival in this group are closely linked to effective medical interventions. Becker and Boyle noted a fall in mortality from testicular cancer among East German men of 50% between 1990 and 1995, suggesting that the rapid increase in the availability of modern pharmaceuticals may be the most likely explanation for this decline (Becker and Boyle 1997).

Conclusion

The process of political, economic and societal transition in central and eastern Europe led to the reform of health care systems by most countries in this region. But, as Wasem has pointed out, "whereas all these countries have to find answers to a huge catalogue of strategic questions, in East Germany these questions were answered through unification" (Wasem 1997a). The process of reform in East Germany thus clearly represents a special case but the experience is an important element of the overall process of transition in eastern Europe in the 1990s and within the framework of European integration. Many aspects of transforming the former GDR were unique, not only the health care sector, and will not apply to the situation in the present candidate countries. However, integrating East Germany into the EU can be seen to have represented an important, if somewhat unusual, step towards enlargement into central and eastern Europe.

References

Anderson, J. (1999) *German unification and the union of Europe.* Cambridge: Cambridge University Press.

Bach, H.-U., Blaschke, D. and Blien, U. (1998) *Labour market trends and active labour market policy in the eastern German transformation process 1990–1997. IAB Labour Market Research Topics 29/1998.* Nürnberg: Institut für Arbeitsmarkt- und Berufsforschung.

Bach, S. and Vesper, D. (2000) Finanzpolitik und Wiedervereinigung – Bilanz nach 10 Jahren, *Vierteljahreshefte zur Wirtschaftsforschung*, 69:194–224.

Becker, N. and Boyle, P. (1997) Decline in mortality from testicular cancer in West Germany after reunification, *Lancet*, 350:744.

Blacksell, M. (1995) Germany as a European power, in D. Lewis and J. R. P. McKenzie (eds) *The new Germany. Social, political and cultural challenges of unification*. Exeter: University of Exeter Press.

Bundesministerium für Gesundheit (1998) *Das Gesundheitswesen in den neuen Ländern*. Bonn: Bundesministerium für Gesundheit.

Bundesministerium für Gesundheit (2000) *Gesundheit in den neuen Ländern. Stand, Probleme und Perspektiven nach 10 Jahren Deutsche Einheit*. Berlin: Bundesministerium für Gesundheit.

Bundesregierung (1991) *47. Bericht der Bundesregierung über die Integration der Bundesrepublik Deutschland in die Europäischen Gemeinschaften. Drucksache 12/217.* Bonn: Deutscher Bundestag.

Commission Decision (1990) Commission Decision 90/481/EEC of 27 September 1990 introducing interim measures relating to the unification of Germany. Official Journal of the European Communities 29/09/1990 L267/37.

Commission of the European Communities (1990) The European Community and German Unification. Supplement /1990. Luxembourg: Office for Official Publications of the European Communities, *Bulletin of the European Communities*, (4).

Council Directive 90/659/EEC of 4 December 1990 relating to the transitional measures applicable in Germany in the field of workers' health and safety. Official Journal of the European Comunities 17/12/1990 L353/77–8.

Council Directive 90/657/EEC of 4 December 1990 on the transitional measures applicable in Germany in the context of the harmonization of technical rules. Official Journal of the European Communities 17/12/1990 L353/65–72.

Council Directive 90/656/EEC of 4 December 1990 on the transitional measures applicable in Germany with regard to certain Community provisions relating to the protection of the environment. Official Journal of the European Communities 17/12/1990 L353/59–64.

Council Directive 90/660/EEC of 4 December 1990 on the transitional measures applicable in Germany with regard to certain Community provisions relating to the protection of the environment, in connection with the internal market. Official Journal of the European Comunities 17/12/1990 L353/79–80.

Freudenstein, U. and Borgwardt, G. (1992) Primary medical care in former East Germany: the frosty winds of change, *British Medical Journal*, 304:827–9.

Kohler-Koch, B. (1991) Die Politik der Integration der DDR in die EG, in B. Kohler-Koch (ed.) *Die Osterweiterung der EG. Die Einbeziehung der ehemaligen DDR in die Gemeinschaft*. Baden-Baden: Nomos Verlagsgesellschaft.

Lehmbruch, G. (1994) The process of regime change in East Germany: An institutionalist scenario for German unification, *Journal of European Public Policy*, 1:1350–763.

Lippert, B. (1993) Die EG als Mitgestalter der Erfolgsgeschichte – Der deutsche Eingungsprozeß, in B. Lippert, D. Günther, R. Stevens-Ströhmann, G. Viertel and S. Woolcock (eds) *Die EG und die neuen Bundesländer*. Bonn: Europa Union Verlag.

Manow, P. (1994) *Gesundheitspolitik im Eingungsprozeß*. Frankfurt/New York: Campus Verlag.

Nolte, E., Brand, A., Koupilova, I. and McKee, M. (2000a) Trends in neonatal and postneonatal mortality in the eastern and western parts of Germany after unification, *Journal of Epidemiology and Community Health*, 54:84–90.

Nolte, E., Shkolnikov, V. and McKee, M. (2000b) Changing mortality patterns in east and west Germany and Poland: II. Short-term trends during transition and in the 1990s, *Journal of Epidemiology and Community Health*, 54:899–906.

Nolte, E., Scholz, R., Shkolnikov, V. and McKee, M. (2002) The contribution of medical care to changing life expectancy in Germany and Poland, *Soc Sci Med*, 55:15–31.

OECD (1992) *The Reform of Health care. A comparative analysis of seven OECD countries. Health Policy Studies No. 2*. Paris: OECD.

Presse- und Informationsamt der Bundesregierung (1990) Vertrag zwischen der Bundesrepublik Deutschland und der Deutschen Demokratischen Republik über die Herstellung der Einheit Deutschlands – Einigungsvertrag. Bonn: Presse- und Informationsamt der Bundesregierung.

Robischon, T., Stucke, A., Wasem, J. and Wolf, H.-G. (1994) Die politische Logik der deutschen Vereinigung und der Institutionentransfer: Eine Untersuchung am Beispiel von Gesundheitswesen, Forschungssystem und Telekommunikation. MPIFG Discussion Paper 94/3. Köln: Max-Planck-Institut für Gesellschaftsforschung.

Singer, O. (1992) The politics and economics of German unification: from currency union to economic dichotomy, *German Politics*, 1:78–94.

Sinn, G. and Sinn, H.-W. (1992) *Jumpstart. The economic unification of Germany*. Cambridge/London: MIT Press.

Spree, H.-U. (1994) *Der Sozialstaat eint*. Baden-Baden: Nomos Verlagsgesellschaft.

Stone, D.A.J. (1991) German unification: East meets West in the doctor's office, *Policy and Law*, 16:401–12.

Toepel, K. and Weise, C. (2000) Die Integration Ostdeutschlands in die Europäische Union: eine Erfolgsgeschichte? *Vierteljahreshefte zur Wirtschaftsforschung*, 69:178–93.

Wasem, J. (1997a) Health care reform in the Federal Republic of Germany: The new and the old Länder, in C. Altenstetter and J. W. Björkman (eds) *Health policy reform, national variations and globalization*. London: Macmillan.

Wasem, J. (1997b) *Vom staatlichen zum kassenärztlichen System: Eine Untersuchung des Transformationsprozesses der ambulanten ärztlichen Versorgung in Ostdeutschland*. Frankfurt: Campus.

chapter seven

The challenges of the free movement of health professionals

Sallie Nicholas

When the candidate countries join the EU they will sign up to legislation allowing the free movement of health professionals and the mutual recognition of their qualifications. What impact will this have on them, and what impact will it have on the current 15 Member States plus those extra countries making up the European Economic Area (EEA)? Are there lessons to be learned before the EU almost doubles in size? The imminent enlargement of the EU has sparked debate among policy-makers and opinion-formers in the health field and seems to be acting as a catalyst for review.

This chapter aims to give a clear understanding of existing legislation in this area and identify the key decision-makers. It will examine the impact of policy so far on EU Member States and the extent of movement among health professionals and will explore some of the problems that have arisen and lessons that might be learned. It will then look at the potential impact on candidate countries and what is being done, or needs to be done, to prepare them and whether now is perhaps the time to iron out problems and improve things for all Member States.

History

International migration of health professionals is now high on the agenda of many countries. When it published the NHS Plan for England (Department of Health 2000), the British Government acknowledged acute shortages of staff in the health service and has since launched a major international recruitment campaign, trawling Europe and beyond. Free movement has become a major news story in the United Kingdom, with regular headlines about the growing numbers of German doctors and Spanish nurses. Meanwhile British patients are travelling to France and beyond for hip and knee replacements. Migration of health professionals is a particular issue for the United Kingdom, in part because of its relatively low production of doctors, but also because the widespread use of English facilitates recruitment from overseas. However, similar stories exist in all industrialized countries. Now, everyone has good reason to be interested in matters such as comparative training standards and language competence, but in fact none of this is new.

The EU has always been about the free movement of goods, services and people. Health professionals are people who provide services. Those governments that signed the Treaty of Rome in 1957 committed themselves to the mutual recognition of qualifications, as it is of little use to professionals to be able to move if they cannot work when they arrive. After many years of negotiations, health professionals were among the earliest and the principal beneficiaries. Two Directives, known as the "Doctors' Directives", were adopted in 1975, supplemented in 1986 by a further Directive on specific training in general practice. All three were amalgamated in a single text in 1993 (European Union 1993). Further Directives followed in 1977 for nurses in general care (European Union 1977), in 1978 for dentists (European Union 1978), in 1980 for midwives (European Union 1980) and in 1985 for pharmacists (European Union 1985), as well as vets and architects. These are known as the "sectoral" Directives; they cover individual professions, so that in theory each profession has its own needs taken into account.

During the 1980s the European Commission, charged with drafting legislation and monitoring its implementation, changed its approach to mutual recognition. In 1989 Member States adopted a Directive setting out a framework for the mutual recognition of professional qualifications involving three years or more of higher (18+) training (European Union 1989). This Directive covers those in regulated professions moving to countries where their professions are also recognized and regulated. Health professionals falling within its scope include specialist nurses, physiotherapists, occupational therapists, speech and language therapists, clinical psychologists, radiographers, optometrists and opticians. It was followed in 1992 by a further Directive for those in professions involving two years' 18+ training (European Commission 1992). Dental hygienists fall into this category. These Directives are known as the "general system" Directives.

The Directives in both categories have been amended at various stages over the years, most recently en bloc in 2001 (European Union 2001). The European Commission has recently published a proposal to amend and amalgamate them all (European Commission 2002).

How the sectoral Directives work

Essentially, the sectoral Directives lay down a system based on mutual trust. Member States agree to recognize each others' qualifications, as long as they are listed in the relevant Directive and as long as those holding them are EEA citizens. Training programmes in all Member States must meet certain minimum standards, which are built in as a protective measure. As an example, doctors who are citizens of Member States, and who have completed basic training in Member States, are entitled to register in other Member States. If they meet both the criteria for registration and have also completed general practice (GP) or specialist training, they also are entitled to have their GP or specialist qualifications recognized.

Language testing may not be made a condition of registration, although there is an assumption that employers will weed out those with inadequate skills. The Doctors' Directive makes the following pronouncement:

> Member States shall see to it that, where appropriate, the persons con-
> cerned acquire, in their interest and in that of their patients, the linguistic
> knowledge necessary to the exercise of the profession in the host country.
> (European Union 1993)

The new draft directive (European Commission 2002), covering all migrant professionals, is more explicit about the need for linguistic knowledge, but still seems to place responsibility with host Member States to ensure that those involved acquire appropriate skills. The Doctors' Directive (European Union 1993) also suggests that countries establish information centres for migrant doctors, but provision seems to vary greatly from one country to another.

When the sectoral directives were adopted, they were accompanied by Council Decisions establishing advisory committees to run alongside them as a means of ensuring that comparable standards were maintained – the Advisory Committee on Medical Training (ACMT) (European Union 1975a) and similarly titled bodies for the other "sectoral" professions. Run by the European Commission, their future has hung in the balance for several years and they appear now to be facing abolition (see below). A similar 1975 Council Decision established a Committee of Senior Officials in Public Health (CSOPH) to oversee the operation of the Doctors' Directives and those that followed (European Union 1975c).

How the "general system" approach works

The general system involves case-by-case scrutiny of applications for registration, but with a built-in assumption that acceptance of qualifications will be the norm. The first general system Directive (European Union 1989) states firmly that competent authorities (the term commonly used for registering and regulatory bodies) may not, on the grounds of inadequate qualifications, refuse to authorize nationals of other Member States to practise in their countries if they hold the diploma required in another Member State for the exercise of the same profession or in certain other circumstances that apply to those from countries where the profession in question exists but is not regulated.

Authorities can, however, ask for evidence of professional experience, where the training involved in the applicant's Member State of origin is at least one year shorter than that required in the host Member State. They can also ask applicants to complete an adaptation period not exceeding three years or to take an aptitude test if the content of their training differs substantially from that required for the diploma in the host Member State or if there are differences between the scope of regulated activities covered by the profession in the host country and the countries from which applicants originate.

Host Member States are supposed to allow applicants themselves to choose between aptitude tests or adaptation periods, except in the case of professions whose practice requires precise knowledge of national law and where the giving of advice and/or assistance on matters of national law is an essential and constant part of professional activity (in effect this means the legal profession). The aptitude test is limited to the professional knowledge of the applicant, which seems to mean that it will not be possible to test language competence. There seem to be uncertainties about the funding of adaptation periods and about the extent to which Member States are obliged to provide top-up training where this might be difficult both to accommodate and to fund.

The operation of the general system is monitored by a coordinating group, made up of one member per country – normally a civil servant.

Advantages and disadvantages

It may be useful here to give a brief summary of what appear to be the advantages and disadvantages of both systems, although some of the points will be covered in greater detail later on.

The main advantages of the sectoral Directives seem to be that they are relatively explicit and give migrants a clear idea of their rights. Administratively they are simpler, and therefore probably cheaper, for Member States to operate. They set out qualitative standards as a safeguard, and it could be argued that they provide an impetus for improving quality as those covered by them strive for comparable standards. The disadvantage, however, is that these arguments fall down if the qualitative standards are set too low, which many believe that they are, and if there are no resources to support updating and improvements. Nor does the "one size fits all" approach always sit comfortably in a Europe characterized by the diversity of its approaches to health care delivery and professional training – diversity that can only increase with enlargement.

The general system approach has attracted interest in some quarters because of its case-by-case approach and the potential to impose aptitude tests or adaptation periods. In reality, however, competent authorities seem to have less room to manoeuvre than might at first appear to be the case (for example, applicants themselves are allowed to choose between aptitude tests and adaptation periods) and, as also mentioned previously, there are many uncertainties about questions such as who funds adaptation periods. The main complaint seems to be that it is complex and expensive to administer, transferring much of the burden from the Commission to Member States. There also seems to be very little to support those who run it in terms of information about training, credit transfer systems and so on, and some scope for confusion about what constitutes a regulated profession and what to do if a profession is regulated in one country and not – or to a different degree – in another.

Recent developments and debates

It is no secret that the European Commission has found the sectoral approach, with its attendant advisory committees, expensive and labour-intensive to maintain, hence the switch to the general system. The advisory committees have complained about the years of cancelled meetings, lack of support and resources and failure to implement their recommendations – although the picture is not all bleak, with the pharmacists and dentists in particular also citing positive experiences (personal communications).

In 1996 the Commission launched the Simpler Legislation in the Internal Market (SLIM) initiative and chose the mutual recognition of qualifications as one of its pilot projects. It set up a focus group involving representatives of the professions and launched a major debate about the future of the sectoral Directives and their accompanying advisory committees. The result was a resounding vote in favour of keeping both, albeit with some streamlining. The response from European-level professional bodies seemed unanimous, and national governments apparently also favoured retention. In the United Kingdom there was a vigorous debate within the medical profession, with dissent in some quarters from the orthodox view. The overall result of a Department of Health consultation exercise involving all the relevant professions, however, seemed to be that the sectoral system was flawed but the lesser of two evils and should be retained and improved. The "general system" approach was held to be less attractive than it might appear at first sight, and those registering bodies with experience of operating both preferred the sectoral system.

With enlargement looming, the Commission continued to look for a system which – from its point of view – would be simpler and cheaper to run and would facilitate freer movement. In 2001 it published a discussion paper on the future regime for professional recognition within the EU, posing a series of questions hinting strongly at a desire for a move to the general system, or at least a closer alignment of the two systems (European Commission 2001). It explored support for replacing the current advisory committee and the Committee of Senior Officials in Public Health structure with a single coordinating body to oversee all matters relevant to all professions. As mentioned previously, it has now published a legislative proposal (European Commission 2002), based on the results of the consultation and bringing all professions, from all sectors and not only health, together in one text. If this is adopted, arrangements for the professions covered by sectoral Directives will remain broadly the same, although medical specialties that are not common to all Member States will move to the general system. Much as expected, the advisory committees are to go. Within the professions opinion seems split between those who continue to resist their abolition and those willing to contemplate a new system as long as there are firm guarantees that their advice will be listened to and acted upon. European professional bodies – whose membership has often overlapped closely with that of the advisory committees and who mostly take a keen interest in training matters – are in some cases asking themselves whether they might do the job in future.

As any change will need the agreement of both national governments and the European Parliament, there will undoubtedly be fierce lobbying in the run-up to the publication of this book. Underlying all these discussions is a tension between free movement, to which the Commission is obliged to give top priority, and the need to ensure quality and guarantee patient safety, which must be the top priorities for the health professions. As was recently pointed out in the British Medical Association's weekly newssheet (Duncan 2002), here is an unusual case – especially when viewed from a British perspective – of European citizens clamouring for greater regulation and interference and a European institution apparently doing its best to avoid providing it.

Who's who: policy-makers, opinion-formers and key players

While national governments (through the Council of Ministers) and the European Parliament are the ultimate legislators, the European Commission is making the running so far on policy formation in this area and is also charged with overseeing preparations for the enlargement of the EU. Responsibility for professional qualifications rests with the Internal Market Directorate-General, in keeping with the emphasis on free movement. Quality and safety campaigners would prefer to see it housed with the Health and Consumer Protection Directorate-General. Meanwhile the Enlargement Directorate-General, with the Internal Market Directorate-General, is overseeing procedures for scrutinizing incoming countries to ensure that they meet the terms of the legislation outlined here. The EU committed itself in the Maastricht Treaty to ensuring that health would be taken into consideration across all policy areas. This commitment was strengthened further in the Amsterdam Treaty and is now incorporated in Article 152 of the consolidated EC Treaty (European Union 1997), which states that *a high level of human health protection shall be ensured in the definition of all Community policies and activities*. We have to hope that this will be a case in point.

Next there are the statutory bodies, funded and administered by the Commission, mentioned previously and currently facing considerable doubt about their future (European Commission 2002). The Committee of Senior Officials in Public Health (CSOPH) was set up in 1975 as a result of the adoption of the "Doctors' Directives" (European Union 1975b; European Union 1993). "Public health" should be interpreted in its broadest sense, as the committee is made up of senior civil servants with responsibility for national health care systems. When first established, its remit was to monitor difficulties with the implementation of the Directives, collect relevant information about the delivery of medical care and provide guidance for the Commission. Its remit expanded as further sectoral Directives were adopted. The Commission now also uses the CSOPH as a "management committee" to update lists of specialties and recommended training durations in the "Doctors' Directive" (European Union 1993). As mentioned previously, the Commission plans to merge it with the coordinating committee which oversees the operation of the general system. While there have been laments in some quarters that few of the CSOPH members are themselves health professionals, once this happens there will be no guarantee that any members will have a background in health workforce policy. Any new structure will need detailed arrangements for consultation and the co-option of appropriate expertise.

Even closer to extinction are the Advisory Committee on Medical Training (ACMT), the Advisory Committee on Training of Nurses (ACTN), Advisory Committee on Training of Midwives (ACTM), Advisory Committee on the Training of Dental Practitioners (ACTDP) and Advisory Committee on Pharmaceutical Training (ACPT) The first to be set up, the ACMT, had a remit *to help to ensure a comparably demanding standard of medical training in the Community, with regard both to basic and further training* (European Union 1975a) and had members drawn from three categories – expressed as the practising profession, university medical faculties and competent authorities. Given the multiplicity of key players in the United Kingdom, competition for seats was fierce. Other committees had similar structures and remits. Between them the committees have produced a wide range of reports over the years and taken varying initiatives with varying degrees of success. At the time of writing, their members express varying degrees of pride in their achievements, despair at their treatment at the hands of the Commission and determination to keep them going by statutory or other means (personal communications)

A conference organized by the English Department of Health in London in July 2001 heard that the ACTM had not met for five years and was effectively moribund. The ACTN, on the other hand, had continued meeting for long enough to complete a pilot project outlining competencies to replace or supplement the core content for nursing training outlined in the nursing directives (European Commission 1998). There has been much interest in recent years in this shift to an "outcome-based" approach, but the question now is whether or when the nurses' work will find its way into legislation and whether the project will be extended to other professions. The ACMT produced reports on both specialist (its fourth) (European Commission 1997) and general practice training (European Commission 1996) during the 1990s; a small proportion of the latter found its way into the 2001 amending Directive (European Union 2001), while the former remains unimplemented. It has not met since early 1999, but nevertheless a working group has – from limbo, if not from beyond the grave – produced a fifth report on specialist training (Twomey and ACMT Working Group on Specialist Training 2001). The ACTDP remained active and met regularly until the end of 2000, producing a wide range of competence-based guidelines for undergraduate and postgraduate dental training. The ACPT also reports many successes. While its recommendations were not enacted in law, consensus-building was so successful that all Member States with one exception apparently implemented its recommendations (personal communications).

There seems to be consensus across the health professions that the advisory committees are essential to support the implementation of the sectoral Directives – they are a form of quality assurance without which the system cannot be guaranteed to be safe. If they cease to exist in their current form, their work must continue by other means. This point has been made repeatedly in national and pan-European submissions to the Commission and in 2001 in *Eurohealth* by Mäkinen and Aarimaa (2001).

This section would be incomplete without reference to some of the many European professional organizations which play a vital role as opinion-formers and whose members, as indicated previously, may have close links with the bodies described above. They are all alive to the challenges and opportunities of

EU enlargement and may offer valuable fora for dialogue and information exchange. Some have representatives of candidate countries as full members, others as associate members or observers. Their membership is likely to include national professional associations and/or registering and regulatory bodies – these being interchangeable in some European countries.

It would be impossible to list all of these organizations, but some of the key players for the "sectoral" professions are set out below. The medical organizations all work closely together, with the CPME (Box 7.1) as the principal EU umbrella organization. The CPME has recently completed a major analysis of the health care systems of the accession countries, working with associate members from those countries (Brettenthaler and Wallner 2001). EFMA-WHO was set up to provide dialogue between the WHO Regional Office for Europe and the national medical associations of the 51 Member States of the WHO European region. Associations from central and eastern Europe and the former Soviet Union are widely represented. Many of the others have published significant work on training and other topics, examples being the recent UEMS Basel Declaration on continuing professional development (UEMS 2001) and two major studies from the PWG on the European medical workforce (PWG 1991, updated 1996).

Box 7.1 European medical organizations

Standing Committee of European Doctors (CPME) – www.cpme.be
European Forum of Medical Associations and the WHO (EFMA-WHO)
European Union of Medical Specialists (UEMS) – www.uems.be
European Union of General Practitioners (UEMO) – www.uemo.org
European Society for General Practice/Family Medicine (ESGP/FM)
Permanent Working Group of European Junior Doctors (PWG) –
   www.pwgeurope.org
Conférence Européene des Ordres der Médecins (CEOM)
European Association of Senior Hospital Physicians (AEMH)
European Federation of Salaried Doctors (FEMS) – www.fems.net

---

Many of the above are thinking about how the work of the ACMT might be continued, by current or other means.

Organizations representing the other "sectoral" health professions are listed in Box 7.2 and Box 7.3.

Box 7.2 European Nursing and Midwifery Associations

Standing Committee of Nurses of the EU (PCN). EU umbrella body for nurses –
   www.pcn.yucom.be
European Network of Nursing Organisations (ENNO). Brings together national
   nursing associations and European specialist nursing groups and has adopted a
   framework for specialist nurse education (European Network of Nursing Organisations (ENNO) 2000).
European Forum of National Nursing and Midwifery Associations and the World
   Health Organization.
European Midwives Liaison Group

Box 7.3 European Dental and Pharmaceutical Groups

Dental Liaison Group. This has four representatives from each EU Member State and observers from accession countries. It has set up a working party to propose a means for the ACTDP, or an alternative body with a similar remit and status, to continue to operate.

The DentEd initiative of visits to dental schools and reports comparing different aspects of the delivery of dental education is run by dental academics has been supported by several EU grants. The Education and Culture Directorate-General has provided €250 000 for the 2002 DentEdEvolves project – www.dented.org.

Pharmaceutical Group of the EU (PGEU) – www.pgeu.org.

There are also European-level groups representing many of the professions covered by the general system.

Theory and practice – how much movement has there been?

Building an accurate picture of the extent of movement over the last 25 years is not easy, and there is little published material. One of the few available studies (Jinks et al. 2000), which focuses principally on EEA doctors in the United Kingdom, confirms that there is little systematic collection of the numbers of people moving throughout the EU. Irwin showed that EU level data on the nursing workforce are practically non-existent (Irwin 2001). Much of the picture is formed by informal studies, anecdotal evidence and studies of registration data, in particular from the United Kingdom where most research has been undertaken (see Chapter 10). A more recent analysis, bringing together material from a range of sources, many for the first time, looks in more detail at movement of physicians. The results are reported in Chapter 9.

In summary, levels of migration have not been enormously high and much of the movement that has gone on has been across neighbouring borders and has probably been influenced by factors such as cultural and linguistic ties between countries. The United Kingdom and to some extent Ireland are, however, exceptions, taking in migrants from a wide range of countries. At least as far as doctors are concerned, it appears to be the largest importer within the EEA. It also appears to be one of the smallest exporters, with its migrating doctors mainly choosing other anglophone destinations.

In an unpublished study prepared for the CEOM in 1999 (and cited with the author's permission), Brearley analyses registration data provided by 13 countries (Brearley 1999). He concludes that the United Kingdom and France are the two largest importers, with movement into all other countries at very low levels. EU registrations in the United Kingdom increased by 75% between 1989 and 1997. The largest overall group of migrating doctors are German. He goes on to say that:

The figures demonstrate the existence of several "regional economies", reflecting historical links or linguistic affinities between groups of countries. Thus Belgian and Luxemburger doctors are most likely to migrate to France. French doctors are most likely to migrate to France, having trained abroad, with some going to Belgium and Luxembourg. There is regular exchange of doctors between Scandinavian countries, between the United Kingdom and Ireland and between Germany and Austria.

The British General Medical Council's (GMC) figures show that the largest groups of European doctors registering in the United Kingdom are German, Greek, Irish, Italian and Spanish. While changes to the GMC computer system mean that the most up-to-date figures are not available at the time of writing, those that are available and personal communications suggest that EEA registrations peaked overall in 1996 and have been in gradual decline since then. Whether the British Government's international recruitment drive will reverse this trend remains to be seen.

What is not clear is how many of the doctors who register remain in the United Kingdom and for how long, but recent figures (*Hansard* 2001) suggest that in 2000 4.97% of the overall National Health Service (NHS) workforce in England had qualified elsewhere in the EEA – 3.9% of GPs and 5.5% of hospital medical and dental staff. Analysed by grade the picture might look rather different. Jinks et al. (2000: 7) point out that up to 10% of senior house officers (the most junior grade following full registration) in England and Wales fall into this category.

A slightly different picture comes from dentistry, where numbers of EEA registrations have been rising steadily year by year from 7 in 1981 to 2019 in 2001 (personal communication). Here again, the United Kingdom is a major importer. Trends in nurse migration are discussed in Chapter 10. Migration among midwives and pharmacists is said to be relatively low.

Factors influencing movement

As already mentioned, language is clearly a significant factor. The diverse range and breadth of sources of migration to the United Kingdom can be explained by the fact that English is widely taught as a second language and is increasingly considered to be the language of scientific literature. Equally, the United Kingdom school system has so far ensured that few of those who study medicine – and probably few who enter other health professions – will have learned a second language beyond the age of 16, thus making it more difficult for United Kingdom professionals to consider working in non English speaking countries. Meanwhile it is a source of intense frustration to non-EEA overseas professionals, including those who have been taught in English, that they are subject to language testing while their EEA counterparts are not.

Perhaps even more significant, however, are levels of unemployment or underemployment in the health professions. There is no EU-level workforce planning and wide variations both in national planning strategy and in doctor:population ratios. OECD figures (OECD 1999) for 1999 show the United Kingdom with a modest 1.8 doctors per 1000, while Germany has 3.5 and Italy a staggering 5.9. Many factors have contributed to the variation – relatively unrestricted access to medical schools in some countries, inaccurate forecasting, and imbalances caused by the increasing popularity of part-time and flexible working among others.

Where there is free movement, one country's overproduction or under-production may distort – or indeed relieve – the employment situation in others. Thus Germany, Spain and Italy have had high levels of medical unemployment in recent years and their doctors have migrated in large numbers to the United Kingdom, which in turn has made no secret of the fact that it needs thousands more. The PWG fired a warning shot that this might not go on for ever by subtitling both its 1991 and 1996 medical workforce studies "from surplus to deficit" (PWG 1991), however, and the GMC's registration figures seem to bear this out. Regional variations are also emerging in countries like France, Spain and Portugal, which are well-supplied with doctors in some areas but have shortages in others.

Other factors identified by Jinks et al. (2000) in interviews with EEA doctors working in the United Kingdom were the reputation of United Kingdom medical education and the more rigid hierarchies in some of their countries of origin. Income levels do not seem to be a significant factor.

The CPME (Brettenthaler and Wallner 2001) reports that there is no oversupply of doctors in the candidate countries it has surveyed and that these have doctor:population ratios lower than the EU average. Irwin (2001) refers to the fears of national nursing associations in eastern Europe about retaining qualified nurses. At the same time Poland was cited by a Department of Health official at a recent meeting as one of the countries from which the English NHS was considering recruiting health professionals.

It follows that those who cannot find work in their own countries will look elsewhere and that doctors from other countries will have little chance in employment markets that are already overburdened. "Political will" is an important factor in European affairs, if difficult to quantify, and lack of it may well lead to the erection of hidden barriers or an unwillingness to dismantle existing ones.

Barriers, problems and lessons learned

Language and labour market conditions, discussed above, can promote or hinder free movement in equal measure. It all depends where the migrant is to start with and where s/he wants to go. A further, more specific, list under this heading could be endless. It may also be dominated by the experience of the medical profession and in particular by the experience of the United Kingdom medical profession as a net importer (the situation with regard to the United Kingdom is looked at in more detail in Chapter 10). Some points have also been raised by other professions, but personal communications have identified few serious problems.

It should be made clear that, while there is much discussion in many meetings about quality, patient safety and comparability of standards, most evidence seems to be anecdotal. There is no evidence from regulatory bodies of disproportionate levels of complaints against EEA practitioners.

Training standards – are they minimal rather than minimum?

Despite the best efforts of the advisory committees and European professional organizations over the years, the standards set out in the various directives are sketchy at best. The doctors' legislation (European Union 1993) was the first to be adopted, and the medical profession was perhaps the "guinea pig". The nurses', dentists', midwives' and pharmacists' directives (European Union 1977; European Union 1978; European Union 1980; European Union 1985) all contain annexes in which lists of subjects to be studied as part of their curricula are set out. Even so, the general view seems to be that these go "so far and no further" and the happiest professions seem to be those which have succeeded in supplementing them by some means. The "Doctors' Directive" (European Union 1993) stipulates of undergraduate training only that it should confer on the graduate:

- adequate knowledge of the sciences on which medicine is based and a good understanding of scientific methods, including the principles of measuring biological functions, the evaluation of scientifically established facts and the analysis of data;
- sufficient understanding of the structure, functions and behaviour of healthy and sick persons, as well as relations between the state of health and physical and social surroundings of the human being;
- adequate knowledge of clinical disciplines and practices, providing him [sic] with a coherent picture of mental and physical diseases, of medicine from the points of view of prophylaxis, diagnosis and therapy and of human reproduction;
- suitable clinical experience in hospitals under appropriate supervision.

In addition it specifies that training should comprise six years or 5500 hours of theoretical and practical instruction given in or under the supervision of a university. As far as specialist training is concerned, the guidance is based almost entirely on its duration, otherwise specifying only that it should comprise theoretical and practical instruction and take place in health establishments approved for the purpose. The requirements for general practice training are similar, and there is no significant shift in the new draft directive (European Commission 2002).

Faced, therefore, with earnest speculation about whether the accession countries meet the standards of the Directives, one might be tempted to ask "What standards?" The danger is that, until there is greater transparency and more support for work to fill in the gaps, the trust on which the sectoral system is supposed to operate will not be there. While Member States may apply the letter of the law, uncertainty about unfamiliar systems may breed prejudice and ultimately undermine free movement. Jinks et al. (2000) drew this conclusion from those they interviewed in the North of England.

> . . . mutual recognition of training is established at a formal level, however, at the informal level, clear ambivalence exists about equivalent theoretical and practical knowledge . . . In the absence of an agreed framework for assessing the degree of equivalence it is easy to adopt a stereotypical

approach based upon previous – and often ad hoc – experiences. An implicit distinction tended to be drawn between doctors from northern or southern countries, which one of the tutors dubbed as "the olive line".

Disparities in undergraduate training

While meeting the standards set out in the Directives, Member States may still take very different approaches to the way in which they organize their training. Different does not mean wrong, as each country has its own culture and traditions and organizes its training to meet the needs of its health system. Free movement will work best, however, if all parties understand this.

One observation often made at medical meetings is that undergraduate training is more practically based in some countries than in others. The United Kingdom is in the former category and has taken in many doctors from countries in the second category. In some cases doctors will have a high level of academic knowledge, but less familiarity with the practical procedures that junior doctors in the United Kingdom perform on a day-to-day basis. The same observations have apparently been made about dental training (personal communication), with exposure to patients said to be particularly low in one country with a substantial overproduction of dentists.

The potential for clinical experience has made the United Kingdom a popular destination for medical students seeking electives, to the extent that there was some concern in the early 1990s that the large intake would overburden the system and reduce the range of experience available to United Kingdom students (Nicholas 1994).

When does a doctor become a doctor?

In the majority of Member States, doctors are given full registration at the end of their undergraduate training. Many, but not all, include in the training a period of "internship", in which graduates work under supervision in approved posts for a certain time before being given full registration – one year as a pre-registration house officer (PRHO) in the United Kingdom, for example, and 18 months as an *Arzt im Praktikum* in Germany. This stage is not covered by the Doctors' Directive, but a 1975 European Community recommendation (European Union 1975b) encourages countries with this arrangement to allow each others' graduates to train in their countries.

In a small number of countries, however, doctors do not become fully registered until they have completed their postgraduate training, either as specialists or GPs. France and Austria are examples. This has posed problems in the United Kingdom in cases where doctors from these countries have not been legally entitled to full registration, which is needed for senior house officer posts upwards, but have been too experienced for PRHO posts. Equally, United Kingdom doctors wanting to train, for example, in France may face difficulties because of their fully qualified status. According to the CPME study (Brettenthaler and Wallner 2001:6) the same system applies in Slovenia and the Czech Republic, and the study highlights this as an area needing attention.

Disparities in specialist training

The question "What is a specialist?" is a difficult one to answer. It is closely linked to the way in which health care systems are organized. The endpoint of United Kingdom specialist training has traditionally been a consultant post in the NHS. In some other countries, where patients have direct access to specialists and many work outside hospitals, doctors may complete their specialist training and set up their own practices, effectively working in ambulatory care. If they remain in hospital medicine, they may spend some time in intermediate posts before reaching the equivalent of consultant level.

The United Kingdom found itself facing infraction proceedings in the early 1990s over what appeared to be a two-tier system of specialist recognition. Until 1996 the General Medical Council issued a certificate of specialist training (CST) to doctors whose training met the minimum standards set out in the Doctors' Directive and who were seeking to practise elsewhere in the EU. This certificate had no legal significance in the United Kingdom, but was issued entirely for European purposes. As a result of the challenge the whole specialist training system was overhauled. The Specialist Training Authority of the Medical Royal Colleges (STA) was formed, a formal specialist register was created and the certificate of completion of specialist training (CCST) became the single endpoint qualification. Doctors with EU/EEA CCST equivalents have access to the specialist register, which is now the prerequisite for a substantive consultant post.

While it has been streamlined, British (and Irish) training still tends to last for longer than in many other countries as it is divided into basic and higher specialist training. Also, some specialists from other EU countries have been known to seek further experience in training posts even though they are legally entitled to be considered for consultant posts.

Disparities in GP training and status

The status of general practice across Europe has risen enormously in recent years, with postgraduate training now compulsory and the minimum duration recently increased from two to three years (European Union 2001). The emphasis in many of the accession countries is shifting from the hospital to the primary care sector. Free movement rules have recently been thrown into confusion, however, by the emergence of a two-tier approach – the "specialist in family medicine" or similar, commonly found in Scandinavia and Germany, and the "Title IV GP", so called after the relevant section in the Doctors' Directive (European Union 1993). Until recently Germany had a specialist tier, *Facharzt für Allgemeinmedizin*, and a second tier, *Praktischer Arzt*, the latter recognized for Title IV purposes. German doctors who had completed GP training in the United Kingdom and sought to return were sometimes annoyed when they were admitted only to the lower tier. They were even more annoyed, however, when Germany abolished this tier completely, leaving them with nowhere to go without further training. The Commission has been alerted to the problem and it is possible that it will issue a formal complaint against Germany in the near future.

The new draft Directive (European Commission 2002) appears to address this problem, stating that Member States cannot ". . . recognise any medical specialism which has a field of professional activity similar to that of general practitioners". At the time of writing, however, the interpretation of this clause is causing a significant amount of confusion.

Recognition of endpoint qualifications only

The sectoral Directives cater for the recognition of endpoint qualifications only – in the case of doctors, basic, specialist or general practice qualifications. There is no table of equivalents for any other qualifications – Royal College membership examinations, for example. Doctors who have done part of their training in one country and then move to another will have no guarantee that they will be able to slot in at a similar level. Some European exchange schemes are in operation, however, and may help to promote understanding.

What about continuing education and revalidation?

The most recent "amending directive" (European Union 2001) acknowledges the importance of lifelong learning for doctors, and states that:

> It is up to Member States to decide how to ensure, by suitable continuing training after completion of studies, that doctors maintain knowledge of progress in medicine.

Current mutual recognition arrangements remain unaffected, however, and there is no mention of continuing education for other professions. While there is increasing agreement about continuing professional development being at least an ethical obligation, the extent to which it is actually obligatory varies from country to country. Some, such as the Netherlands, already operate a revalidation system for doctors and the United Kingdom is now implementing such a scheme. While doctors (and other health professionals) must adapt to the requirements of the countries in which they work, no-one yet seems sure to what extent this area should be addressed at European level.

The proposed new Directive (European Commission 2002) seems to move a step further by stating that "continuous training shall ensure, in accordance with the procedures specific to each Member State, that persons who have completed their studies are able to keep abreast of medical progress". Once again, the requirement appears to be exclusive to doctors.

Different approaches to specialty recognition

Leaving aside differing approaches to training, some problems can be caused just by the different ways in which specialties are classified. This is principally a problem for medicine, which houses such a vast array of disciplines. To achieve automatic recognition with no further assessment or top-up training, specialists must be qualified in a specialty that is also recognized as such in the country to which they wish to move. The Doctors' Directive (European Union 1993) has a relatively short list of specialties that are common to all Member States and a much longer list of those that are common to two or more. The latter is constantly in need of updating, as specific groups lobby for the inclusion of their specialties. There may be difficulties because a particular discipline is a full specialty in one country and a subspecialty of a different discipline in another. Or there are cases such as dermatology and genito-urinary medicine, distinct specialties in the United Kingdom and Ireland but amalgamated everywhere else as dermato-venereology.

The ACMT has done its best to rationalize the classification system, in its unimplemented fourth report on specialist training (European Commission 1997:6) and in its as yet unpublished fifth report (Twomey and ACMT Working Group on Specialist Training 2001). As mentioned previously, however, the Commission has addressed the problem by proposing to move specialties that are not common to all Member States to the general system (European Commission 2002).

"Acquired rights"

All of the Directives make provision for those who may not meet their requirements to the letter because they qualified before the rules were adopted. Before 1986 there were several EU countries that had no compulsory postgraduate training for general practice. The requirement for such training to be compulsory came into full effect on 1 January 1995, and those already in practice on 31 December 1994 were given "acquired rights". Some countries conferred these on all medical graduates who might notionally have been entitled to work in general practice on that date. Some of these doctors moved to the United Kingdom and fought to be included in vocational training programmes, arguing – no doubt rightly – that they did not feel equipped to practise without appropriate training. Because of their "rights", the system for a while did not allow their training to be funded, although this problem has now been resolved. There may well be many doctors in the accession countries in a similar position.

Exchange of information about disciplinary procedures

In recent years a strong consensus has developed that registering and regulatory bodies should exchange information on a regular basis about disciplinary procedures. Doctors who have faced proceedings in one country should not be able to move to another in a way that conceals their records. Information from the

CEOM (unpublished study) indicates that there are variations between countries in the operation of the machinery for withdrawing the right to practise on grounds of professional misconduct, between different countries' responses to particular types of misconduct, and in the provision of information to other countries, both in terms of the meaning of "certificates of good standing" and responses to direct requests for information. Apparently only France, Ireland and the United Kingdom routinely send details of fitness to practise findings to other EEA countries, while some will do so on request and others are prevented from doing so by domestic data protection legislation.

EEA citizens with "third country" qualifications

There has been an enormous amount of discussion – mostly within the medical profession – about the position of those who are EEA citizens and who are registered in and practise in the EEA, but who originally qualified outside the EEA. So far they have not enjoyed the same rights as their EEA-qualified counterparts to have their qualifications recognized elsewhere, a situation perceived as unjust and discriminatory. While the British Medical Association has lobbied hard for a change in the law, with strong support in some quarters, the overall response has been cautious. The 2001 amending Directive (European Union 2001:2) built on recent case law and introduced an obligation for countries to examine the experience of professionals in this position. One country's decision cannot be binding on another, however. The general system approach is slightly different in that it makes provision for those with non-EEA qualifications but three years of practice in a Member State to be treated in the same way as those with EEA qualifications. The new draft Directive (European Commission 2002) appears to extend this provision to all professions within its scope – sectoral and general. As many professionals in some central and eastern European candidate countries will have trained in the former Soviet Union, with its very different model of undergraduate medical training, this may be quite a significant issue to be tackled (Brettenthaler and Wallner 2001), but will be addressed if the above-mentioned proposal is adopted.

"Third country" nationals with EEA qualifications

In contrast, those who are not EEA citizens but who have completed all their training in EEA Member States may find themselves treated as overseas professionals while those with identical training are admitted automatically. This has certainly been the situation for some doctors in the United Kingdom and has caused much confusion and frustration. While European law discriminates in favour of European citizens, rather than against others, more thought is now being given to the rights of "third country" nationals resident in the EEA. Given the large international medical training programmes undertaken by some candidate countries (such as the English and German language courses in Hungarian and Czech medical universities) this is likely to become an important issue.

Language (again)

Language has been covered previously, but is worth mentioning again. While language testing may be a barrier to free movement, inadequate language skills are a barrier to safe practice. It is discussed too often, in particular in United Kingdom meetings and in the British media, to pretend that there is no degree of unease about it. Perhaps the most positive approach would be to ensure that language training is at least offered to migrants, even if it cannot be imposed. Interestingly, the United Kingdom Health Professions Council (formerly the Council for Professions Supplementary to Medicine) which has extensive experience of operating the general system Directive, has decided to "stick its neck out" as one official put it, and test incoming speech and language therapists. It has decided to risk possible objections because linguistic knowledge is such an essential part of the profession concerned (personal communication).

Availability of information and advice – for migrants and competent authorities

As indicated previously, lack of information about training content can breed distrust in a system supposed to be based on trust. Competent authorities operating the general system Directives face particular difficulties with access to accurate and up-to-date information. Migrants themselves need clear information from easily identifiable sources. One suggestion to emerge from several sources during the European Commission's recent consultation (European Commission 2002) is for a central website with detailed country-by-country information. The new draft Directive (European Commission 2002) would require each Member State to designate a contact point to provide information and help citizens to exercise their rights.

Bureaucracy

While Member States are obliged to meet their obligations under the various directives, there is no centralized registration procedure and each has its own formalities. Some of these may be quite daunting, and there is anecdotal evidence from more than one profession of what seem to be unreasonable demands. "Red tape" may sound trivial, but should not be underestimated as a barrier to free movement. A nursing representative at a recent meeting organized by the English Department of Health identified a need for common paperwork. Whether this could ever happen is open to doubt, but some form of audit of what is required in each country would not be out of place. Some intent to streamline bureaucracy is expressed in the new draft Directive (European Commission 2002).

Induction and support

All of the above points indicate the need for formal induction and support mechanisms for EEA health professionals. The interviews conducted by Jinks et al. (2000) in the North of England demonstrated a lack of systematic support and absence of advice about training and career options. For doctors, the United Kingdom now has a formal induction programme leading to a certificate of United Kingdom induction (CUKI) which might serve as a model of good practice.

Defining roles – what is a doctor and what is a nurse?

Doctors in the United Kingdom use the title "Dr" as a courtesy title as soon as they take up PRHO posts. German doctors, on the other hand, cannot call themselves Dr. med. until they have written a thesis – the Doktorarbeit. Until then they are named Arzt (Ärztin). Movement between countries offers some scope for confusion, but all are recognizably medically qualified so what's in a name?

At least the sectoral system, for all its problems, is relatively clear cut. Doctors, dentists, general care nurses, midwives and pharmacists are sufficiently identifiable and similar enough in each Member State to be covered by one piece of legislation per profession. Different as their day-to-day roles may be if one looks beneath the surface, those who run the general system probably have the best picture of the sheer multiplicity of health professions. Osteopathy and chiropractic are now fully regulated professions in the United Kingdom, for example, and therefore notionally covered by the first Directive (European Union 1989). Representatives at a recent meeting pointed out, however, that the practice of both disciplines remains illegal in some Member States. Where chiropractic is legal, it may mean quite different things in different countries. Different approaches to psychology and psychotherapy were also cited. A vast array of non-conventional medicine flourishes in some countries with little regulation, whereas in others its practice may be restricted to doctors. The German *Heilprak-tiker* is apparently unique, and other "medical assistant" posts are little known elsewhere. Enlarging the EU can only add to the richness and increase the complexity.

Cultural differences are inevitable in a Europe stretching from the Baltic to the Mediterranean, taking in countries with diverse political, economic and religious backgrounds and diverse health care systems. The American journalist Lynn Payer compared medical practice in France, Germany, the United Kingdom and the United States (Payer 1989). She linked French practice to the cartesian thought system of Descartes, German to the romantic tradition of the early nineteenth century and British practice to the empiricist tradition of Locke and Hume. The "hands-on" emphasis of United Kingdom medical training fits this picture. There are different approaches to disease and treatment – witness, for example, the continuing popularity of spa treatments in many European countries – and very different approaches to issues such as patient autonomy, confidentiality and multidisciplinary teamworking. Any time spent in a

European gathering will demonstrate these differences. French practice is closely regulated, often by statute, whereas there are strong elements of pragmatism in the British approach, practice in controversial areas being guided by case law rather than code and ethical guidelines placing greater emphasis on doctors' judgement and ability to justify their actions.

The organization of health care systems, and the way in which health professionals work within them, are also important. European health care systems can be divided very roughly into two types, albeit with many variants:

- "National health service", funded centrally by government from general taxation;
- Insurance-based, managed by sickness funds with contributions by individuals and employers, with varying degrees of government subsidy.

In the insurance-based systems there is a strong tradition of "liberal practice". Patients often have access to specialists without GP referral and may see several doctors rather than one who takes an overall coordinating role. In countries such as the United Kingdom, Ireland and the Nordic countries, and more recently Spain, GPs have traditionally been "gatekeepers" to specialist care and have assumed overall coordination of care of patients on their lists. Will the work of a GP working alongside primary care specialists in paediatrics and gynaecology, for example, differ from that of the "gatekeeper" GP? How does the paediatrician with a practice outside hospital compare with the United Kingdom consultant? And so on . . .

Nurses and other health professionals in the United Kingdom have developed their roles to an extent that might well be unthinkable in some other countries, taking on many tasks previously carried out by doctors. Multidisciplinary teamworking is essential in a hard-pressed NHS. In a relatively centralized system where most professionals are salaried or hold contracts involving capitation fees and the like, these developments are less likely to be perceived as a threat than they are in countries where doctors may perceive other health professionals as competing for fees.

The picture in many of the central and eastern European accession countries seems to be of health services dominated by specialist practice, with a need to build up the primary care sector. Further differences – and similarities too – will no doubt soon become evident. It would be impossible to standardize the roles of health professionals and senseless to try. Some degree of diversity is inevitable and indeed desirable. At the same time, increasing familiarity will also bring with it a degree of convergence as colleagues share experience and learn from each other.

Impact of accession

The European Commission points to research that suggests that there will be no dramatic increases in migration, and that the impact on the EU labour market should be limited (European Commission 2001a). It goes on to suggest that the main factors influencing migration will be the income gap between the countries concerned and the labour market situation in the country of destination.

Other factors include geographical proximity, culture and language. The highest number of migrant workers would be expected to go to Germany and the second highest number to Austria. The governments of these two countries have taken the lead in enlargement negotiations in calling for transitional measures to delay the full application of free movement rules to the candidate countries. The general impression is that they have done so in response to the fears of their electorates rather than an overwhelming evidence base.

The agreed position, as confirmed by the United Kingdom Foreign and Commonwealth Office (personal communication), is that there will be a maximum transition period of seven years before the central European candidate countries benefit from full free movement rights. The basic transition period, during which current Member States will not be required to open their labour markets, is five years. Member States may decide to suspend the transition period after two years, however (which the United Kingdom expects to do, subject to labour market developments), or to extend it by a further two years if there is a serious threat of disturbance to their labour markets. There is nothing, meanwhile, to prevent Member States from using national legislation to admit citizens of the accession countries as soon as they join, and several Member States have already expressed their willingness to do so.

Whether the Commission's predictions will apply to the health sector remains to be seen, but current shortages in countries like the United Kingdom mean that movement could well extend beyond the two countries mentioned above. Income gaps might be a significant factor as things stand. While income levels need to be viewed in the context of purchasing power in the country concerned, doctors and other health professionals in the former communist countries generally enjoyed lower prestige and incomes in relative terms than their western European counterparts and will take time to close the gap.

The CPME (Brettenthaler and Wallner 2001) has highlighted the risk of "brain drain" among doctors and Irwin (2001) among nurses. Irwin (2001) refers to the potential conflict between individual nurses' freedom to choose where they work and the need to deliver health care in the countries they leave, going on to ask "How might the Commission respond to this issue?". This is an interesting question, given the emphasis so far on unfettered free movement, and is probably more a matter for discussion between national governments. The Czech Government has apparently raised concerns informally with the English Department of Health (personal communication), presumably because of the current international recruitment campaign.

A common view expressed by health professionals in candidate countries is that "those who wanted to go have gone already". While anecdotal evidence suggests that England, Norway, Sweden, France and some parts of eastern Germany are already recruiting from some candidate countries, doctors' representatives at least do not seem to be expecting a seismic shift.

One further aspect worth mentioning is that patients may also move (see also Chapter 11). At a recent European meeting, one delegate referred to the large numbers of Austrians in border regions who go to Hungary for dental treatment – presumably because of the lower costs. On a cycling holiday in Austria/Hungary a few years earlier, the author had noticed this herself and was interested to hear it confirmed by an "official" source.

In terms of process, the United Kingdom Health Professions Council expects its workload post-accession to be "business as usual". It is already used to processing applications from accession countries and foresees little change once these are covered by the general system directive. Because of the way in which the sectoral directives operate, far more detailed preparation is going on this area.

The Internal Market and Enlargement Directorates-General, together with the Office for Technical Assistance and Information Exchange (TAIEX) have launched a major programme of "expert mobilization" whereby teams of experts from the professions concerned are visiting the accession countries and reporting on progress already achieved in implementing the relevant *acquis communautaire*, action still needing to be taken and timetables for the latter. The scrutiny programme for health professions is very detailed and covers two main areas:

- Training: To include basic training, additional training in general medical practice (doctors only), additional specialist training and continuing education, with detailed questions to be answered about each.
- Practice of the profession: To include "organization of the profession" (trade unions and professional associations), access to practice, disciplinary rules and scale of penalties and status of practitioners within different sectors (employed, independent contractor and so on).

This exercise is particularly interesting because in the past applicant states have been asked to submit information on relevant areas themselves, but seem not to have been the subject of such direct scrutiny. Perhaps not surprisingly, the scale of the project seems to be posing problems, with one commentator querying the feasibility of covering a whole country in three days and others raising a variety of practical and organizational issues (personal communications). Nevertheless, if similar reports were compiled on all Member States and made easily available, this might go a long way towards increasing confidence in the system.

The CPME, in its study (Brettenthaler and Wallner 2001) has concluded that medical training at least in the applicant countries complies in principle with the standards set out in the Doctors' Directive. The only caveat is that some eastern European countries previously followed a Soviet model whereby specialist training was carried out in two stages, with specialist certificates being awarded after the first stage lasting three years. This practice has now been discontinued, but may need examination in the light of "acquired rights" or transitional provisions. This means quite simply that doctors trained under previous systems may, if seeking to move within the EU, need to provide evidence of satisfactory practice or supplementary training, or that the EU may decide to confer "acquired rights" on all those in a certain category – this last arrangement is often known as a "grandfather clause". Negotiations on these arrangements are taking place at the time of writing. They are a normal part of the process, however, and similar arrangements have been made in the past when other countries have joined the EU. They are not unique to this enlargement round.

Will there be overall winners or losers? There is a fierce debate raging about agriculture, where there is much to win or lose for many countries. The debate about the health care sector is taking place in a somewhat lower key, however.

Most predictions seem to indicate that there will be no major changes. When the author put this question to a doctor from one of the central European countries, he echoed this point, but also believed that the acceding countries would gain from the general impetus to reform that is already taking place.

Conclusions

It is often said that debates about European matters involve a clash between conceptualism and pragmatism – or in other words, between those with a vision and those concerned with how to implement it. The United Kingdom is usually to be found among the pragmatists, sometimes to the frustration of its fellow members. Free movement was one of the great visions of the EU's founders and remains an article of faith today. Enlargement is a challenge, because it will change the scale at which we all operate, but it also offers an opportunity to reflect on experience so far and to decide what has worked well and what could be improved. The Commission is certainly doing this although, with its relatively small secretariat, its first concern is probably about reducing its own administrative burden. The candidate countries, for their part, seem to be undergoing a scrutiny process on an unprecedented scale.

The sectoral system seems to have run relatively smoothly from an administrative point of view, but there are some problems to iron out and steps to be taken to increase the trust on which it depends. Those operating the general system seem to need better and more up-to-date sources of information.

The immediate requirements for the accession countries seem to be:

- Clearly designated competent authorities for basic, specialist and continuing training;
- Transparent registration procedures indicating different levels of training;
- Training at all levels to measure up to the requirements in the various directives in terms of curriculum, delivery and duration. Training in general practice may need particular attention in some countries where primary care has been less developed in the past;
- Arrangements for those with "acquired rights", that is those professionals qualified before the requirements imposed by the various directives came into force.

Further options might include an "inventory" of health professions likely to try to migrate under the general system directive.

Points to be taken into account for everyone include the following. First, there is a need for robust mechanisms for consultation with the professions concerned, whatever form these take in the future, and guarantees that advice will be taken and acted upon. Second, training criteria in the sectoral Directives need to be updated and expanded. Information about training content and organization in different Member States should be available centrally. The work of expert professional organizations may usefully be harnessed for this purpose, and initiatives such as visiting programmes should be encouraged. The use of outcome-based measures should be explored further. Third, other sections, such as lists of specialties in the Doctors' Directive (European Union 1993), also need regular updating.

Fourth, confusion arising from definitions needs to be ironed out – for example, different categories of general practitioner, or different approaches to full registration as a doctor – and the general system needs to be supported by regularly updated databases with information about training in different countries. Fifth, migrants should have access to clear information about registration, perhaps on a central EU website directing them to appropriate bodies in each Member State.

Sixth, as the organization of health care, ethical and legal requirements may vary widely from one European country to another, Member States should offer structured induction programmes and continuing support to doctors new to their countries. The needs of European doctors should not be overlooked because their qualifications are recognized automatically. Finally, there should be formal arrangements in place for competent authorities to exchange information about disciplinary procedures.

Further thought should also be given to the following issues. First, further development of exchange programmes and credit transfer systems, to supplement the "endpoint" recognition guaranteed by the sectoral system and to strengthen the operation of the general system. Second, how to formalize the mutual recognition of continuing training and how to deal with the impact of revalidation mechanisms now being introduced in some countries. Third, the rights of EEA citizens holding non-EEA qualifications and of "third country" nationals with EEA qualifications, numbers of which are likely to increase post-enlargement. Fourth, shifting responsibility for matters concerning the training of health professionals to the European Commission Health and Consumer Protection Directorate-General.

Finally, the following may be politically sensitive, but Member States may also wish to explore exchange of information on workforce planning, to help to identify potential movement trends and allay concerns about "brain drain", and the potential for some degree of harmonization in registration paperwork – starting perhaps with a "bureaucracy audit".

As the EU grows still further in size and diversity, now is the time to improve the system for everyone.

Acknowledgements

The author acknowledges the assistance of the Department of Health, Foreign and Commonwealth Office, General Medical Council, British Dental Association, General Dental Council, Royal College of Nursing, United Kingdom Council for Nursing, Midwifery and Health Visiting, Royal College of Midwives, Royal Pharmaceutical Society of Great Britain and the Health Professions Council, all of which provided background information and briefing. The chapter also draws on research and discussions which have taken place within the British Medical Association, other United Kingdom medical organizations and the wide range of European medical bodies cited in the text. The views expressed are the author's own.

References

Brearley, S. (1999) Medical Migration within the European Economic Area. Unpublished study for CIO.

Brettenthaler, R. and Wallner, F. (2001) Analysis of the health care systems of the accession countries and the possible consequences for the accession negotiations. Standing Committee of European Doctors, http://www.cpme.be/en/news.htm. 5 March 2002.

Department of Health (2000) *The NHS Plan: A plan for investment, a plan for reform*. London: HMSO.

Duncan, B. (2002) Off the record: Europe, *BMA News*. 16 February.

European Commission (1997) Advisory Committee on Medical Training: Fourth Report and Recommendations on the Conditions for Specialist Training XV/E/8306/4/96 final. Brussels: Internal Market DG.

European Commission (1996) Advisory Committee on Medical Training: Report and Recommendations on the Review of Specific Training in General Medical Practice XV/E/8443/1/95. Brussels: Internal Market DG.

European Commission (1998) Advisory Committee on Training in Nursing: Report and Recommendations on the competencies required to take up the profession of nurse responsible for general care in the European Union XV/E/8481/4/97. Brussels: Internal Market DG.

European Commission (1992) Council Directive 92/51/EEC of 18 June 1992 on a second general system for the recognition of professional education and training to supplement Directive 89/48/EEC, http://www.europa.eu.int/eur-lex/en/lif/reg/en_register_0610.html accessed 5 March 2002.

European Commission (2001) European Commission staff working paper on the future regime for professional recognition, MARKT/D/8131/3/2001. Brussels: Internal Market DG.

European Commission (2001a) Information Note: The Free Movement of Workers in the Context of Enlargement 6 March 2001. Brussels: European Commission.

European Commission (2002) Proposal for a Directive of the European Parliament and of the Council on the recognition of professional qualifications. COM (2002) 119 final. Brussels: Internal Market DG.

European Network of Nursing Organisations (ENNO) (2000) Recommendations for a European Framework for Specialist Nursing Education. Paris: ENNO.

European Union (1975a) 75/364/EEC: Council Decision of 16 June 1975 setting up an Advisory Committee on Medical Training, http://www.europa.eu.int/eur-lex/en/lif/dat/1975/en_375D0364.html accessed 5 March 2002.

European Union (1975c) 75/365/EEC: Council Decision of 16 June 1975 setting up a Committee of Senior Officials on Public Health, http://www.europa.eu.int/eur-lex/en/lif/dat/1975/en_375D0365.html accessed 5 March 2002.

European Union (1975b) 75/367/EEC: Council Recommendation of 16 June 1975 on the clinical training of doctors, http://www.europa.eu.int/eurlex/en/lif/dat/1975/en_375H0367.html accessed 5 March 2002.

European Union (1997) Consolidated version of the Treaty establishing the European Community, http://www.europa.eu.int/eur-lex/en/treaties/dat/ec_cons_treaty_en.pdf accessed 6 March 2002.

European Union (1977) Council Directive 77/452/EEC of 27 June 1977 concerning the mutual recognition of diplomas, certificates and other evidence of the formal qualifications of nurses responsible for general care, including measures to facilitate the effective exercise of this right of establishment and freedom to provide services and Council Directive 77/453/EEC of 27 June 1977 concerning the coordination of provisions laid down by Law, Regulation or Administrative Action in respect of the activities of nurses responsible for general care, http://www.europa.eu.int/eur-lex/en/lif/reg/en_register_062050.html accessed 5 March 2002.

European Union (1978) Council Directive 78/686/EEC of 25 July 1978 concerning the mutual recognition of diplomas, certificates and other evidence of the formal qualifications of practitioners of dentistry, including measures to facilitate the effective exercise of the right of establishment and freedom to provide services and Council Directive 78/687/EEC of 25 July 1978 concerning the coordination of provisions laid down by Law, Regulation or Administrative Action in respect of the activities of dental practitioners, http://www.europa.eu.int/eur-lex/en/lif/reg/en_register_062050.html accessed 5 March 2002.

European Union (1980) Council Directive 80/154/EEC of 21 January 1980 concerning the mutual recognition of diplomas, certificates and other evidence of formal qualifications in midwifery and including measures to facilitate the effective exercise of the right of establishment and freedom to provide services and Council Directive 80/155/EEC of 21 January 1980 concerning the coordination of provisions laid down by Law, Regulation or Administrative Action relating to the taking up and pursuit of the activities of midwives, http://www.europa.eu.int/eur-lex/en/lif/reg/en_register_062050.html accessed 5 March 2002.

European Union (1985) Council Directive 85/432/EEC of 16 September 1985 concerning the coordination of provisions laid down by Law, Regulation or Administrative Action in respect of certain activities in the field of pharmacy and Council Directive 85/433/EEC of 16 September 1985 concerning the mutual recognition of diplomas, certificates and other evidence of formal qualifications in pharmacy, including measures to facilitate the effective exercise of the right of establishment relating to certain activities in the field of pharmacy, http://www.europa.eu.int/eur-lex/en/lif/reg/en_register_062050.html accessed 5 March 2002.

European Union (1989) Council Directive 89/48/EEC of 21 December 1988 on a general system for the recognition of higher-education diplomas awarded on completion of professional education and training of at least three years' duration, http://www.europa.eu.int/eur-lex/en/lif/dat/1989/en_389L0048.html accessed 5 March 2002.

European Union (1993) Council Directive 93/16/EEC of 5 April 1993 to facilitate the free movement of doctors and the mutual recognition of their diplomas, certificates and other evidence of formal qualifications., http://www.europa.eu.int/eur-lex/en/lif/reg/en_register_062050.html. 2002.

European Union (2001) Directive 2001/19/EC of the European Parliament and of the Council of 14 May 2001 amending Council Directives 89/48/EEC and 92/51/EEC on the general system for the recognition of professional qualifications and Council Directives 77/452/EEC, 77/453/EEC, 78/686/EEC, 78/687/EEC, 78/1026/EEC, 78/1027/EEC, 80/154/EEC, 80/155/EEC, 85/384/EEC, 85/432/EEC, 85/433/EEC and 93/16/EEC concerning the professions of nurse responsible for general care, dental practitioner, veterinary surgeon, midwife, architect, pharmacist and doctor (Text with EEA relevance), http://www.europa.eu.int/eur-lex/en/lif/dat/2001/en_301L0019.html accessed March 2002.

Hansard (2001) 10 December 2001, col. 722. London: HMSO.

Irwin, J. (2001) Migration Patterns of nurses in the EU, *Eurohealth*, 7:(4).

Jinks, C., Ong, B.N. and Paton, C. (2000) Mobile medics? The mobility of doctors in the European Economic Area. *Health Policy*, 54(1):45–64.

Mäkinen, M. and Aarimaa, M. (2001) The challenge of professional freedom, *Eurohealth*, 7(4).

Nicholas, S. (1994) Mobility of Doctors – the Theory and the Practice, in P. Neale (ed.) *Creating European Professionals*. Leeds: University of Leeds.

OECD (1999) *Practising Physicians – Density/1000 population*. Paris: OECD.

Payer, L. (1989) *Medicine and Culture*. London: Victor Gollancz Ltd.

PWG (1991, updated 1996) *Medical Manpower in Europe by the Year 2000: From Surplus to Deficit*. Copenhagen: PWG.

Twomey, C. and ACMT Working Group on Specialist Training (2001) Draft Fifth ACMT Report and Recommendations on the Conditions for Specialist Training. Unpublished but partially available at http://www.uems.be/acmt5-s.doc accessed 6 March 2002.

UEMS (2001) Basel Declaration: UEMS Policy on Continuing Professional Development, http://www.uems.be/d-0120-e.htm accessed 2002.

chapter eight

Free movement of health professionals: The Polish experience

Monika Zajac

Introduction

In 1999, 14.6% of the total workforce in Poland was employed in the health sector (World Bank 2001). Health professionals – defined as those whose status is regulated by legislation – in Poland are organized by statute into three associations, or chambers, with mandatory membership: physicians (including dentists), nurses and midwives, and pharmacists. Each association has the same structure and is divided into district chambers with headquarters in Warsaw. The numbers of doctors, nurses and pharmacists in Poland relative to population are similar to those in western European countries, although there has been a small decline in their overall number since 1996 (Table 8.1). However, the aggregate figures conceal the pattern of distribution. Three-quarters of total health care staff are employed in urban areas that account for only 65% of the

Table 8.1   Health care professionals in Poland (per 10 000 population)

Year	Physicians	Dentists	Nurses	Midwives	Pharmacists
1996	23.5	4.6	55.7	6.4	5.2
1997	23.6	4.6	56.2	6.4	5.3
1998	23.3	4.5	55.1	6.3	5.3
1999	22.6	3.4	51.0	5.9	5.2

Source: Statistical Yearbook 2000, Ministry of Health, Centre of Information Systems in Health Care, Warsaw.

population and there are shortages of physicians in family medicine (Zaborowski and Rebandel 2001) as well as specialized nurses.

The process of the accession of Poland to the EU has various elements that also affect health. Topics that are the responsibility of the Ministry of Health can be found in 11 out of 29 chapters of the negotiation papers and require 191 legal acts to be screened (Department of European Integration and International Affairs at Ministry of Health 1999), one of which being the mutual recognition of qualifications of health professionals. Adoption of the *acquis communautaire* in relation to health professionals will have consequences for the Polish health care system. This chapter outlines the main changes in Polish legislation that seek to bring training and regulation of health professionals into line with European law. It will show that the impact of enlargement will be both positive and negative, in some cases with different consequences for Poland and the rest of the EU.

Legislation

Poland's negotiation position regarding "free movement of persons"

On 21 December 2001 Poland announced the (provisional) closure of negotiations with the EU within the chapter "free movement of persons". This means that all agreements within the Polish and EU negotiation position (in this area) are considered settled, although they can be changed up until the closing date of all other areas of negotiation. The final closure of all areas of negotiation takes place at the last stage of the procedure, having enacted the legislation required to comply with the *acquis communautaire* and subject to verification by both sides. On accession, EU citizens will have equal rights in the Polish labour market (Government Plenipotentiary for Poland's Accession Negotiations to the EU at Chancellery of the Prime Minister of the Republic of Poland 2001a); Polish citizens will be entitled to employment in Member States after a flexible transitional period. Transitional arrangements are set from two years (Denmark, France, Greece, Spain, the Netherlands, Ireland, Sweden) to a maximum of seven years (Germany, Austria).

The chapter's compliance with the *acquis communautaire* received a relatively good evaluation in the European Commission's Regular Report 2001 (European Commission 2001a). Poland undertook to implement the *acquis communautaire* concerning "free movement of persons" so that the relevant laws may operate, with reciprocity, between Poland and the other Member States as of 1 January 2003 (Government Plenipotentiary for Poland's Accession Negotiations to the EU at Chancellery of the Prime Minister of the Republic of Poland 2000).

Mutual recognition of professional qualifications

A key issue in the chapter on "free movement of persons" is mutual recognition of professional qualifications, which allows every citizen of a EU Member State to practise their profession in another Member State. According to Poland's position paper, Poland accepts the *acquis communautaire* in the area of "mutual recognition of professional qualifications". It declares that Polish law will be in accord with the *acquis* as of the date of Poland's membership of the EU (Government Plenipotentiary for Poland's Accession Negotiations to the EU at Chancellery of the Prime Minister of the Republic of Poland 2000) and transposition of Polish legislation will be ready in time for accession.

The *acquis communautaire* concerning mutual recognition of professional qualification contains:

- Directives (89/48/EEC and 92/51/EEC) dealing with the general system for recognition of higher-education diplomas and qualifications required to exercise "regulated professions";
- sectoral Directives covering recognition of qualifications of lawyers, architects, physicians, dentists, nurses, midwives, pharmacists and veterinary surgeons.

Poland's negotiation position on "free movement of persons" in the paragraph "mutual recognition of professional qualifications" includes medical and paramedical activities, dealing with physicians, dentists, pharmacists, nurses and midwives (and veterinary surgeons, who are not considered in this chapter).

Approximation of Polish legislation

The full approximation of Polish law to the *acquis* on doctors, dentists, pharmacists, nurses and midwives was effected by the introduction of the principle of equal treatment of Polish citizens and those of EU Member States in licensing including, especially, the lifting of the Polish citizenship requirement. Procedures were developed for the recognition of qualifications according to the relevant Directives. All procedures are regulated by legal acts covering the respective major health professions (see below); bodies governing recognition of professional qualifications and required documents are defined by law. Executive acts are still to be developed such as the supplementary acts listing the medical diplomas that will be recognized after Poland's accession. These are essential for effective mobility and are expected to be ready in time to provide the regulatory bodies with the necessary working frameworks.

Polish law imposes obligations on service providers concerning health professionals who are nationals of EU Member States and are covered by the various sectoral directives (see Chapter 7).

For each profession, these Directives cover detailed training programmes (hours and areas of study), types of specialization and degrees offered. In general, existing training programmes complied with EU standards. One exception was training for nurses, which is discussed later in the chapter. Expert groups (including national specialists and representatives from the Centre for Medical Postgraduate Training) were created to screen programmes and ensure compliance of Polish curricula with EU Directives. However, the most important changes concerned equal treatment of EU and Polish citizens. The requirements for foreigners wishing to practise a health profession in Poland have been lifted in respect of citizens of other Member States although they remain for those from outside the EU.

TAIEX (the Technical Assistance Information Exchange Office of the Phare Programme) organized peer review conferences in all candidate countries to look at training programmes. In Poland this took place between 11 and 14 March 2002. However, considerable uncertainty remains as, apart from the minimal requirements, mainly listing of hours of study, there are no agreed standards, in particular with regard to content of curricula.

The *acquis* provides for mutual recognition of diplomas and qualifications by means of a fast-track procedure. The Act on the Recognition of Qualifications for Regulated Professions acquired in EU Member States was adopted by Poland in May 2001 and enters into force upon accession (European Integration Committee Office – UKIE 2001). At that time, Poland will be obliged to recognize medical diplomas from each Member State. Using a list of approved diplomas, issued by the Minister of Health, regional chambers of professionals will be responsible for issuing rights to practise in Poland. In order to scrutinize applications rapidly, regional bodies will require training to be able to answer possible questions and be informed about the documents required. It is likely that the system will take some time to work efficiently and there may be problems with information flow.

As noted above, prior to accession, Polish legislation on health professions complied partially with EU Directives. Amendments adopted by the Polish Government during the negotiation process included changes in training programmes and standardization of diplomas. The requirement that members of the medical profession are able to speak Polish was maintained. In the following paragraphs the main amendments to Polish legislation concerning particular professions will be discussed, including those regulatory acts that have been changed in response to the accession procedure.

The professions

Physicians

An amendment to the Act on the Profession of Medical Doctor (1996) and the Act on Chambers of Physicians (1989) was adopted in September 2001. Its provisions will enter into force gradually. After Poland's accession to the EU, physicians with diplomas acquired in EU Member States will have the right to:

- provide services in Poland;
- be a member of professional bodies;
- establish themselves in private practice.

The crucial change is equalization of Polish and EU citizenship (Table 8.2). The amendment bans discrimination, specifically with regard to establishing a medical practice, registration and membership of professional bodies. For instance, the requirement that foreigners undertake an obligatory internship has been cancelled if they are EU citizens with the right to practise in another Member State. Moreover, the amendment guarantees automatic equalization procedures

Table 8.2 Key harmonization issues

Mutual recognition of qualifications	Freedom to provide services
Equalization of Polish and EU citizenship	Automatic "temporary" registration by the chamber of physicians
Recognition of EU diplomas and certificates	Providing services within the social security scheme (Sickness Funds)
Provision of the law on the profession of physician concerning foreigners – to apply to non-EU citizens	Requirements related to establishment of individual medical practice cannot apply to EU professionals

for diplomas and other documents giving evidence of qualifications acquired in other Member States. The amendment requires that the Minister of Health will announce the list of information centres where EU citizens can obtain full information on the requirements necessary to practise as a medical doctor. The Minister is also obliged to announce the list of required certificates and the equalization procedure must not take longer than three months. In addition, a EU citizen applying for the right to practise as a medical doctor in Poland is obliged to submit a written statement confirming that they are sufficiently competent in the Polish language to provide services. Levels of Polish language proficiency will be set out in a separate amendment.

Medical doctors from Member States who wish to practise in Poland for short periods (up to three months) can acquire a "temporary right to practise the profession of medical doctor" in a fast-track procedure with the chamber of physicians. They would be obliged to submit a written statement specifying the location and duration of practice and a document proving entitlement to practise in another EU Member State. The amendment retains all rights to exercise a profession that existed previously.

While the legal position is clear, its practical application may be less straightforward. While discrimination is illegal, it would be naïve to deny the possibility of problems contracting with Sickness Funds. It is also possible that some patients might discriminate against foreign doctors in certain situations (for example in the case of family doctors) although foreign specialists may be preferred if they are seen as offering more innovative treatment methods.

Although training programmes for physicians in Poland generally conformed to the requirements of the relevant Directive, the amendment created a new system of medical education. A Medical Examination Centre (CEM) will be created; this will be independent of the existing Postgraduate Medical Education Centre (CMKP – Centrum Medycznego Kształcenia Podyplomoweg). The CEM (located in Łodz), accountable to the Minister of Health, is responsible for oversight of syllabuses, appointments to medical academies, speciality examinations and continuing professional development. Separate legal acts regulate the supervision and control of education and educational standards, under bodies such as the National Accreditation Council, the Ministry of Health, the National Board of Physicians, and the National Board of Medical Examination.

These are independent bodies with different areas of responsibility but coordinated by the Ministry of Health.

The new regulations enter into force on different dates, with those dealing with continuing medical education on January 2003 while others relating to EU citizens working as physicians in Poland linked to the date of Poland's accession to the EU.

Dentists

All the changes mentioned in the previous section also apply to dentists, who are covered by the Act on the Profession of Medical Doctor. However, negotiations concerning dentists were quite difficult with Directive 78/686/EEC requiring three years of practical training. The Commission questioned whether the Polish training programme complies with this regulation and suggested that Polish dental graduates should acquire the title of "dentist" (lekarz dentysta) rather than the current "doctor in dentistry" (lekarz stomatolog).

It must be emphasized that there are many different models of dentistry training across the EU. The Polish system takes six years: five years of regular dental studies in combination with general medical subjects (for example internal medicine, ear and eye sciences, paediatrics; a total of 550 hours of study) as well as more general subjects (for example chemistry or physiology). Practical training on patients starts in the third year (under supervision in university clinics). The sixth year is an obligatory internship, working with patients, for a total of 2400 hours. Graduates may undertake further specialist training as part of their employment.

The German model is similar to that in Poland. Five years of studying dentistry and success in an exam allows graduates to practise as dentists and establish themselves in independent practice (Fortuna 2001). In Belgium prospective dentists study in a separate university department (dental sciences) to become Bachelors of Dentistry. Theory is covered in the first two years of the five year course and practical work begins in the third year. The title of doctor of dentistry is awarded after seven years of regular medical studies and five years of specialization in dentistry.

Polish experts in dentistry participating in the commissions equalizing foreign diplomas argue that education of dentists in Poland is at least equal to EU standards, if not higher. Moreover, representatives of the EU Commission who visited three Polish Medical Academies (Cracow, Lodz, Warsaw) confirmed that training programmes for dentists met EU standards. Polish experts emphasized the increasing medical content of training programmes for dentists in many countries. Therefore, they suggest it would not be reasonable for Poland to go in an opposite direction (Fortuna 2001).

In December 2001 Poland's Government adopted a new version of the negotiation paper "free movement of persons" containing changes concerning dentists in the paragraph "mutual recognition of qualifications" (Government Plenipotentiary for Poland's Accession Negotiations to the EU at Chancellery of the Prime Minister of the Republic of Poland 2001b). Poland agreed to change the title "doctor of dentistry" (lekarz stomatolog) to "dentist" (lekarz dentysta) following EU confirmation that training programmes for Polish dentists comply with *acquis communautaire* (on the basis of additional information supplied by Poland). The same condition concerns the right to use the title dentist and to practise the profession by those who have or will acquire qualifications with the title "doctor of dentistry". The change of title will affect people starting university education after the adoption of this solution.

Nurses and midwives

Training programmes for nurses and midwives in Poland were not consistent with Community standards as they required fewer hours of study. A new training programme for nurses that conforms to Community standards has been introduced gradually in Poland. Most of the relevant amendments to the Act on the Professions of Nurse and Midwife (1996) have been in force since March 2001, except for the regulations concerning accreditation, which have been in force since January 2002. Regulations allowing provision of services by nurses and midwives from other Member States come into force following Poland's accession.

Two major areas were addressed in the amendment. First, nationals of Member States are permitted to work as nurses or midwives in Poland, with specific conditions that should be fulfilled depending on whether registration is to be temporary or permanent. Second, the amendment implemented the new training system for nurses and midwives, corresponding with EU standards and Directives.

On accession, citizens of other Member States wishing to work as nurses and midwives in Poland must produce documents confirming the right to pursue these professions in another Member State; the Ministry of Health will publish the list of required certificates. An additional requirement will be proficiency in the Polish language to a level necessary to provide services; the Ministry of Health will set standards of Polish language proficiency in a separate amendment. The registration procedure in the Chamber of Nurses must take no longer than three months. A nurse or midwife wishing to provide services temporarily is obliged to inform a relevant Chamber of Nurses and submit the required certificates showing the right to practise in a Member State.

The regulations requiring two years' experience before setting up in independent practice were removed for EU nationals. Nurses or midwives from Member States who satisfy the above requirements will acquire full rights to practise the profession within the Polish health care system.

The EU Directives require training programmes for nurses to include 4600 hours of study. The Polish training system has been transformed to require three years (equal to 4600 hours) of higher education for nurses (Bachelor) with possible extension to five years (Masters Degree). The previous education system for nurses and midwives was based on a five year vocational training course, which began after primary school or two to three years vocational training after secondary school. The amendment contains detailed guidelines on the organization of the training system for nurses and midwives. All these changes were implemented as part of a general reform of the education system in Poland. The amendment will allow automatic recognition of nurses' and midwives' diplomas.

During Poland's efforts to harmonize nurses' and midwives' training systems with the *acquis communautaire* and WHO recommendations, the following key actions have been carried out:

- Parliament adopts Act on Professional Self-Government (1991) and Act on Professions of Nurse and Midwife (1996), both regulating matters relating to the training, practice and supervision of these professions;
- 1998: Collegium Medicum of Jagiellonian University, Cracow, begins training nurses at Bachelor level (licencjat);
- 1999–2000: minimum programme requirements for nursing education at Bachelors and Masters level developed and approved by the Higher Education Council;
- February 2001: amendment to Act on Professions of Nurse and Midwife signed;
- 2001: Ministry of Health develops "programme of transformation of nurses' and midwives' education system for 2001–2005" – national strategy with detailed plan of action;
- October 2001: Ministry of Health appoints National Accreditation Council of Medical Education (responsible for accreditation procedures of schools with training programmes for nurses and midwives);
- Since the academic year 2001/02, all Medical Academies and some Higher Vocational Schools have been offering a Bachelors degree in nursing and midwifery. Recruitment to vocational schools will cease in 2003/04.

Higher education for nurses will be expanded by incremental growth of new university departments. At the same time, vocational schools will progressively be closed. The facilities of these schools and their staff will be absorbed into the new system and used as the basis for Bachelor and Masters training. The Ministry of Health has guaranteed financial and organizational support to these new departments in Medical Academies. As of 16 April 2003 new requirements for recognizing nursing qualifications in Poland were implemented within the framework of the Accession Treaty. A Bachelor of Nursing qualification requires training for three consecutive years during the five years prior to the date of issue of the certificate. This model of training only began in 2001 so the numbers involved are still small. A nursing qualification based on post-secondary non-university education requires training for at least five consecutive years during the seven years prior to the date of issue of the certificate. 2003/2004 is the last year of recruitment to post-secondary medical schools. Similar requirements apply for midwives.

By 2005 the Government envisages the establishment of 40 training programmes for nurses and midwives. However, some projections indicate that the Polish health care system will need an annual inflow of 10 000 to 17 000 nurses until 2010, implying a need for around 60 programmes, on the basis of current scales of provision (Kadalska 2001).

Pharmacists

Training programmes for Polish pharmacists' generally conform to the relevant Community standards. However, the present requirement of one year internships for graduates of pharmacy departments in Poland will be lifted. Accordingly, graduates of pharmacy departments will be able to practise independently upon graduation.

The Act on the Chambers of Pharmacists (1991) does not technically belong to the group of legal acts adjusting Polish law to the *acquis communautaire*. However, its amendment includes regulations dealing with the professional responsibilities of pharmacists. In that sense it corresponds with Article 9 of Directive 85/433/EWG, which says that the Polish Chamber of Pharmacists can provide information about disciplinary measures against a pharmacist to the relevant authorities in another EU Member State where appropriate (Banasinski 2001).

The Council of Ministers adopted the project on the Act on the Profession of Pharmacist on 23 May 2001. The Act complies with relevant EU Directives and covers the following areas:

- qualifications and education necessary to exercise the profession;
- conditions and regulations for acquiring the right to exercise the profession;
- conditions to be fulfilled to establish individual pharmaceutical practice;
- activities performed while exercising the profession.

It should be emphasized that in Polish legislation the scope of activities performed while practising as a pharmacist is broader than that defined in Article 1 of Directive 85/432/EWG (European Integration Committee Office – UKIE 2001).

The main goal of the project is to enable equivalence of qualifications of pharmacists in Poland and the rest of the EU. According to requirements included in Directive 85/432/EWG, the condition for recognition of the diploma is a minimum of six months' training in a pharmacy. This requirement was incorporated in the project adopted by the Polish Government. Accordingly, a pharmacist in Poland would hold either a Masters degree in Pharmacy from Poland (with minimum of six months' training in a pharmacy, unless included in the university curricula) or a degree in pharmacy acquired in a Member State. The Ministry of Health is required to provide the list of documents and certificates that are acceptable as evidence of the latter. Moreover, pharmacists from Member States will have the right to use titles acquired in these States in the language where the diploma was issued, even if these could be confused with other titles, which in Poland require additional training. The Ministry of Health will announce the catalogue of titles and university degrees that will be accepted in Poland (from Polish or EU citizens).

As well as relevant education and qualifications, EU citizens applying for the right to practise as pharmacists in Poland are obliged to declare that they can use the Polish language (spoken and written) to the extent necessary to provide services. Levels of Polish language proficiency will be set out in a separate amendment. Regulations concerning the obligation to take up professional activities within five years of acquiring the right to practise do not apply to EU citizens.

In summary, the project on the Act on the Profession of Pharmacist approved by the Polish Government on 23 May 2001 entirely corresponds with relevant *acquis* (Saryusz-Wolski 2001). The project was adopted by Parliament at the end of 2002. A subsequent Act on Chambers of Pharmacists was published in July 2002. All regulations concerning EU citizens will enter into force on Poland's accession to the EU.

After accession

Labour market and enlargement

The future implications of accession for health professionals may be considered as part of wider changes in the labour market in both the EU and Poland. Transition periods aim to ensure a gradual introduction of free movement of workers but without excessive delay while at the same time providing sufficient guarantees for Member States. Although transitional agreements were settled, it is worth mentioning previous experiences of migration of workforces following earlier enlargements.

Very modest migration flows were recorded after the Spanish and Portuguese accessions (European Commission 2001a). In 1991 the Council examined the effects of the transition period, on the basis of a Commission report and found that the achievement of free movement was not likely to damage the various national labour markets. Consequently the Council decided to shorten the transition period. A recent analysis (EUROSTAT 2000) concludes that there has been no clear, common or consistent relationship between changing patterns of population and workforces attributable to the accession of Greece, Spain or Portugal. Although predicting labour flows is not straightforward, research suggests that the freedom of movement of workers after further enlargement should have limited impacts on the EU labour market (European Commission 2001a). One of the more detailed studies produced for the Commission by a consortium of EU research institutes (Brücker and Boeri 2000) seems to confirm that the overall impact on the European labour market should be limited, both negatively and positively. Enlargement should not affect wages and employment significantly. However, it is important to note that, according to this study, labour migration would be concentrated in a few Member States only.

Nevertheless, there are still concerns about the impact of free movement based on considerations such as geographical proximity, income differentials, unemployment rates and propensity to migrate. As well as geographical differences, sectoral differences may be noteworthy although it is difficult to assess with any certainty such potential differences. Many sectors in both the EU and in candidate countries will benefit from increased cross-border labour movements, for example, where the supply of certain specialist staff (for example health care or information technology) on the national market cannot meet demand.

Shortages in health care personnel in many EU countries has forced governments and private health care providers to seek additional staff abroad, including candidate countries. In Poland, during the last two years, there have been significant increases in offers of work from abroad, including current Member States. Advertisements have been placed in newspapers, web-services for health professionals, career opportunity sites and distributed by professional bodies of nurses and physicians. In a few cases even the Government was involved. Although there are incomplete statistics of trans-border movement of health care staff in the EU, they seem to be at a relatively low level (see also Chapters 9 and 10). A review of the first ten years of implementation of free movement of persons found that the number of physicians moving abroad was only 0.21% of the overall workforce (Hurvitz 1990).

Advantages and disadvantages of accession

The overall influence of the accession process can be considered in terms of advantages and disadvantages for both Polish and EU health care labour markets. Although health care professionals are a specific group in this market, in most cases they follow the same trends as other groups of well-qualified personnel. In the following paragraphs we will try to analyse what the Polish health care system and health professionals can gain or lose on Poland's accession to the Union, together with the implications for the EU.

Advantages for polish health professionals and health care system

The primary advantage from enlargement arises from the process of accession itself. This forced a review of Polish legislation pertaining to the health professions and brought it up to European standards. Many long-standing issues now have been resolved; the completely new Act on the Profession of Pharmacist is a perfect example.

A major advance is the implementation of a new training system for nurses, which was finalized in an amendment to the Act on the Professions of Nurse and Midwife. Upgrading nurses' education will improve their position in both Polish and EU labour markets. Improved education and qualifications for nurses should lead to improvement in the status of nursing (previously devalued) and encourage new candidates to take up the profession. Furthermore, professional relations between nurses and doctors may be expected to improve as nurses increase their scope of competencies and help to restrict doctors' duties to those where it is necessary to have a medical qualification. Improved skills among nurses and midwives will improve quality of, and accessibility to, health care services.

The process of negotiation has seen an increase of interest in, and knowledge of, other health care systems, especially among physicians. The prospect of working legally in other Member States may be seen as the key benefit of free movement of workers and mutual recognition of qualifications. Equal status in the labour market, once the transitional period has ended, presents new opportunities for Polish nurses and doctors interested in working abroad.

Improvements in qualifications, work experience and economic status could be beneficial for individual Polish health professionals and have long-term advantages for the Polish health care system. Those who choose to work abroad temporarily and return to Poland could act as conduits for the transfer of increased knowledge and new technologies. These new skills could enhance the development and modernization of the health sector in Poland; in the long term it will strengthen the health care system. Recent evidence suggests that potential migrants prefer short-term, temporary work to permanent emigration.

The possible inflow of EU health professionals may generate increased competition in the provision of health services. This could benefit the Polish health care system through quality improvement.

Advantages for the European Union

The provision of highly qualified professionals, especially in areas with significant shortages, might be seen as an important advantage for EU countries. Nurses and doctors with compatible diplomas and proficiency in foreign languages (but where the host country has not had to pay for the education) will be sought after workers in European health systems. Some Member States may be tempted to change their training policies by restricting medical training, relying on trained personnel from abroad.

There are shortages of health care staff in many EU countries, in particular the United Kingdom and Sweden, many international posts are offered in the Polish media and through professional bodies. For instance, one of the regional Chambers of Nurses and Midwives (Dolnośląska) has been engaged in the process of helping nurses to seek jobs abroad. The Chamber received offers from Italy (palliative care nurses) and Germany (operating theatre nurses). National initiatives contribute to such procedures, for example the Swedish preference policy that encourages Polish doctors to practise in Sweden.

Freedom of practice might create another benefit for Member States, especially in border areas such as the Polish–German border. Practices established by Polish doctors are likely to charge lower prices (especially dentists) that may encourage EU citizens to use these services and corresponding cross-border demand by German citizens has already been observed. This could improve access to services for some population groups. Competition in the market for health services may improve quality.

At the horizontal level, the principal advantage is derived from the legalization of employment for Polish citizens in the 15 Member States. This will lead to additional revenue from taxes for national budgets. Moreover, immigrants would increase consumption of goods and services and support local economies (Stepniak 2001).

An additional benefit of workforce migration is the increase in professionally active human resources supporting the EU labour market. Statistical data indicate a likely decrease in the professionally active workforce in the Member States after 2005. Between 2001 and 2010 Poland anticipates an increase in this group, although between 2001 and 2005 the increase will be in the less mobile group (over 45). Thus, there should be no danger of increased migration to EU states at the moment of enlargement in 2004 (Department of International Integration Strategies in Governmental Centre of Strategic Studies 2001). After 2005 there is likely to be an increase in younger groups of professionally active workers – which could supplement shortages in the Member States.

Disadvantages for Polish health professionals and health care system

As mentioned above, the freedoms of movement and practice may result in emigration of health professionals and thus the loss of one of Poland's real assets. This risk of brain drain could be the most important disadvantage of enlargement for the Polish health care system. Moreover, the group of potential emigrants most likely to leave would be the youngest and the best qualified nurses (Box 8.1) and doctors. The last two years has seen increasing interest in international work opportunities among health care staff, taking advantage of existing agreements.[1]

There are some disadvantages for individual professionals working abroad such as taking up positions for which they are overqualified. There are examples of fully qualified nurses working as assistant nurses, or physicians as nurses. However, many countries operate positive initiatives against such discrimination practices, with, for example, the publication of NHS guidelines by the United Kingdom Government concerning the recruitment of nurses and physicians from abroad in 2001 (see Chapter 10).

Another possible disadvantage could be an inflow of doctors from other Member States (Solecka 2001). It could be argued that professionals from states with medical unemployment, with an estimated 200 000 unemployed physicians in the EU, may seek a career in Poland. This, combined with transitional periods (and unequal rights in the labour market) might be perceived as a risk to the Polish health care sector. A new group of professionals would increase competition and could cause difficulties in employment of Polish professionals (Gwiazdowicz 2001). Although this is unlikely, since future shortages of doctors are predicted throughout Europe, it is a particular concern of the National Chamber of Physicians in Poland.

Disadvantages for the European Union

The evidence so far suggests that the impact on the EU labour market of freedom of movement of workers after accession should be limited. However, EU officials expect the predicted labour migration to be concentrated in certain Member States, resulting in disturbances of their labour markets. Concerns are based on considerations such as geographical proximity, income differentials, unemployment and propensity to migrate (European Commission 2002a).

One concern is that Polish migrants might take jobs from citizens in the current Member States. Usually the positions offered to workers from abroad are those that have not been accepted by home citizens (Ciechomska 2001). A high

Box 8.1 Enlargement and the nurse profession in Poland (Department of Science and Medical Staff at Ministry of Health 2001)

Recent data (1999) show that Poland has about 200 000 active nurses and midwives (public and private sectors); a further 15 000 are registered as unemployed. Data on nurses who have changed profession due to unemployment or any other reason are not available but may be estimated at 10–20% of the active nursing population (Department of Science and Medical Staff at Ministry of Health (2001)). These numbers relate to registered, fully qualified nurses. Poland ceased training assistant nurses long ago (assistant nurses account for less than 1% of the total nurse population). Along with the changes in nurse training, preparations have begun for the introduction of a new profession of auxiliary nurse. Implementation of education for auxiliary nurses is planned for 2004.

Analysis of quantitative indicators concerning nurses and midwives indicates that Poland does not have an excessive number of nurses. There has been a decline in both the overall number of nurses (55.1 per 10 000 population in 1998, 51.0 in 1999) and in the number of candidates for nursing schools (reducing the supply of new human resources). In combination with increasing demand for nursing services (for example an ageing society) within the next few years it is likely that Poland will join most other European countries in facing a shortage of nursing personnel.

Nurse unemployment in recent years has been due to economic problems, a consequence of the health care reform process and difficulties in general public finances, rather than an excess of nurses. Difficult financial conditions in health care facilities have meant that payment and conditions of nurses are unsatisfactory and extremely low compared to other professions. Moreover, the disproportion between health sector wages and costs for accommodation make migration impossible inside the country. Unemployment is worsening in rural areas and small towns at a time of shortages in urban areas.

These factors may pose incentives for the best-educated and qualified (especially young) nurses to seek other career opportunities. Professionally active nurses have various options such as enrolling for another university degree, that is change profession, improving proficiency in foreign languages with the prospect of seeking a job abroad or taking up formal and legal procedures required to obtain a licence to practise abroad (about 1000 nurses/midwives during 2001). It is difficult to assess how many nurses who apply to seek professional careers abroad will do so. This will be influenced by two factors, first, the pace of further structural changes to the Polish health care system and related strengthening of nurses' position within the system and, second, job opportunities in EU Member States.

level of unemployment in the country of origin (high in Poland – 16.1% in 2000) can push migration. Equally, high levels of unemployment in the destination country can also have a strong effect, deterring work-seeking immigration. The current unemployment rate in Poland is comparable with that in some Member States (for example Spain – 14.1% in 2000). Furthermore, even where there are high levels of unemployment, labour shortages in specific sectors may exert a pull on labour migrants with the right skills. This may be the case for qualified health care professionals. Another concern is the effect on wage levels. The legal migrant's willingness to accept a lower wage is of limited importance in the regulated EU labour market as labour agreements tend to protect the social *acquis* from downward adjustments. In many EU countries there are national pay-rates for health care professions (for example the United Kingdom). Migrants have to take account of often higher costs of living. Highly skilled staff hoping to offset the costs of migration would be very unlikely to accept a lower than average wage.

Summary

The recent changes in Polish legislation on regulated health professions allowed Poland to close negotiations on the chapter "free movement of persons". As discussed above, the advantages and disadvantages of enlargement for both Poland and present Member States are linked mainly to the potential increase in mobility of health care staff following accession. However, a large scale inflow of labour is modified by barriers to migration. Major factors that would discourage movements of labour include migration costs, cultural and linguistic barriers, expectations and lack of information.

Migration costs (social and economic) are very important since the wages of health care personnel are critically low (Table 8.3). Box 8.1 illustrates how nurses' mobility can be very restricted even within the country, not to mention internationally. Migration abroad is an investment that not many nurses can afford. Apart from foreign language training and travel costs, there are the costs of adaptation to a foreign country. Moreover, low wages often lead to reliance on the financial support of a spouse whose chosen career could be a major barrier to migration, or possibly permit only temporary migration alone. The risk of reduced professional status may also be a discouragement. A well-qualified, experienced physician with foreign language proficiency would probably not accept a lower grade; a high status operating theatre nurse would probably not wish to work as an assistant nurse. It must be remembered that, especially in the health sector, one's place in the hierarchy is important for highly qualified staff who have invested much into education and qualifications.

Often those who have the money to do so are those who tend to migrate. Some might argue that health care staff would like to improve their economic status but formal and informal payments that are widespread in Poland can combine to give a decent salary that does not encourage migration (Box 8.2). The question is whether it is worth exchanging the familiar (with the benefits of informal payments) for the job abroad without these bonuses and in totally new surroundings (legal, economic, social and so on). After detailed calculation of the costs it may be that few will decide to do so.

Socio-psychological and cultural factors play a major role in the decision to work abroad, especially for a longer period. The need to learn a foreign language usually is a great obstacle for many people, although crucial to the provision of health services. Even within Poland where linguistic and cultural differences do not exist labour mobility is relatively low. Optimistic economic expectations in the potential migrant's own country also reduce the propensity to migrate.

Table 8.3 Selected payments among health care staff in Poland (2000)

Position and working experience	Elements included in the payment	Salary (gross) in Polish currency (zloty)	in Euro
Physician without speciality, 4 years' experience, outpatient clinic	salary	850	236
Physician with speciality, 10 years' experience, PhD, city hospital	salary; additional bonuses for PhD and working experience	1130	315
Physician with speciality in dermatology, deputy director of city hospital department; 35 years' experience	salary; bonus for experience	1300	362
Surgeon with speciality, 10 years' experience, emergency medicine course	salary; shifts in emergency room	2400	668
Physician, PhD, speciality, director of hospital department	salary; shifts; outside consultations; private practice	4700	1309
Nurse, intensive care unit, city hospital, course in anaesthetics, 8 years' experience	salary	820	228
Nurse, 10 years' experience, city hospital	salary, night shifts	930	259
Midwife, 20 years' experience, outpatient clinic	salary	1150	320
Nurse in ambulance team; 20 years' experience	salary; night shifts	1440	401
Nurse in private clinic in one of the biggest cities; 10 years' experience	salary	2500	696

Source: Gazeta Wyborcza – Lista plac sluzby zdrowia – 2000

Accession itself, or the prospect of it, may have an important influence on expectations. EU accession-induced growth prospects in Spain and Portugal are sometimes cited as one reason for low emigration. Health care reform continues and the Polish government is working to improve the position of health care staff in the labour market, for example through the creation of new opportunities in the health care market such as self-employment or the creation of over 100 palliative care units in 2001. Recent international investment in health care also may support the development of the sector. Migration of pharmacists is least likely because of the development of a successful pharmaceutical market in Poland. Pharmacists are the only group permitted to own and run pharmacies, and there have been many investments in services. Dentists also are unlikely to

Box 8.2   Health care staff income – formal and informal payments

Incomes in the public health sector are fairly low in comparison to the national average, with the average salary being approximately 2050 zloty (€570) (2001). Due to the diversity of salaries in the health sector (there are no fixed payments) this average can be compared with some of salaries in the health sector, as shown in Table 8.3.

Historically, wages for health sector workers in the former communist countries were lower than average and this has remained the case in Poland. However, the increase in informal "envelope" payments may have offset the salary drop for some. Doctors in particular now aspire to salary levels closer to their western European counterparts (Karski and Koronkiewicz 2000). Informal payments pervade the Polish medical and health care system and range from small gifts *ex post*, through "speed money" for faster treatment, to extortion of large bribes on an informally established tariff for surgery and other treatments (World Bank 1999).

Informal payments might be considered as a form of systemic corruption. A report on corruption in public health care issued in Warsaw seems to confirm this assumption (Kubiak 2001). However, the report stresses that neither patients nor doctors perceive informal payments as bribes, but rather as expressions of gratitude for treatment. More than 80% of doctors deny receiving money from patients; those who confirmed taking "an envelope" perceived it as an expression of gratitude. There seems to be less rigidity towards presents; almost 70% admitted to receiving presents from patients. A majority of these consider presents as thanks for their service.

The average informal payment reported by patients interviewed in the survey was 500 zloty (€139); over 10% reported higher payments. Although the underlying reason for accepting informal payments may be a low salary, the report showed that the majority of staff involved belonged to the higher salaried groups, such as directors of hospital departments (63%), experienced physicians (31%) and directors of hospitals (24%). Nurses and less experienced physicians were mentioned less often (14% and 9% respectively). Moreover, as long as there are patients willing to give money in gratitude there will be staff willing to take it. Among respondents who have visited a doctor during the last year, over 40% admitted to giving an informal payment; among respondents who had been hospital patients during the last ten years (four times and more) over 53% admitted doing so.

Informal payments are present in the majority of central and eastern European countries (Lewis 2000); discussion continues on the possible solution. Nevertheless all economic solutions might miss the point, which is the patient giving "the envelope". In the report over 25% of respondents do not agree that co-payment will eliminate the problem of informal payments.

If the average informal payment was added to the formal salary it would (usually) double. Although unofficial, they must be considered as additional sources of revenue for health care staff. As mentioned before, not all professionals benefit from these informal payments; usually the least paid professions (nurses, young doctors) receive little or nothing and have few opportunities to find another source of revenue such as private practice. The nurse with children cannot easily work night shifts. Therefore, the situation of health care staff varies with their position, power and practice setting (urban rural areas, public/private facilities). There are well-paid doctors and nurses but the majority have salaries below the national average.

emigrate for economic reasons. Most dentists work in private practices with higher economic status than the average physician.

Lack of clear information about the procedures for professional registration might discourage potential migrants (Box 8.3). Although long advocated there are no official sources of information for professionals wishing to work in other Member States. Lack of information combined with bureaucratic barriers may discourage even the most desperate candidates; in Greece, nurses who wish to practise must pay for and pass complicated exams.

Finally, although many health professionals may declare a wish to work abroad, intention and action can differ considerably. Most people can see opportunities but are too risk-averse to pursue them. The Polish borders have been open for more than a decade and there are not many convincing

---

Box 8.3   Are there problems with following the *acquis communautaire* on health professions in the Member States?

There are many requirements to be fulfilled by candidate countries. However, there are also problems regarding the implementation of the *acquis communautaire* concerning health professionals and EU legislation among current Member States (European Commission 2002b), for example:

- Austria – The Commission questioned Austria's compliance with the EU Directives on dentists and other medical professions as it demands additional internships or training before recognition of qualifications.
- Greece – The Commission has decided to refer Greece to the European Court of Justice (ECJ) due to non-conformity with the Directive in its legislation concerning mutual recognition of qualifications.
- Portugal – Reasoned Opinion by the Commission stressing that there are mechanisms that hinder the free movement of health professionals. Portugal did not implement the Directive concerning medical speciality diplomas (deadline for implementation passed December 1999).
- France – Reasoned Opinion concerning the non-conformity with Community law in its legislation on the mutual recognition of diplomas and the legislation's application to access to the profession of pharmacist.
- Spain – The Commission has decided to refer Spain to the ECJ because its legislation does not comply with the Directive on the qualification of general nurses, that is minimum training requirements, which is stipulated at 4600 hours. However, Spanish law requires that general nurses train for 3900 hours only. Spain has taken action to bridge the gap but a substantial difference still exists.

However, conformity with the *acquis communautaire* is not the only problem. Some sections of other important directives are hardly followed by any of the Member States, for example Article 20 of Doctor's Directive[2] regarding the establishment of information centres for professionals seeking to work in Member States other than their home countries. This legislation was transferred into Polish legislation although there are hardly any such centres (Belcher 2000). Despite Council suggestions it remains difficult for a migrating specialist to obtain the necessary information (see also Chapter 7).

arguments to support the idea that after enlargement labour migration will suddenly increase. Research conducted after previous accessions appears to reject such sudden increases. Indeed, there is a new phenomenon, professionals returning to Poland after long migration overseas. Physicians who left the country during the "Cold War" are returning to the home country, with some 500 000 persons returning to Poland in the 1990s. However, the true impact of enlargement will be known in the next few years.

Notes

1 In February 2001, the Norwegian and Polish National Labour Offices signed an agreement about cooperation in employing Polish health care staff in Norway. Although not an EU Member State, this is a useful example as it was widely discussed in the media in the context of labour migration of health care staff.
2 Council Directive 93/16/EEC, Article 20.1. Member States shall take necessary measures to enable the persons concerned to obtain information on the health and social security laws, where applicable, on the professional ethics of the host Member State. For this purpose Member States may set up information centres from which such persons may obtain the necessary information.

References

Banasinski, C. (2001) Uzasadnienie dostosowawczego charakteru projektu ustawy o zawodzie farmaceuty z dnia 25 maja 2001 (Argumentation on the EU legislation approximation character of The Act on the Profession of Pharmacist project from 25 May 2001). Warsaw: Urzad Komitetu Integracji Europejskiej. Kncelaria Prezesa Rady Ministrow (European Integration Committee Office, Chancellery of the Prime Ministry of the Republic of Poland).

Belcher, P.J. (2000) Rola Unii Europejskiej w opiece zdrowotnej (The role of the European Union in healthcare). Warsaw: National Centre for Health Information Systems.

Brücker, H. and Boeri, T. (2000) The impact of Easter Enlargement on Employment and Labour Markets in the EU Member States. Commissioned by the Employment and Social Affairs DG of the European Commission. Berlin and Milan: European Integration Consortium.

Ciechomska, G. (2001) Emigracja zarobkowa. Kariera czy harówka? (Labour migration. Career or hard job?), Gazeta Lekarska, (3).

Department of European Integration and International Affairs at Ministry of Health (1999) Informacja dla Sejmowej Komisji Zdrowia – na temat przystosowania polityki zdrowotnej Polski i harmonizacji prawa z zakresu ochrony zdrowia do wymogów Unii Europejskiej (Information note for Parliamentary Health Commission – on adjustment of Polish health policy towards EU requirements and transposition of legislation in the area of healthcare). Warsaw.

Department of International Integration Strategies in Governmental Centre of Strategic Studies (2001) Dostep do Unijnego Rynku Pracy – Obawy i argumenty (Access to European Union labour market – fears and arguments). Warsaw.

Department of Science and Medical Staff at Ministry of Health (2001) Pielegniarstwo w Polsce (Nursery in Poland). Warsaw.

European Commission (2001a) The Free movement of workers in the context of enlargement – Information Note. Brussels.

European Commission (2001b) Regular Report on Poland's Progress Towards Accession. Brussels.

European Commission (2002a) Enlargement and Negotiations. Chapter 2 – Freedom of movement for persons. Brussels.

European Commission (2002b) Free Movement of People and Individual Rights – Infringements. Brussels.

European Integration Committee Office – UKIE (2001) Bilans dzialan negocjacyjnych 2000–2001 (Balance of negotiation actions 2000–2001). Warsaw.

EUROSTAT (2000) Patterns and trends in International Migration in Western Europe Eurostat Studies and Research. Luxembourg.

Fortuna, A. (2001) Wymogi Unii Europejskiej u stomatologów (European Union requirements for dentists), *Gazeta Lekarska*, (1).

Government Plenipotentiary for Poland's Accession Negotiations to the EU at Chancellery of the Prime Minister of the Republic of Poland (2000) *Poland's negotiation position on chapter "Free movement of persons"*. Warsaw.

Government Plenipotentiary for Poland's Accession Negotiations to the EU at Chancellery of the Prime Minister of the Republic of Poland (2001a) *Glosariusz negocjatora (Negotiator's Glossary)*. Warsaw.

Government Plenipotentiary for Poland's Accession Negotiations to the EU at Chancellery of the Prime Minister of the Republic of Poland (2001b) *Zmiana stanowiska negocjacyjnego Polski w obszarze "Swoboda przeplywu osób" przyjeta na podstawie decyzji Rady Ministrów z dnia 15 listopada 2001 oraz 18 grudnia 2001 (The change of Poland's Position Paper in the chapter of "Free movement of persons"* adapted by the Council of Ministers from 15 November 2001 and 18 December 2001). Warsaw.

Gwiazdowicz, E. (2001) Nowa ustawa dla Europy (The new legislation act for Europe), *Gazeta Lekarska*, (6).

Hurvitz, L. (1990) *The free circulation of physicians within the European Communities*. Aldershot: Avebury.

Kadalska, E. (2001) Regulacje prawne zawodu pielegniarki i poloznej w swietle dyrektyw Unii Europejskiej (Legal regulations on the professions of nurse and midwife with reference to European Union directives), *Zdrowie i Zarzadzanie*, III(5): 8–14.

Karski, B. and Koronkiewicz, A. (2000) *Health care systems in transition: Poland*. Copenhagen: European Observatory on Health Care Systems.

Kubiak, A. (2001) Pacjenci i lekarze o korupcji w publicznej sluzbie zdrowia – Raport z badan (Patients and doctors about corruption in healthcare – the report from survey). Warsaw: Fundacja im. Stefan Batorego, Program przeciw korupcji. 2002.

Lewis, M. (2000) Who is paying for health care in Eastern Europe and Central Asia? Washington, DC: The World Bank.

Saryusz-Wolski, J. (2001) Opinia o zgodnosci projektu ustawy o zawodzie farmaceuty z prawem Unii Europejskiej z dnia 22 maja 2001 (The Opinion on approximation of The Act on the Profession of Pharmacist project to European Union legislation – 22 May, 2001). Warsaw: European Integration Committee.

Solecka, M. (2001) *Sliska sciezka europejska (A slippery European path)*. Rzeczpospolita.

Stepniak, A. (ed.) (2001) *Swobodny przeplyw pracownikow w kontekscie wejscia Polski do Unii Europejskiej (Free movement of workers in the context of Poland's membership in the European Union)*. Warszawa: Government plenipotentiary for Poland's accession negotiations to the European Union, Chancellery of the Prime Minister of the Republic of Poland.

World Bank (1999) *Corruption in Poland: Review of priority areas and proposal for action*. Warsaw.

World Bank (2001) *The World Bank Country Study – Poland's Labour Market – the challenge of job creation*. World Bank.

Zaborowski, P. and Rebandel, H. (2001) Sytuacja stanu lekarskiego w Polsce. Próba analizy demograficznej (The profession of physician in Poland. Demographic analysis approach), *Gazeta Lekarska*, (4).

chapter nine

The market for physicians

Elke Jakubowski and Rainer Hess

Introduction

As shown in Chapter 7, physicians and other health professionals who are citizens of the EU and meet certain criteria can register to practise in every EU Member State. This policy also applies to other countries in the European Economic Area (Norway, Iceland and Liechtenstein). Thus, at a formal level there is mutual recognition of diplomas, certificates and other evidence of qualifications enabling the free movement of physicians across EU borders. Yet there is limited information on the actual scale of movement of physicians within the existing 15 Member States of the EU, making it difficult to predict what may be expected after the current round of enlargement.

At the same time, there is growing public, professional and political interest in cross-border movement of physicians and other health professionals. For example, national workforce planners in Member States may wish to make allowances for conditions in labour markets in the EU when developing national workforce plans. Politicians, professionals and the public may be concerned about access to and quality of care, for example where the scale of migration might impact on the ability to deliver health care or where migrating health professionals are not considered to possess equivalent professional qualifications. Countries that are net donors of health professionals may be concerned about the use of national resources spent on training professionals who will no longer contribute to the national health system. This "brain-drain" may also impact on health care provision in the country that is loosing them. Health professionals and health administrators will be interested in the opportunities arising from greater mobility of persons and services within the EU, such as new job opportunities and a wider pool of human resources for health care, as well as its risks, for example downward pressure on wages.

Labour markets for health professionals in Member States are affected by trends in demography, economics, social norms and alternative sources of employment. These must be taken into account in speculating how the process of enlargement will affect cross-border movement of health professionals and consequently provision of health care in the future. Several factors suggest that there is likely to be a growing demand for physicians in the next few decades. First, in the current 15 Members States those of working age will increase steadily as a proportion of the overall population until 2011 and will then drastically decline as the post-war "baby-boom" moves into retirement (Jennet 2001). This will have consequences for the medical workforce, which is also ageing. For example, a study of German physicians in independent practice, undertaken in 2001 by the Federal Association of Social Health Insurance Physicians (*Kassenärztliche Bundesvereinigung*, or KBV) reported that, between 1995 and 2000, the proportion of physicians aged over 59 years increased by 40% and the proportion of those under 35 declined from 27.4% in 1991 to 18.8% in 2000 (Kopetsch 2002).

Second, an ageing population can be expected to place new demands on health care provision and consequently on the number of physicians and other health professionals needed. A major factor will be increasing survival with chronic diseases, especially in candidate countries where life expectancy has risen markedly in the past decade.

Third, the proportion of female physicians has been increasing steadily, especially in the countries of western Europe where the medical profession has traditionally been predominantly male (Figure 9.1). Unless there are substantial changes in gender roles within families, this is almost certain to lead to a reduction in the number of hours worked by physicians over the course of their careers, reflecting greater use of part-time working and career breaks by female physicians.

Fourth, although the numbers of physicians leaving medicine has been stable over recent decades (Bundesanstalt für Arbeit 2002; Goldacre et al. 2002), there

Figure 9.1 Proportion of female physicians: 1985–1998

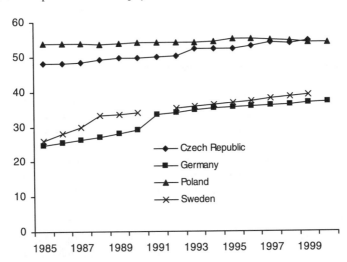

Source: OECD health database 2002

are concerns that this may not be the case in the future, as younger physicians make different choices about work–leisure balance. This is examined for Germany below.

Fifth, European hospitals will face major changes as a consequence of the application of the Working Time Directive to doctors in training in 2004, with a transition period of five years (with the possibility, in some circumstances, of being extended by two to three years). Earlier assumptions about the impact of this measure have been overturned by the ruling of the European Court of Justice in the SIMAP case that time spent on-call in hospitals would count as working time. After 1 August 2004 average weekly working hours will be limited to 58 hours in the first three years, reducing to 56 hours and then to 52 hours, finally falling to 48 hours when the Directive is fully implemented. Additional requirements relate to the length of shifts and rest periods. However, the European Commission, in January 2004, began to pave the way for a liberalisation of the Working Time Directive so that Member States would be allowed to revert to more flexible arrangements for working times of physicians and others employed in the public sector.

It is widely believed that these changes will have profound implications for the pattern of hospital services. If current work profiles were to be maintained many more physicians would be required. German trade unions have called for the recruitment of a minimum of 15 000 additional doctors (Bundesanstalt für Arbeit 2002). In practice, the Directive will force the implementation of new methods of working, with many tasks traditionally undertaken by physicians being done by other health professionals. Nonetheless, the consequences will be considerable.

One response to these growing demands will, as in the past, be to import physicians from other countries. Inevitably one source will be the candidate countries, in particular the countries of central and eastern Europe. This chapter explores the possible consequences of these changes, focusing on the potential for movement between two candidate countries, Poland and the Czech Republic, and certain EU Member States, in particular Germany but also other northern European countries.

Scale and determinants of physician migration

As noted earlier, mutual recognition of medical qualifications already applies throughout the European Economic Area. On accession to the EU this will extend to the candidate countries. Member States are not allowed to demand additional evidence of ability to practise from migrant physicians. Each physician wishing to practise in another EEA country must register in the country of destination. There is no centralized system of registration, so each migrant physician must undergo a registration procedure that is unique to each Member State (Klemperer 1996).

As noted in Chapter 7, migration is driven by several factors, such as the absorptive capacity of labour markets in the countries of destination, employment rates in both countries of origin and destination, the transaction costs borne by migrants and by differences in national characteristics such as language, culture differences and standard of living. Taken as a whole, there is a widespread consensus that most movement is likely to be from east to west rather than the other way round. The following sections will examine in more detail aspects of the labour market and income differentials as possible driving forces behind migration.

Absorptive capacities of countries of destination

Germany is a country with a relatively high level of health care provision, compared to other industrialized countries. Within the countries that are members of the Organization for Economic Co-operation and Development (OECD), Germany has the fourth highest density of physicians with 355 practising physicians per 100000 inhabitants, following Italy, the Netherlands and Belgium. The density of physicians in Germany is nearly double that in the United Kingdom.

However, in spite of the comparatively high numbers of physicians, recently, German media have increasingly conveyed dramatic warnings about looming shortages of physicians. These have often originated from physicians' organizations but increasingly also from health care administrators. A particular concern relates to the situation in the eastern part of Germany, with some calls for a "green card" for physicians (Bundesanstalt für Arbeit 2002).

In reality, however, the number of physicians practising independently under contracts with the statutory health insurance system has steadily increased until 2001 (Klose et al. 2003), with the year 2001 seeing further increase in the number of active physicians in Germany of 1.1% (Bundesärztekammer 2001). However, this aggregate figure conceals large regional differences with many *Länder* (federal states) in the western part reporting steady increases, for example a 10% growth in physicians working in hospitals in North-Rhine-Westphalia in 2001. However, others such as Berlin and Bremen as well as the eastern Länder Sachsen, Sachsen-Anhalt and Thüringen reported falling numbers. There have also been declining numbers of physicians working independently in Hamburg, Mecklenburg-Vorpommern and Sachsen-Anhalt. These recent developments have caused concern about the ability to deliver comprehensive health care in some of the eastern Länder (Maus 2002).

An important factor is an increase in the number of physicians leaving medicine. A study by the KBV reported that of 11 500 medical students, only 7200 applied for posts as *Arzt im Praktikum* (AIP), which lasts for 18 months following completion of basic medical education and is required for full registration as a physician. Numbers of these junior physicians (AIPs) have declined significantly in nearly all of the eastern Länder in 2001, by 8% in Thüringen to 17.6% in Brandenburg. In addition, the KBV study projected that some specialities will soon experience net losses of independent physicians. These include ophthalmologists from 2004, radiologists from 2005 and general practitioners from 2006 (Kopetsch 2002).

The number entering medical school has remained stable, but the number of graduates is declining as ever more discontinue medical studies (Kopetsch 2002). It has been suggested that this reflects various factors. They include reduced prestige of medicine as a career (Maus 2002), a growth in administrative workload, unwillingness to work long hours, over-hierarchical structures and increasing financial risks facing those setting up private practices (Bundesanstalt für Arbeit 2002; Flintrop 2002). As a consequence several Länder are reporting substantial increases in vacancies for junior house officers (*Assistenzärzte*), including Bremen (+39%), Saarland (+35%) and Sachsen (+24%) (Bundesanstalt für Arbeit 2002). Vacancies for specialists have increased countrywide, with the number of posts advertised in the *Deutsche Ärzteblatt* ("German Physician Journal", published jointly by the Federal Physicians' Chamber and the KBV) in 2001 being twice the number advertised in 1997. Finally, as noted earlier, the Working Time Directive is likely to have a profound effect on demand for physicians in German hospitals.

In summary, although Germany has traditionally had a high physician:population ratio it is likely that it will increasingly seek to recruit physicians from other parts of Europe to maintain the current levels of supply. This may have important consequences for some candidate countries, in particular those where German is widely spoken.

Future demand for physicians will not be confined to Germany, however. As was noted in Chapter 7, the United Kingdom, long an active importer of physicians, is seeking to recruit even more. Similarly the Nordic countries, with traditionally low numbers of physicians are becoming active recruiters. This is particularly true of Norway. During the 1980s it has experienced a continuous shortage of physicians while its neighbours have had alternating periods of surplus and shortage. Staffing forecasts in the early 1980s underestimated future growth in health care provision. In the mid-1990s Norway actively recruited foreign physicians, increasing its numbers sharply but it continues to face shortages in many specialities, including radiology, anaesthetics, surgery, internal medicine and psychiatry.

In the mid-1990s, Sweden experienced a temporary oversupply of physicians, owing to steep increases in training between 1980 and 1987. The rate of growth has since slowed and Sweden has begun to recruit physicians from abroad. The Swedish Medical Association and the National Board of Health and Welfare have recently published a guide for physicians wishing to work in Sweden (*http://www.ronden.se/slf/*). The Swedish Medical Association also has an action programme to recruit doctors from the outside the EU/EEA area (Swedish Medical Association 2001). The greatest demand is for those with specialist qualifications. Within the Nordic region Iceland remains an exception. It has long had a surplus of physicians who have sought work in other Nordic countries, although their total numbers are small relative to the workforce in the Nordic countries.

Levels of employment in countries of origin

Historically the countries of central and eastern Europe were seen as potential sources of health professionals by western European countries facing shortages. On several occasions western countries had absorbed waves of emigrants, for example from Hungary in 1956 and Czechoslovakia in 1968. Moreover it was known that these countries had a large medical workforce, reflecting the communist policy of training large numbers of doctors. However, by the 1980s, entry to medical schools was reduced reflecting changing priorities. In particular, there was a greater emphasis on banking and industrial sectors to meet the emerging challenges of economic transition. Some countries, such as Slovenia, are now reporting a shortage of physicians.

Income differences

There are few recent comparative data on incomes of health professionals although public sector wages usually correlate well with national income and in this respect differentials between the current Member States and the candidate countries are substantial. However, there are numerous reports that the official incomes of physicians in candidate countries compare poorly with those obtained in other sectors with the exemption of Slovenia, where physicians' average earnings were reported to be 2.5 times the average salary in 2001 (Albreht et al. 2002).

What data exist suggest that incomes of physicians working in Germany and in the Czech Republic may vary by a factor of roughly around five (Table 9.1). However, the disparities become less pronounced when differences in purchasing power are taken into account. Moreover, experience in current Member States suggests that considerable convergence is likely following accession (Boeri and Brückner 2000). For example, in 2000 it was projected that the Polish

Table 9.1 Employment indicators

	Germany	Czech Republic	Poland
Population (million)	82.0	10.3	38.6
Physicians per 100 000 population (1999)	355	308	226
% Physicians working in hospitals (1999)	47.3	25.6	n/a
General practitioners per 100 000 population	102.9 (1998)	68.2	n/a
Specialists per 1000 population (1999)	2.2 (1997)	2.2	1.9
Physicians graduating per 100 000 population	10 (2000)	7.9 (2000)	9.7 (1993)
			8.8 (1996)
Dentists per 100 000 population (1999)	76.2	62.5	34.3
Proportion of female physicians	36% (1997)	54.5%	54%
Net average physician income per year	€45 000–55 000 in ambulatory care (2002)	€3586 (1993) €6924 (1999)	Estimated €4800–6000

Continued

Table 9.1 continued

	Germany	Czech Republic	Poland
Number of registered unemployed doctors	6582 (9/2001)	292 (9/2003)	1200
Unemployment rate of doctors	2.2% (9/2001)	0.8%	1.4%
Retirement age of employed doctors	65 years	60–62 male 57–60 female	65 male 60 female
Restriction to medical school entry	Yes	No	Yes, since 1995
Minimum duration of medical studies	6 years	6 years	6 years
Minimum duration of postgraduate general practice training	4 years	3 years	4 years
Duration of postgraduate specialist training	4–6 years	3–5 years	4–8 years
Special licence needed for self-employment in private practice	No (only if practising under statutory health insurance)	Yes (requires an additional training period of 3 years)	Yes (requires proof of an established private practice facility)
Basic payment method in general practice/specialist self-employment	Fee for service	Fee for service	Capitation/NA (not applicable)
Granting of medical licence	Medical approbation after 1.5 years of postgraduate training	Only after specialization as general practitioner or as specialist	Only after postgraduate training of 1.5 years
Licensing authority	Regional physicians chambers	Physicians chambers	Regional physicians chambers

Sources: WHO European Health for all database 2002; Health Care Systems in Transition profiles (European Observatory on Health Care Systems (Busse 2000a; Busse 2000b; Karski and Koronkiewicz 2000); OECD Data; EUROSTAT; International Labour Organisation)

economy would grow two to three times more quickly than the German economy (Budnikowski 2000). Yet despite much higher rates of growth in the Czech Republic and Poland, the gap with Germany remains substantial.

Differences in other aspects of employment may also be important, such as social security for their families, or enhanced pensions. However, expectations may not always be realistic. There is evidence that, notwithstanding shortages, employment opportunities for migrant physicians compares adversely with their German counterparts: unemployment among migrant physicians in Germany is 12% compared with 2.2% among German trained physicians (Bundesanstalt für Arbeit 2002).

In summary, several factors may be conducive to migration of physicians from Poland and the Czech Republic to Germany. Income is clearly one motive and language may not be a significant barrier because teaching of German is ubiquitous in schools in both countries. In addition, a small, but significant number of physicians in both countries have attended medical schools in Germany or Austria, at least for some time.

Actual and projected cross-border migration in the enlarged European Union

Projections on general labour migration

It is estimated that 850 000 people have already migrated from the countries of central and eastern Europe to western Europe since 1990, of whom some 300 000 are in employment, including temporary and seasonal workers. These figures equate to 0.2% of the EU population and 0.3% of the Member States workforce, respectively. About 80% of these migrants reside in Austria or Germany, with the majority having migrated before 1993. Since 1993 the level of migration to the EU has been negligible as receiving countries have erected new barriers.

It has been suggested that the present round of enlargement will lead to an initial inward migration of about 335 000 people per year, 35% of whom will be seeking employment (Boeri and Brückner 2000). After the first decade it is projected that this figure will fall to 150 000 per year. Germany is expected to receive about 220 000 migrants from the new Member States, assuming stable employment conditions. However, as Table 9.2 shows, other projections by labour market economists wary widely, from 41 000 to 200 000 persons per year.

Assumptions about future migration trends reflect demographic patterns. Thus, the rapid decline in birth rates in Poland from the mid-1980s underlies the estimated fall in the Polish workforce between 15 and 44 years of 570 000 while those aged over 45 will increase by 1.42 million (Budnikowski 2000). As younger workers are more likely to emigrate, this trend may have a substantial impact on migration. It has also been argued that the existence of similar patterns of

Table 9.2 Projections of levels of migration of residents on EU enlargement

Source	Estimated potential number of migrants	Countries included
Deutsches Institut für Wirtschaftsforschung (1997)	680 000 at the time of accession; 340 000 in 2030	Poland, Czech Republic, Hungary, Slovenia, Slovakia
Polish Academy of Science (1998)	771 000 from all CCEE; 380 000 from Poland	Poland
Austrian Academy of Science (1997)	700 000 from all CCEE; 390 000 from Poland	Poland, Czech Republic, Hungary, Slovakia
European Integration Consortium (2000)	335 000–150 000 estimated potential for 10 CCEEs; Migration to Germany: 220 000	10 CCEEs

Source: Budnikowski 2000

employment in Poland and Germany (especially in border regions) will inhibit migration. On the other hand, at least in some sectors of the economy, Poles increasingly face competition from workers recruited from the former Soviet Union as Russians and Ukrainians accept lower wages (Budnikowski 2000). It is as yet not clear whether this phenomenon, exacerbated by illegal employment, is translatable to skilled employment in health care. One pointer can be gained from the experience of the 2001 German green card campaign to recruit people from the countries of central and eastern Europe for the information technology industry. The limited success of this scheme suggests that that labour migration tends to be overestimated.

Migration from and to Germany, and between East and West Germany

Returning to physicians, the number of foreign physicians in independent practice in Germany has increased steadily from 2484 in 1991 to 3390 in 2000 (Figure 9.2 and Figure 9.3). Out of Germany's 350000 physicians, about 5% (15 143 on 1 January 2003) are foreign citizens. Of these, about one-quarter (4187 on 1 January 2003) migrated from another EU country. Most foreign physicians come from the Russian Federation. However, only about 50 per cent of the Russian physicians living in Germany practise their profession. Iran is another country of frequent origin (1478 on 1 January 2003), followed by Greece (1014 on 1 January 2003). The KBV estimates that about 2000 physicians from the current candidate countries have migrated to Germany in recent years, although not all eventually practise their medical profession. In January 2003, 2041 foreign physicians from EU Member States practised in German hospitals, and 1183 physicians practised as free practising physicians in ambulatory care. The proportion of foreign physicians in independent practice from a non-EU country is significantly lower (less than 30%). This difference reflects the more

Figure 9.2   Number of foreign physicians in independent social health insurance practice in Germany 1991–2001

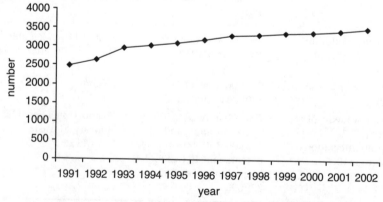

Source: Statistisches Bundesamt, online (*http://www.destatis.de/themen/d/thm_gesundheit.htm*)

Figure 9.3 Number of foreign physicians working in German hospitals 1991–2001

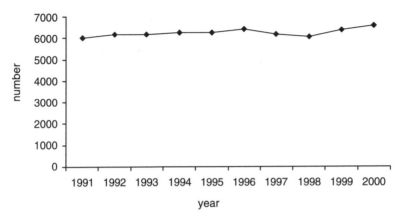

Source: Statistisches Bundesamt, online (*http://www.destatis.de/themen/d/thm_gesundheit.htm*)

restricted procedure for licensing physicians for free practice under contract with the statutory health insurance system for physicians from non-EU countries. In reality, licences to practise will only be granted to physicians from non-EU countries in special circumstances, for example when undersupply of ambulatory care services has been proven. In these cases, physicians can be granted temporary licences to practise.

The number of physicians moving from Germany to central and eastern European countries, other than those working short-term in international donor projects, is negligible. In contrast, there have been significant flows from Germany to other EU countries. For example, from 1997 to 2001, Norway recruited 268 German general practitioners, 101 specialists and 19 dentists. Over the same period 100 German physicians were recruited in Sweden. In 2002, more than 2000 German physicians worked in the United Kingdom NHS (Bundesanstalt für Arbeit 2002). France has recently begun to recruit specialist physicians from Germany, with particular demand for anaesthetists, surgeons, gynaecologists and emergency medicine specialists. The Netherlands is recruiting German physicians for work in occupational health, social care homes and work in health insurance funds. Interestingly, these roles do not exist to the same extent in Germany. Ireland is recruiting German physicians specializing in anaesthetics and emergency medicine, especially for private hospitals. In this area the Irish authorities are working with the German Central Office for Labour (*Zentralstelle für Arbeitsvermittlung*) and an Irish private recruitment company (Kelly 2002).

Movement has also taken place within Germany, between the former eastern and western parts after unification. This has been attributed to the lower incomes of physicians both in hospitals and in private practice in the east of Germany: salaries of physicians working in hospitals in eastern Länder earn still only about 75 per cent of levels in the western Länder. The scale of movement from the east to the west has been substantial whereas migration of physicians from west to east has been largely limited to top-level positions in academic hospitals. An analysis of personnel registries and other publications between 1990 and 1997 in the eastern Länder showed that of 815 university chairs in university hospitals (C4 professorships), 183 were filled by physicians from the western part. Of these, only 67 held the academic title *Privatdozent*, which is usually an obligatory prerequisite for such positions in the west. In contrast, of the 575 physicians obtaining the title *Privatdozent* in the eastern part of the country, only 14 were nominated for top-level positions in medical institutions. This suggests that, in the unification process physicians from the west were privileged over those from the east.

Migration between EU Member States

As noted in Chapter 7, the United Kingdom has long been a major importer of physicians. Its efforts to attract physicians from abroad is likely to increase over the next decade at a time when general practitioner numbers would otherwise fall markedly because of the imminent retirement of many who came from the Indian subcontinent in the 1960s. The NHS plan envisages that, to achieve these targets, it will be necessary to recruit physicians from abroad, in particular from other EU countries. An international recruitment programme has been established and, since 2001 the United Kingdom has increasingly advertised internationally for physicians. The British media report that this has led to criticism by several Member States including Austria, Germany, Greece, Italy and Spain and also in some candidate countries such as Bulgaria, Czech Republic and Poland, as well as in countries elsewhere in the world (Deutsches Aerzteblatt 2002). Under pressure from some overseas governments, such as South Africa, the English Department of Health has undertaken not to recruit from certain developing countries facing shortages of physicians, although there are many examples of individual hospitals disregarding this agreement. However, despite these efforts, the number of physicians from the European Economic Area registering in the United Kingdom declined by 45% between 1996 and 2000, with the number of German physicians registering declining from 950 in 1996 to 340 in 2000 (Jennet 2001).

Large mobility between the Nordic countries is partly attributed to the similarity of the languages and a shared culture (Skoglund and Taraldset 2000). However, as noted earlier, each country is now recruiting from outside the region.[1] In early 2002 Sweden initiated a recruitment campaign in Poland, leading to the employment of 30 Polish physicians.

Predicting future trends

Freedom of movement of people within an enlarged EU will inevitably lead to changes in patterns of migration of physicians. Classical economic theory predicts that integration of economies will provide gains for all of the countries involved, although the gains and losses may not be distributed unevenly within each country (Boeri and Brückner 2000). In reality it is unlikely that countries will benefit to the same degree from enlargement, so placing pressures on labour markets and health systems.

Unfortunately, the many factors involved make it difficult to predict what the overall impact of accession will be. It is apparent that many countries in western Europe face shortages of physicians, shortages that will increase in the near future. They also offer relatively high incomes and other employment benefits. Yet it is also apparent that there are many obstacles to migration, so that the long-standing imbalances in supply of and demand for physicians among current Member States have persisted despite the opportunities for physician mobility. On the other hand, the current round of enlargement is quite different from earlier ones in terms of the scale of income differentials. Thus, the one former communist country to have acceded so far, the former German Democratic Republic, has experienced substantial losses of physicians, albeit in the face of unique circumstances.

Much will depend on future economic growth in the candidate countries. Judged by the past decade, there is likely to be continuing convergence, although the history of economic forecasting does not inspire confidence in the power of prediction. On balance, however, it seems unlikely that predictions of massive migration of skilled workers, including physicians, will occur from the candidate countries, although the scale of movement is likely to increase to some extent and it seems likely that there will be selective loss of certain individuals with particular skills.

Note

1 Schweden braucht dich. *Berliner Zeitung*, 17 September 2001; Norwegen wirbt verstärkt um Ärzte aus Deutschland. *Berliner Morgenpost*. 28 February 2001, p. 2.

References

Albreht, T., Cesen, M., Hindle, D. et al. (2002) *Health Care Systems in Transition: Slovenia.* Copenhagen: European Observatory on Health Care Systems.

Boeri, T. and Brückner, H. (2000) European Integration Consortium: DIW, CEPR, FIET, IAS, IGIER: The impact of Eastern Enlargement on Employment and Labour Markets in the EU Member States. Final report.

Budnikowski, T. (2000) Effects in the area of migration, in A. Stepniak (ed.) *Enlargement of the European Union to the East. Consequences for prosperity and employment in Europe.* Warsaw, Government Plenipotentiary for Poland's Accession Negotiations to the European Union.

Bundesanstalt für Arbeit (2002) Zentralstelle für Arbeitsvermittlung (ZAV) Arbeitsmarkt-Informationen für qualifizierte Fach- und Führungskräfte. 3/2002. Bonn: Arbeitsmarktinformation.

Bundesärztekammer (2001) Ärztestatistik der Bundesärztekammer zum 31.12.2001 (www.bundesaerztekammer.de/30/Aerztestatistik/).

Busse, R. (2000a) *Health Care Systems in Transition: Czech Republic.* Copenhagen: European Observatory on Health Care Systems.

Busse, R. (2000b) *Health Care Systems in Transition: Germany.* Copenhagen: European Observatory on Health Care Systems.

Deutsches Aerzteblatt (2002) Ausland. Grossbritannien: 19 Länder protestieren gegen die Abwerbung von Aerzten, *Deutsches Aerzteblatt*, 1 July.

Flintrop, J. (2002) Niederlawung: Zunehmend weniger attraktiv, *Deutsches Aerzteblatt*, 99(3):A-78.

Goldacre, M.J., Lambert, T.W. and Davidson, J.M. (2002) Loss of British-trained doctors from the medical workforce in Great Britain, *Medical Education*, 35(4):337–44.

Jennett, N. (2001) Medical Employment in the EU in 2022. Implications for the UK. Health Trends Review Conference. London: HM Treasury.

Karski, B. and Koronkiewicz, A. (2000) *Health care systems in transition: Poland.* Copenhagen: European Observatory on Health Care Systems.

Kelly, M. (2002) Personal communication with Dr Michael Kelly, State Secretary, Department of Health, Ireland on 21 May 2002, Department of Health.

Klemperer, F. (1996) How to do it: work in the European Union, *British Medical Journal*, 312:567–70.

Klose, J., Uhlemann, T. and Gutschmidt, S. (2003) Ärztemangel – Ärzteschwemme? Auswirkungen der Alterstruktur von Ärzten auf die vertragsärztliche Versorgung. Wissenschaftliches Institut der AOK (WidO 48).

Kopetsch, T. (2002) KBV-Studie zu Arztzahlen: Überaltert und zu wenig Nachwuchs, *Deutsches Ärzteblatt*, 99(9):A-544.

Maus, J. (2002) Neue Bundesländer: hausärztliche Versorgung vor grossen Problemen, *Deutsches Ärzteblatt*, 99(7):A-402.

Skoglund, E. and Taraldset, A. (2000). Legemarkedet i Norden 1980–2000, *Tidsskr Nor Lægeforen*, 120:2030–4.

Swedish Medical Association (2001) Immigrant doctors – a Swedish health care resource (http://www.ronden.se/slf/).

chapter ten

Not from our own backyard? The United Kingdom, Europe and international recruitment of nurses

James Buchan and Anne Marie Rafferty

Introduction

The United Kingdom is a large net importer of health professionals in the EU. As such, conditions in the British labour market have a disproportionate effect on rates of migration from other countries. It is also the Member State in which migration of health professionals has been studied in most detail.

This chapter examines the connections between the United Kingdom and other EU nursing labour markets, and places these in the broader context of international recruitment of nurses. Specific attention is given to the implications of the accession states becoming part of a pan-Europe labour market for registered nurses.

The chapter has three main objectives:

- to examine trends in inward recruitment of nurses to the United Kingdom;
- to assess, from a United Kingdom perspective, the impact of free mobility of registered nurses within the EU;
- to explore the implications of the accession states entering a single labour market for nurses.

The United Kingdom nursing labour market

The key current feature of the United Kingdom nursing labour market is skill shortages. The United Kingdom Health Department in 2001 acknowledged that "the biggest constraint on the NHS's capacity to deliver was the need to increase the number of staff" (Department of Health 2001a). An official survey in 2001 (Office of Manpower Economics Annual Survey 2001) reported that 78% of NHS employers in England and Wales reported that they had "quite a problem" or a "major problem" in recruiting nurses and midwives, up from 69% in the previous year.

These shortages have occurred as a result of a combination of factors. Some are demographically driven, with increased demand for health care related to an ageing population. More patients are being treated, and patient care has become more "intense", with higher dependency patients requiring more care in a shorter time period. Various supply-side factors, including increased competition from the private sector for skilled nurses, and the ageing of the nursing profession, are also further exacerbating short- and mid-term recruitment difficulties (Buchan and Seccombe 2002).

Most nurses in paid employment in the United Kingdom work in the National Health Service (NHS). In total, there were about 400 000 registered nurses, midwives and health visitors employed by the NHS in the four countries of the United Kingdom in September 2000. Nurses are also employed in primary care, as practice nurses working with general practitioners; in private sector nursing and residential homes, independent hospitals and clinics; in independent hospices; with nursing agencies; and in other public sector services (prison service, defence medical service, higher education, police service, local authorities). Table 10.1 shows the best estimates of the overall number of registered nurses in all types of nursing employment in the United Kingdom, which total approximately 518 670.

Since 1998 the implementation of NHS strategies for nursing and human resources, and NHS modernization plans ("The NHS Plan" (NHS Executive 2000)), have symbolized a fundamental policy shift in the NHS. It is recognized that achieving health gain targets depends, in part, on achieving plans to increase NHS nurse numbers throughout the United Kingdom.

Table 10.1 United Kingdom employment of registered nurses, midwives and health visitors, 2000

	NHS nursing	GP practice nursing	Nursing homes, independent hospitals and clinics	Other	Total
England	256 280	10 710	54 830	n/a	321 280
Scotland	35 600	1 123	4 728	n/a	41 451
Wales	16 920	698	2 410	n/a	20 028
NI	11 500	100	1 425	n/a	13 025
Total (wte)	320 300	12 631	63 393	n/a	395 784
TOTAL (heads)	395 430	21 410	82 330	19 500*	518 670

*estimate

Note: non-NHS data for Northern Ireland is from 1999

Source: Buchan and Seccombe 2002

The NHS Plan targets for nurse staffing growth are based on four areas of intervention:

- attracting more applicants to nurse education;
- encouraging "returners" to nursing employment;
- improving retention through improved career structures and flexible working practices;
- recruiting nurses from other countries.

Government action is underway in the first three areas. All pre-registration nurse education in the United Kingdom is funded and provided in the public sector and the number of nursing and midwifery students has increased significantly in the last three years. Funding has also been allocated to attracting back "returners" – qualified practitioners returning to paid nursing employment after a career break. There has been an increased emphasis on the provision of flexible working hours, action to reduce violence against staff, a commitment to increased funding for lifelong learning (Department of Health 1999b), and plans to introduce a new pay and career structure for nurses and other NHS staff.

The fourth area for intervention, the active recruitment of nurses from other countries, has become a significant element of British policy in recent years. The English Department of Health has been explicit that international recruitment will be part of the solution to meeting its staffing targets: "we shall build on our successes in recruiting staff, particularly nursing staff, from abroad to help us, in the short term at least to deliver the extra staff we need to deliver the NHS Plan" (Department of Health 2001b).

It has set up "a network of international recruitment co-ordinators . . . to speed up the recruitment process" (Department of Health 2001c). This network connects with "NHS Professionals", the nationwide temporary staffing organization recently set up by the NHS in England. The United Kingdom Government has also initiated government to government "concordats" on nurse recruitment with other governments, such as those in Spain and the Philippines. The overall effect of these initiatives has been a significant growth in the numbers of nurses recruited from other countries to work in the United Kingdom. The next section will examine this trend in detail.

International recruitment of nurses to the United Kingdom

A historical perspective

There has been a long tradition of United Kingdom recruitment of nurses from other countries. In the earlier part of the twentieth century this owed much to colonial policies and the attitude towards "empire" as a supplier of goods and services to the imperial centre.

During the inter-war period the Aliens Act of 1920 allowed United Kingdom hospitals to employ foreigners under certain restricted conditions. These included where:

- the foreigner came from a country in which the hospital provision was poor and there was no opportunity for proper training;

- there was definite evidence that the hospital in Britain could not obtain British applicants;
- such trainees returned to their native countries after completing training.

Matrons had to submit applications to employ foreign nurses to the Ministry of Health, which would then decide whether or not to issue a permit. There was an entry quota of foreign nationals into nursing of 3% (Ministry of Health 1935). There are few data on numbers of non-United Kingdom nurses working in the United Kingdom in the inter-war period. Census returns correlating occupation with nationality were only made erratically. In 1921, for example, there were 718 foreign-born nurses from 28 different countries, the majority coming from the USA (82 female nurses) and France (206 female nurses). The largest single category of male nurses was Italian.

By 1935 the Ministry of Labour in England was advocating a more restrictive policy on recruitment of foreigners as the shortage of British applicants for training began to wane. Permits for foreign probationers were to be limited to approximately 3% of total probationer posts and furthermore the foreigner was expected to return to her own country after completion of training (Ministry of Health 1935). The situation was to change with the war and the introduction of the NHS.

There was an upsurge in recruitment of nurses during and after the Second World War. One major source of recruits was Ireland. In 1947, the Wood Committee, set up to consider the nursing needs of the new NHS estimated that some 15 000 (12%) of the total hospital nursing workforce had been born in Ireland; their distribution throughout various specialities was uneven. The recruitment of Irish nurses had intensified throughout the war: the Ministry of Labour had a recruitment liaison office staffed by technical nursing officers in Dublin. The numbers peaked in 1946 at 2561 female recruits, and fell to 80 in 1954 (Ministry of Health et al. 1947).

In contrast, recruitment of European foreign nationals for training steadily increased from 584 in 1946 to 2234 in 1957. Surprisingly perhaps, given the prevailing anti-German sentiment after the war, it was German nurses who constituted the largest single group of overseas workers during this period (Ministry of Health et al. 1947). Volunteers were subject to conditions not imposed on home nationals. Those accepted could enter on a permit valid for only three years, register with the police and enter employment specified by the Ministry of Labour and National Service. They were not allowed to leave their employment without the consent of the Ministry of Labour. This was the de facto direction of labour, which had operated during the war and was feared by some nurse leaders as the price of the introduction of the NHS (Dingwall et al. 1988).

Small numbers of nurses from former British colonies were also recruited after the war but their numbers only became significant in the 1960s. The origins of recruitment from former colonies is complex but derives in part from the early export of British-born nurses to far-flung corners of the empire from the late nineteenth century to provide care and subsequently training for so-called "native" patients and nurses in government hospitals. Momentum in this policy only began to develop with changes during the inter-war period in colonial development policy itself, with a noticeable shift towards enlightened self-interest and reciprocal registration schemes for nurses throughout the British Commonwealth.

In 1957 the Ministry of Labour handed its recruitment and "placing" functions in nursing over to the Ministry of Health which then became responsible for statistics on nursing services, recruitment campaigns and matters related to publicity. The rise in recruitment from overseas resulted from what Thomas and Morton-Williams refer to as a "marriage of convenience" between the nursing shortage in the NHS and Commonwealth citizens keen to enter the United Kingdom to train as nurses (Beishon et al. 1995). By 1971 there were 15 000 overseas student nurses, of whom 40% were West Indian, 29% Asian and 27% African (Beishon et al. 1995). Recruitment from non-Commonwealth sources had tended to rely upon nurses from Ireland, where a long tradition had built up of recruitment to mental health hospitals. In the early 1970s it has been suggested that overseas nurses represented some 10% of the NHS workforce (Beishon et al. 1995).

International nurse recruitment: The current situation

The previous section has highlighted how the United Kingdom has placed a heavy reliance on international recruitment of nurses at various times through the last century, primarily as a reaction to skills shortages. In recent years this reliance has been reaffirmed. This section assesses the current level of inflow of nurses to the United Kingdom.

There are two sources of data that can be used to assess trends in the inflow of nurses to the United Kingdom; work permits and the professional register. Neither gives a complete picture, but in combination they enable an overview to be established.

One main source of data is applications for work permits. All non-United Kingdom applicants from countries outside the EU/European Economic Area (EU/EEA) who wish to take up employment in the United Kingdom are required to obtain a work permit. Work permit data can therefore be used as another source of information on trends in inflow of nurses from non-EU/EEA countries. Work permit data are presented primarily in terms of numbers of new applications and applications for extension approved in calendar years. Because data on new applications and applications for extension are reported separately, there is some scope to use data to assess the numbers of non-EU nurses already working in the United Kingdom who wish to continue working after their initial permit has expired (usually a two year permit is granted). Some occupations and professions are designated as "shortage occupations". These occupations have been acknowledged to be particularly difficult to fill, and their designation means that there is a simplified procedure for applicants, in order to "fast track" the work permit application process. The designation of shortage occupations is under continuous review, but at the current time "all registered nurses and midwives" are listed as facing a shortage in the United Kingdom.

Table 10.2 shows the work permit data for 2001 for the job title "nurse" (see Box 10.1 for details). It shows the overall data, main countries of nationality of applicants and applicants from accession states. There were a total of 23 603

Table 10.2 Total numbers of work permits approved for nurses, UK, 2001, by category and selected country of nationality, including accession countries

Country	Total, all applications	*Composition of total applications:*					
		First permission	In country change of employment	In country extension	In country technical change	Work permit	Work permit extension
TOTAL of which	23 063						
Philippines	10 050	210	1433	952	26	7422	7
India	2612	105	646	92	9	1759	1
South Africa	2514	149	669	490	33	1163	10
Zimbabwe	1801	851	527	146	13	261	1
Nigeria	1110	217	424	104	11	354	0
Australia	601	149	69	99	4	277	3
Poland	56	13	4	5	0	34	0
Czech	61	25	6	3	0	27	0
Cyprus	2	0	0	0	0	2	0
Estonia	1	0	0	0	0	1	0
Slovenia	1	0	0	0	0	1	0
Hungary	14	9	1	2	0	2	0
Bulgaria	72	5	6	11	0	50	0
Latvia	1	1	0	0	0	0	0
Lithuania	6	2	2	1	0	1	0
Malta	3	0	0	0	0	3	0
Romania	37	10	2	5	2	17	1
Slovakia	35	23	6	3	0	3	0

Source: Work Permits United Kingdom; provisional, up to 17 December 2001 only.

applications recorded, up to 17 December of the year, of which 12 762 (54%) were recorded as "work permit" – in other words over 12 700 new work permits were issued to individuals who had not previously been working as nurses in the United Kingdom.

These work permit data highlight the significant numbers of applications from non-EU countries, particularly the Philippines, South Africa and other British Commonwealth countries, with the Philippines alone accounting for nearly half (44%) of the overall total, the majority of which were new work permits (7422). In contrast, candidate countries accounted for only 289 applications (or just over 1% of applications), of which 141 were for new work permits. The five main candidate countries from which applications were processed were Poland, Bulgaria, the Czech Republic, Romania and Slovakia. However, no single accession state accounted for 100 or more applications.

The other main source of data is the professional register of the United Kingdom Central Council for Nursing Midwifery and Health Visiting (UKCC). These data can be used to assess trends in the number of applications and admissions from non-United Kingdom nurses. Individual judgements are made by the

Box 10.1 Work permit definitions

"First permission." Records that the applicant has been given permission to work in the United Kingdom, subject to Home Office approval, that is the applicant has not yet entered the United Kingdom.

"In country change of employment." Records that an applicant already in the United Kingdom has been granted a change in type of employment. One example would be an individual working as an auxiliary during an adaptation period who has now been granted a change of status to nurse on successful registration with the UKCC.

"In country extension." Records that an applicant already in the United Kingdom has been granted an extension to the time period of their work permit – for example a nurse working on a two year period applying for and being granted a further two year extension.

"In country technical change." In a small number of cases there will be a technical change to permit details – for example if the employer for whom the nurse is working changes their location or the title of the organization.

"Work Permit." Records the first time issuing of a work permit to the individual applicant.

"Work permit extension." Records the issuing of an extension to a work permit, for an applicant currently not located in the United Kingdom.

UKCC on each application, on the basis of the duration and type of training and previous work experience of the applicant. Because the UKCC deals differently with applications from EU and non-EU countries, it is possible to track the relative importance of these two sources.

Individuals with general first level nursing or midwifery qualifications from the other countries of the EU/European Economic Area (EU/EEA), have the right to practise in the United Kingdom because of mutual recognition of qualifications across the countries of the EU/EEA (see Chapter 7). As such, they can register with the UKCC via the European Community Directives. All other nurses from non-EU/EEA countries have to apply to the UKCC for verification of their qualifications in order to be admitted to the Register. Most nurses from outside the EU will also have to apply for, and be granted, a work permit to take up paid employment in the United Kingdom.

There are limitations in using the data to monitor inflows to the United Kingdom. Registration data only record the fact that a nurse has been registered, they do not show when a nurse actually enters the United Kingdom, nor do they indicate what the nurse is doing. As such, it is a measure of intent to practise in the United Kingdom, rather than necessarily an indicator that the nurse is actually working in the United Kingdom. Figure 10.1 shows the trend in annual number of non-United Kingdom trained nurses that were accepted onto the United Kingdom nursing register. Without registration, a nurse cannot practise in the United Kingdom, so the data give a broad indication of trends in inward mobility of nurses to the United Kingdom.

In 2000/2001 a total of 9694 entrants were recorded as entering the Register from abroad (provisional data); of these, 8403 (87%) were from non-EU/EEA countries. The three most important source countries were the Philippines

Figure 10.1 Admissions to the UKCC Register from EU Directive/Non-EU Sources 1993/
94–2000/01 (Initial Registrations)

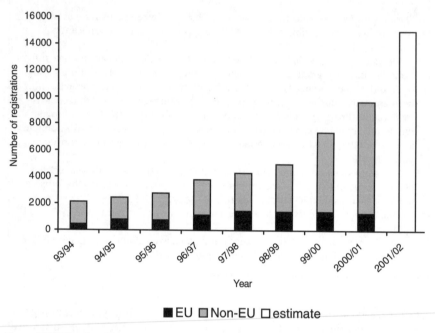

Source: UKCC/Buchan 2002

(3396), South Africa (1086) and Australia (1046). An estimate for 2001/02 suggests that admissions will have increased further this year, to almost 15 000
(Buchan 2002).

The number of nurses from EU Member States has flattened off. In the mid-
1990s they accounted for between one-quarter and one-third of annual total
overseas admissions, but by 2000/01 this had dropped to only 13% of the total.
In 2000/01 the total number of nurses registering from all EU countries was
1291, little more than from either Australia or South Africa, and much less than
the numbers registering from the Philippines.

The European Union

First level registered nurses from EU Member States have a right to free mobility
within the countries of the EU under Directives that guarantee mutual recognition of nursing qualifications (see Chapter 7). Yet relatively few nurses from
elsewhere have been exercising this freedom to move to the United Kingdom,
compared to the inflow of nurses from other countries, whose entry is complicated by the need to apply for a work permit.

The EU was also highlighted in the 1999 guidance from the Department of
Health as being an "acceptable" source of recruits. The Department has reached

agreement with the Government of Spain to undertake systematic and structured recruitment of cohorts of Spanish nurses to designated NHS employers in England. However, as noted above, all the recent growth in the numbers of overseas nurses on the United Kingdom Register has been accounted for by an increase in inflow from non-EU countries. The overall contribution of EU countries reduced from 33% to 13% of total inflow of overseas registrants between 1997/8 and 2000/01 (Table 10.3).

Spain reportedly has a surplus of nurses, so there is an apparent "win-win" situation, with vacant nursing posts in the United Kingdom being filled by nurses currently unemployed in Spain. The initial projections were to recruit several thousand nurses from Spain. There is as yet little sign of an inflow of this magnitude. Media coverage has suggested that some of the Spanish nurses already recruited to the United Kingdom have had English language difficulties (Akid 2002). Under EU law a language test cannot be applied to EU nationals, but it is reported that potential recruits from Spain will now be assessed on their language capabilities prior to travel to the United Kingdom. The United Kingdom nurse regulation council has also announced that all non-EU nurses (including those whose first language is English) will now have to pass a standard English test administered by the British Council (Lipley 2002).

Although not a large increase, the number of Spanish nurses registering in the United Kingdom has gone up as a result of the NHS recruitment initiative, but the number of registrants from some other EU counties reduced (Table 10.4). For example, in the late 1990s some United Kingdom employers were active in recruiting Finnish nurses at a time when there was a relative oversupply of nurses in the Finnish nursing labour market. This situation has now adjusted, and the inflow from that country has reduced. The traditional flow of nurses from Ireland to the United Kingdom has reversed as the Irish government attempts to solve its nursing shortages by recruiting in the United Kingdom and elsewhere. It is apparent from the UKCC data that the EU Member States have not been a growing source of nurse recruits for the United Kingdom in recent years. While there is some indication of a growth in recruitment from Spain, the most significant long-term trend is the link between the United Kingdom

Table 10.3   EU registrants as a percentage of all overseas registrants, 1993/4–1999/2000

Year	No. of EU registrants	EU registrants as a percentage of all overseas registrants
1993/4	456	21
1994/5	798	33
1995/6	763	28
1996/7	1141	30
1997/8	1439	33
1998/9	1413	28
1999/2000	1416	19
2000/2001	1295	13

Source: UKCC

Table 10.4 Numbers of new registrants on United Kingdom Register from selected EU countries

Country	1998/9	1999/2000	2000/01
Finland	312	279	127
Sweden	148	108	79
Germany	258	259	202
Spain	126	213	260
Ireland	232	234	315
(Total)	(1412)	(1416)	(1295)

Source: UKCC

and Anglophone Ireland. Ireland, once a major source of nurses for the United Kingdom, has now become a major destination of United Kingdom registered nurses.

International recruitment: The policy dimension

One key policy issue is the extent to which there is a common understanding of what is meant by a "nurse", and whether there is mutual recognition of nursing qualifications. This relates to how the profession and its members are defined; the scope of practice is determined; and standards of education and of ethical and competent practice are set. Systems of accountability are established through these means. This is no easy task and it is often difficult to develop agreed and officially recognized standards of practice and education. This can lead to confusion when the title "nurse" is applied to such a heterogeneous range of personnel, from those requiring only six years of general education prior to entry into a nursing programme, to nurses with a university level preparation. The need for regulation is critical in bringing some regularity to the enormous diversity of professional practice. In this regard guidelines produced by the International Council of Nurses (ICN) (International Council of Nurses 1998) through international consensus workshops have provided an important framework to help national nursing organizations implement legislative changes.

There are a series of constraints to international mobility of nurses that must be considered in any policy analysis. These include the individual circumstances of nurses, language differences, variations in push and pull factors related to relative pay levels and roles, and regulatory differences (see Box 10.2 for summary).

One policy challenge is the question of whether national governments or international agencies should intervene in the process of international recruitment to moderate or "manage" it, or introduce an ethical dimension if there is concern that developing countries are losing scarce nursing skills. In November 1999 the Department of Health in England reacted to concerns about accusations of creating "brain-drain" from developing countries, by issuing guidelines

Box 10.2 Potential constraints on international nurse mobility

- Differences in organization and structures of health systems;
- Variations in nurses pay/status;
- Variations in career opportunities/promotion opportunities;
- Variations in nurses' roles, responsibilities and working relationship with other groups of health workers;
- Lack of recognition given to nursing experience in other countries;
- Variations in levels of access to continuing professional development/ educational opportunities;
- Variations in perceived social and economic standing of nurses;
- Language differences;
- Professional/national/international regulatory frameworks;
- Broader economic conditions/employment prospects, stability, security;
- Gender issues – nurses'/women's status.

Source: Buchan et al. 1994:16

on international recruitment of nurses to National Health Service employers (Department of Health 1999a). The guidelines indicated specifically that NHS employers should avoid direct recruitment from South Africa and the West Indies, and set out good practice guidelines in international recruitment. It also highlighted that the countries of the EU were an appropriate place to target for recruitment. This was one of the first attempts at national level to set out some guidelines for "ethical" behaviour in international recruitment, and as such it warrants some examination. Analysis of registration data (Buchan and Seccombe 2002) suggest that the guidelines had some short-term effect in reducing the level of recruitment from designated countries, but that this recruitment effort may then have been displaced to other developing counties not covered by the guidelines.

The Department then updated and strengthened the 1999 guidance when it published a new Code of Practice (Department of Health 2001d) in September 2001. The new Code attempts to put right some of the limitations of the 1999 guidance. It covers issues of working with recruitment agencies, working in developing countries, advertising, fair recruitment and English language proficiency. It is too early to assess the effect of the new Code. It only covers NHS employers, and while it will put more pressure on NHS employers to comply with national policy, it is not intended to end the practice of international recruitment – its objective is to make international recruitment more effective. The English Department of Health has developed a NHS Plan with targets for increased numbers of NHS nurses; this will continue to act as a significant "pull" factor and therefore it is likely that there will continue to be high levels of recruitment of nurses, at least over the next couple of years.

It is likely that the need to maintain an ethical dimension, while continuing to promote recruitment, will lead to the United Kingdom Department of Health encouraging more country to country "concordat" or contracts. In this scenario the United Kingdom would recruit a specified number of nurses from the partner country, perhaps for a defined time period, with the "win-win" potential being that these nurses would return home with new skills or qualifications. There has been some pressure from some countries for monetary compensation for the "loss" of their skilled health professionals, but at the time of writing this does not appear to be on the policy agenda. The other area of official action in relation to improving the effectiveness of international recruitment in the NHS has been to set out more detailed guidance for employers on the provision of supervised practice and adaptation for nurses, when this is required by the UKCC (Department of Health 2001e). The independent (private) health care sector employers have also issued similar documents, aimed at supporting the process of recruitment and induction of nurses recruited from other countries (Independent Healthcare Association et al. 2002).

Conclusions: The United Kingdom, Europe and the candidate countries

The United Kingdom is currently heavily reliant on international recruitment of nurses to meet staffing targets and combat skills shortages. In 2001, approximately four in ten new nurses on the United Kingdom Register had been recruited from abroad. The main source countries in recent years have been the Philippines, South Africa and Australia. Most of these nurses enter the United Kingdom on work permits; as such they will be eligible to work for a specified period (usually two years). They will then have to renew their permits. This means that there is the potential for a high level of turnover of these staff, either because they have no intention of staying on, or if their permit is not renewed.

In contrast, first level registered nurses from EU Member States have the right of free entry to practise in the United Kingdom, but there has not been any growth in inflow of nurses from these countries to the United Kingdom in recent years. Freedom to enter is not in itself sufficient. One key "barrier" is language; the United Kingdom has tended to recruit from countries where English is the first language. A second factor is the absence of any significant and continuing imbalance of "push" and "pull" factors between the United Kingdom nursing labour market and other EU nursing labour markets. Pay, career opportunities and working conditions do not vary significantly enough among Member States for nurses to be motivated to overcome barriers to migration in significant numbers. It is where these longer-term imbalances have persisted that migration of nurses has been at a more significant level. One example is the much lower standard of living experienced by nurses in the Philippines, South Africa and the West Indies being a "push" factor in motivating nurses to move. Another push factor is historical links, such as the tradition of the young Australian nurse "backpacker" coming to the United Kingdom for a year to explore Europe.

Where do the accession states fit into this picture? Currently there are only small numbers of nurses from these countries who have moved to the United Kingdom. This has been primarily because of individual contacts between United Kingdom based managers and specific candidate countries (for example, hospitals in the East Midlands of England have recruited Bulgarian nurses because of personal contacts). The lack of inflow of nurses from current Member

States has been linked to language differences, and to a lack of "push/pull" imbalance. In contrast, nurses in the candidate countries are paid much lower salaries and some are experiencing very poor working conditions (International Labour Organization 2001) and so are more likely to be motivated to move. The younger ones from the "MTV generation" are also more likely to speak English. This suggests a potential for increase in recruitment to the United Kingdom once the candidate countries have entered the EU, in terms of the existence of major push factors (low pay and limited career opportunities) and a key United Kingdom "pull" factor (the continuation of staffing shortages).

Any growth in recruitment of nurses from candidate countries to the United Kingdom would be from a virtually nil current base, and would have to overcome concerns in the United Kingdom that some candidate countries do not provide adequate training for their nurses. It is unlikely that United Kingdom employers will invest heavily in attempting to open up these new nursing labour markets in eastern Europe unless they are experiencing difficulties in recruiting from their current "preferred providers" in the Philippines, Australia and so on. What is more likely is that United Kingdom employers would target individual post-basic qualified nurses with good English capabilities and advanced nursing skills. In contrast to the "bulk" recruitment from the Philippines, where a United Kingdom employer will recruit 50 or 100 nurses at a time, the candidate countries may be regarded as fertile territory for individualized recruitment to meet a specified skills need.

The main policy message from this analysis is that providing an EU framework for freedom of movement of nurses does not necessarily mean that many nurses will exercise that freedom. Other factors, such as language skills, cultural and post colonial ties, and push/pull imbalances are the main drivers. The short term "pull" factor of meeting the United Kingdom NHS staffing targets is likely to continue to be a dynamic in the interaction of the United Kingdom with international nursing labour markets. The United Kingdom will continue to be active in international nursing labour markets, and there may be an increased focus on some candidate countries as a source of some skilled nurses. However, it is likely that a bigger "pull" will come from some of the other current Member States that are experiencing nursing skills shortages, and who are "closer" to the candidate countries, in terms of language, culture or geographical proximity.

Acknowledgements

The paper draws from other research on nurse mobility, funded by WHO, ICN and RCN (Buchan 2002). The authors also acknowledge the assistance of informants at the Department of Health, England; Work Permits (UK); United Kingdom Central Council for Nursing Midwifery and Health Visiting (UKCC); Royal College of Nursing (RCN); NHS Professionals; two private sector recruitment agencies; and management and nurses at two NHS Trusts who all provided background information. The views expressed in the report are those of the authors.

References

Akid, M. (2002) Recruits' poor English putting patients at risk, *Nursing Times*, 98(9):4.

Beishon, S., Virdee, S. and Hagell, A. (1995) Nursing in a multi-ethnic NHS. Policy Studies Institute.

Buchan, J. (2002) *International Recruitment of Nurses: United Kingdom Case Study* WHO/ICN/RCN. London: Royal College of Nursing.

Buchan, J. and Seccombe, I. (2002) *Behind the headlines: A Review of the UK Nursing Labour Market*. London: Royal College of Nursing/Queen Margaret University College.

Buchan, J., Seccombe, I. and Ball, J. (1994) The international mobility of nurses: A UK perspective, *International Journal of Nursing Studies*, 31:143–54.

Department of Health (2001e) *Code of Practice for NHS Employers involved in international recruitment of healthcare professionals*. London: Department of Health (www.doh.gov.uk/international-nurse/).

Department of Health (2001d) *Guidance for the provision of supervised practice for nurses and adaption of midwives in London*. London: Department of Health (www.doh.gov.uk/nurseguidance.pdf).

Department of Health (1999a) *Guidance on International Recruitment*. London: Department of Health.

Department of Health (1999b) *Improving Working Lives*. London: Department of Health.

Department of Health (2001b) *Investment and Reform for NHS Staff – Taking Forward the NHS Plan*. London: Department of Health.

Department of Health (2001c) *NHS Emergency Pressures: Making Progress*. London: Department of Health.

Department of Health (2001a) *Review for 2002. Written Evidence from the Health Departments for Great Britain. Review Body for Nursing Staff, Midwives, Health Visitors and Professions Allied to Medicine*. London: Department of Health.

Dingwall, R., Webster, C. and Rafferty, A.M. (1988) *An Introduction to the Social History of Nursing*. London: Routledge.

Independent Healthcare Association, Registered Nursing Home Association and Voices (2002) *Supervised Practice Programme for Internationally Qualified Nurses: Independent Sector Recommendations*. London: Independent Healthcare Association.

International Council of Nurses (1998) ICN on Regulation: towards 21st Century Models. Geneva: International Council of Nurses.

International Labour Organization (2001) East European Healthcare in Crises. Press Release ILO/01/3, 10 December. Geneva: ILO.

Lipley, N. (2002) UKCC introduces English test for non-EU applicants, *Nursing Standard*, 16(26):4.

Ministry of Health (1935) Letter, Ministry of Labour to the Secretary, PROMH55/447, 6 September 1935.

Ministry of Health, Ministry of Labour and National Service and Department of Health for Scotland (1947) Report of the Inter-departmental Committee on Nursing Services (Chairman: Earl of Athlone). London: HMSO.

NHS Executive (2000) *The NHS Plan*. London: Department of Health.

Office of Manpower Economics Annual Survey (2001) Nineteenth Report. Office of Manpower Economics, London.

chapter eleven

Free movement of patients

Martin McKee, Laura MacLehose and Tit Albreht

Introduction

Since their inception, all health care systems have placed limitations on what they will cover. Countries differ in the approach taken, although all involve a combination of explicit limitations, for example the exclusion of procedures for which there is little evidence, and implicit ones, such as constraints on supply leading to waiting lists. However, one explicit limitation that is common to virtually every system is the principle of territoriality (Cornellisen 1996). In other words, health care usually will only be provided in facilities that are on the national territory. Of course there have always been some exceptions, in particular in smaller countries where a decision has been made that, because the volume of cases that would be treated each year would be small it makes more sense to purchase care abroad. For example, there is a long tradition of Maltese and Cypriot patients receiving treatment in the United Kingdom, in the same way that Luxembourg patients have long received treatment in neighbouring countries. In countries outside the EU, however, the decision to pay for the treatment abroad has generally been made by the organization paying for it.

The situation within the EU is different. The principle of free movement of people has always implied that an individual should not face financial obstacles in obtaining health care abroad if that would prevent him or her travelling to other Member States for professional reasons. Otherwise the fear of falling ill, and the financial consequences that would result, would act as a barrier to mobility and thus to a common employment market.

The first part of this chapter will review the circumstances in which an individual may obtain treatment in another Member State. Before doing so, however, it is important to note that the situation is far from straightforward. For many years a set of procedures, agreed by Member States, had tightly circumscribed the conditions under which treatment abroad had to be covered by the organization responsible for paying for that person's care. This situation has changed rapidly since 1998, when the European Court of Justice (ECJ) gave two rulings that had important implications for the existing arrangements, effectively introducing a new set of rules. Specifically, the ECJ ruled that the earlier procedures remained valid but were not an exhaustive exposition of the possibilities that were available to someone seeking care in another Member State. Since then a series of subsequent rulings have built on these rulings, clarifying some ambiguities but leaving others unresolved.

These developments have been subject to many differing interpretations but it is necessary to understand how the current situation arose if one is to anticipate developments in the future. Consequently the first part of this chapter will describe the situation that existed until 1998 before looking at more recent developments. Only then will it be possible to explore the implications of EU enlargement.

Regulation 1408/71

Early in its existence the European Community enacted a series of provisions to ensure that certain groups could obtain health care abroad in certain carefully defined circumstances. Initial regulations, issued in 1958, gave way in the early 1970s to Regulation 1408/71, later supplemented by Regulation 574/72.

These Regulations have until recently set out the legal position in respect of social security provision across borders within the EU. It is important to note that the regulations explicitly did not seek to harmonize social security systems but just to coordinate them (Department for Work and Pensions 2002). Article 152 of the Amsterdam Treaty clearly limits the role of the Commission or other EU-wide bodies in the field of health care stating that "community action in the field of public health shall fully respect the responsibilities of the Member States for the organisation and delivery of health services and medical care".

The scope of the legislation has extended steadily, originally covering only "workers" in employment and their families but subsequently encompassing the self-employed and then students and others not in gainful employment so that now they cover almost everyone living within the EU, with the exception of citizens of non-EU countries (Van Raepenbusch 1997; Fillon 1999). When issues of cross-border care arise, one state is designated as "competent". This is the state in which the individual, or the head of his or her family where applicable, pays contributions or is otherwise provided with health insurance.

Clearly the situation is complicated by the great diversity of health care systems within Europe, with some reimbursing expenditure made by the patient, to varying degrees, while others provide benefits in kind, in other words the patient does not pay directly for the health care received but the facility providing it is reimbursed by the insurer. However, the principles underlying cross-border care are relatively straightforward, even if the implementation can be extremely complicated. Where a right to cross-border care is established, it is the relevant institution in the competent state that is responsible for paying for it, providing the individual concerned meets the criteria for entitlement to benefits in the competent state. The individual obtaining treatment in a second country should receive it on the same terms that he or she would if insured in that country. This, inevitably, creates numerous anomalies. For example, a person may be required to pay a co-payment in the country in which they are insured, but if this is not required in the country in which they are treated, then none is payable. As a consequence, those responsible for administering payments in health care systems require a detailed understanding of procedures in other Member States.

So who is entitled to obtain health care abroad? Two issues are relevant. First, has the illness arisen during a temporary stay abroad or is the individual travelling abroad for the purpose of obtaining treatment? Second, if the stay abroad is temporary, is the patient's condition urgent, defined as requiring immediate and necessary investigation and treatment?

Temporary stays abroad

The following summary is inevitably a simplification of what is a very complex set of rules. A more detailed guide can be found at *http://europa.eu.int/comm/ employment_social/soc-prot/schemes/guide_en.htm#6*. In brief, people entitled to receive treatment in a country other than the competent state regardless of whether their condition is urgent include:

- pensioners entitled to a pension and their families;
- persons who have been employed or self-employed but are not currently in employment, and their families, who go to another Member State to seek work;
- employed or self-employed persons exercising their professional activity in another Member State;
- frontier workers (although their families must obtain prior authorization for non-urgent treatment if there is no specific agreement between the countries concerned);
- students and those undertaking professional training and their families (since October 1997).

Anyone else seeking treatment while temporarily abroad must meet the condition of urgency of treatment, although a precise and internationally consistent definition of "urgency" remains elusive. However, one aspect was recently clarified by an ECJ ruling that an individual suffering from a long-standing illness may use the E111 mechanism to claim for emergency care if his or her condition deteriorates, even though the underlying condition preceded travel abroad (Case C-326-/00 *Ioannidis*).

The E111 procedure is the most common mechanism covering those seeking health care while temporarily abroad. It is necessary to obtain, in advance, the relevant form issued by the competent organization in the home state. In addition, there is a range of specific mechanisms covering particular groups. Frontier workers (people living in one country but employed in another) are, in addition, entitled to treatment using the E106 mechanism, regardless of its urgency, in both countries. The E109 mechanism covers students attending educational establishments abroad, the E119 covers those travelling to another country to seek work, and the E110 covers those working in international transport. Finally, other provisions cover those who would be unable to travel if they did not have access to specific life-sustaining treatments, such as renal dialysis, or other necessary services such as antenatal care for women who are pregnant (European Commission 2002). In all cases the individual concerned must obtain the necessary form in advance.

Recognition of the limitations of the E111 scheme, together with the growth of entitlement cards of various types in many national health systems, has given rise to a proposal to implement a European Health Insurance Card. It is envisaged that this card will begin to be issued from June 2004 (European Commission 2003).

In addition, however, many people, in particular those on holiday, pay for any treatment they require while in another Member State through travel insurance policies or, in some cases, private health insurance. The scale of this activity is unknown but likely to be substantially larger than that covered by the E111 and related mechanisms.

Planned treatment abroad

The second set of circumstances in which an individual may be entitled to health care abroad is where the necessary treatment cannot be provided in the competent state. The clear goal of the Member States has been to limit these circumstances to situations in which the organization in the competent state required to pay for funding gives authorization for treatment to take place, issuing an E112 form. This was first challenged in two rulings by the ECJ in the late 1970s, requiring that the relevant institution must give such authorization in all cases where it would improve the medical state of the patient, regardless of any other considerations (ECJ; C-117/77, Judgement of 16 March 1978, *Bestuur van het algemeen Ziekenfonds Drenthe-Platteland Pierik I*; ECJ, C-182/78, Judgement of 31 May 1979, *Pierik II*).

This was not what the Member States had intended (Council of the European Communities 1981; Kesteloot et al. 1995). In particular it was seen as a means by which patients could avoid waiting lists (Van der Mei 2001), which were a consequence of policies in some countries to constrain supply as a means of limiting increases in health care costs.

Shortly afterwards, a new regulation was agreed (Council of the European Communities 1981), specifying that treatment abroad would only be made available:

- when the treatment required by the interested party is part of the health care package covered by the social protection system in the area of health care; and
- this treatment cannot be given to him or her in his or her state of residence within the period that is normally necessary, in view of his or her current state of health and the probable course of his or her disease.

It should, however, also be noted that, notwithstanding more recent developments that will be discussed in the next section, the existence of the E112 mechanism does not preclude other arrangements, of which there are a variety that take place independently of any EU provisions. For example, the Dutch

Zeeland-Flanders and West Brabant Sickness Fund formed contracts with two Belgian hospitals as long ago as 1978 although even in this well established scheme few Dutch patients (around 4% insured under the scheme) appear to take advantage of the available cross-border care (Busse et al. 2002).

A more recent example is the decision to promote cross-border provision of health services in Ireland as a means of facilitating peace and reconciliation (Jamison et al. 2001). Recent initiatives by the English Department of Health to reduce waiting times by means of block contracts for non-urgent surgery with hospitals in France, Germany and Belgium have also taken place outside the E112 system.

Overall, however, even when these additional movements are included, the scale of cross-border movement for planned treatment abroad is small in relation to overall health care budgets, with one estimate that it accounts for under 0.5% of public expenditure on health care (Mossialos and McKee 2002).

A new situation: The *Kohll* and *Decker* rulings

As noted previously, Member States felt that, in Regulation 1408/71, they had taken control of the circumstances in which patients could obtain treatment abroad. Their complacency was shaken by two rulings by the ECJ in 1998. The rulings concerned two people insured under the Luxembourg social security system who had obtained treatment abroad, in one case without seeking authorization, and in the other after it was rejected when it was deemed not to be urgent. Neither case involved admission to hospital and in both, the providers were paid directly by the patients, who then sought to reclaim the sums from the Luxembourg insurance fund. The patients argued that the restrictions placed on them contravened free movement of services (provision of orthodontic treatment) and goods (spectacles).

The Luxembourg Government, which was supported by several other governments, initially argued that the rules on the free movement of goods and services did not apply to matters of social security. However, the ECJ decided that, while Member States had considerable flexibility in how they organized their social security systems, those systems were not exempt from rules on the free movement of goods and services or, as the Advocate General put it, that "the social security sector constitutes an island beyond the reach of Community law and that, as a consequence, all national rules relating to social security fall outside its scope".

In interpreting the implications of these rulings it is necessary to consider the arguments used by the Luxembourg Government against issuing authorizations and the ECJ's responses to them. It argued that prior authorization was needed to:

- Ensure the financial balance of the social security system and to enable the Government to provide a balanced medical and hospital service open to all insured persons;
- Protect the public health of the population since there would be no way of ensuring the quality of the goods and services provided by orthodontists and opticians in other Member States.

The ECJ rejected these arguments. First, it noted that, as both patients had only requested what would have been paid had they sought care in Luxembourg there was no adverse impact on the financing of the Luxembourg system and so there could be no justification for the claim that they would destabilize it. Second, the ECJ rejected the argument that the claims should be rejected as they would damage Luxembourg's ability to protect its medical infrastructure and so threaten public health, as this hardly applied to provision of spectacles or orthodontic treatment.

Third, it denied that these actions prevented the Luxembourg authorities from ensuring that the quality of care provided was adequate. It referred to the mutual recognition of diplomas and the work that had taken place in the 1970s to harmonize training requirements (Council of the European Communities 1993) and concluded that "the purchase of a pair of spectacles from an optician established in another Member State provides guarantees equivalent to those afforded on the sale of a pair of spectacles by an optician established in the national territory". Consequently, the ECJ concluded that the requirement for prior authorization meant that Luxembourg's national rules created an unjustified impediment to the free movement of goods and services within the EU. Echoing landmark rulings in the 1970s, in which the ECJ established the concept of direct or indirect, effective or potential, barriers to trade and to the freedom to provide services (Bosco 2000), it established that simply showing how free movement of goods and services might be prevented was sufficient to be considered incompatible with the EC Treaty.

The implications of these rulings have been debated extensively, and in some cases have been overtaken by subsequent cases. For the present purposes, however, the main point is that the Luxembourg Government had relied upon its national rules that had incorporated Regulation 1408/71 into domestic law. The ECJ noted that this could not take legal precedence over the EC Treaty itself and, while the Regulation (Nickless 2001) was valid, it was not the only way in which an individual could obtain medical goods and services in another Member State, but was only one possible option.

The *Kohll* and *Decker* rulings pose some important challenges for health policymakers. It has been argued, for example, that contrary to the view taken by the Court, it cannot be assumed that there is a similar standard of health care throughout the EU (Nickless 2001), an issue that takes on even greater significance in an expanded Union in which some health care systems have experienced long periods of very low levels of investment. Furthermore, this position contrasts with emerging initiatives in some countries on accreditation and revalidation (Nickless 2001). These are a departure from the implicit assumption in the relevant EU regulations that once a qualification has been obtained it is valid for life.

At a more practical level, however, by establishing a dual system of social protection for non-urgent health care received in another Member State, EU citizens now have a choice of two mutually inconsistent options if seeking health care abroad. The classic E112 procedure, involving prior authorization, establishes that patients receiving care in a second country do so "as though [they] were insured with it" (Article 22.1.c). In other words, they are subject to the same arrangements for cost-sharing or gate-keeping and the cost of treatment is determined by the tariffs in the country in which it was delivered.

In contrast, the *Kohll and Decker* procedure establishes that a patient can freely choose a provider abroad without seeking prior authorization in their home state. They can then claim reimbursement from their home health care system "as if they received the treatment there". In other words, there are now two quite different sets of rules for reimbursement in existence. Some clarification was given in the *Vanbraekel* case. Ms Descamps (Vanbraekel), a Belgian national insured under the Belgium social security system, requested authorization from her sickness insurance fund to undergo orthopaedic surgery in France. Belgian law allowed treatment abroad to be reimbursed if it could be provided there more effectively and has been considered necessary (prior to treatment), as certified by a specialist at a Belgian university hospital. Her application was refused because she had not obtained the opinion of a specialist at a university hospital. However, she then obtained treatment in France without authorization and launched a successful appeal in the Belgian Courts against the refusal to authorize her treatment. However, the Belgian court could not decide whether she should be reimbursed according to the Belgian or the French tariffs. Under the E112 system she would have been reimbursed according to the French tariff (FF 38 608), whereas under the *Kohll* and *Decker* procedure she should have been reimbursed according to the Belgian tariff (FF 49 935).

The ECJ held that if an insured person was incorrectly refused authorization to receive hospital treatment in another Member State, he or she should be guaranteed reimbursement according to the rules applicable in the Member State in which treatment was provided, although this would not prevent the insuring state from reimbursing according to its own tariffs when they would appear to be more favourable. The ECJ then considered whether such a "top-up arrangement" would be necessary to ensure free movement of services, concluding that, if a patient received a lower reimbursement than if treated in his or her home state, this would deter, if not prevent him or her from looking to foreign health care providers. Consequently, the Belgian fund was required to give the patient additional reimbursement to compensate for the difference.

Developments since *Kohll* and *Decker*

Inevitably, the rulings raised as many questions as they answered as the ECJ was only able to rule on the precise circumstances of the cases before it. Did they apply to hospitals as well as to care provided in an ambulatory setting (Palm et al. 2000)? Clearly a few people travelling abroad to obtain spectacles or orthodontic treatment would not affect the viability of health care facilities but at what stage would this arise if large numbers of people sought care in a nearby hospital that happened to be across a national frontier? Did they apply to individuals insured in countries where costs were not reimbursed but instead paid directly to the provider, with the patient receiving benefits in kind?

As a consequence, there was considerable discussion in national governments about how to respond. Luxembourg, Belgium and Denmark rapidly amended their legislation to establish administrative procedures for unconditional reimbursement of certain outpatient services and health care products purchased in another Member State. Austria had already allowed this to take place, with patients entitled to reimbursement of costs of care from a provider who did not have a contract with a sickness fund, regardless of whether they were in Austria or abroad, at a rate of 80% of the amount paid for the same treatment from a contracted provider (Palm et al. 2000). Other countries were more cautious, and in some cases, demonstrated apparent confusion. The United Kingdom, for example, used the case to argue that it would allow local health authorities to make the decision to send their patients abroad, rather than requiring them to get approval from the Health Ministry, ignoring the fact that the matter was one for the individual patient.

Since then, a series of further ECJ rulings have introduced other new concepts that must now be taken into account. In July 2001 the Court ruled in the cases of *Smits-Peerbooms*. Both were insured under the benefits in kind system of the Dutch social health insurance system. In this system, authorization to obtain treatment from non-contracted providers abroad is only granted if:

- the required treatment falls within the scope of what is regarded as "usual in the professional circles concerned";
- the required treatment is necessary and is not available without undue delay in the Netherlands.

Mrs Geraets-Smits received treatment for Parkinson's disease from a specialized clinic in Germany without obtaining prior authorization. She paid the clinic directly and then requested reimbursement from her Dutch sickness fund using the procedure established by *Kohll* and *Decker*. The sickness fund refused to reimburse her, arguing that the treatment involved was not "usual", that satisfactory and adequate treatment for her symptoms was available in the Netherlands from a contracted provider and that the treatment provided in Germany conferred no additional advantage. Mr Peerbooms fell into a coma after a traffic accident. His specialist neurologist asked for him to be sent to a university hospital in Austria where he received intensive therapy and recovered consciousness. This therapy was only available on an experimental basis in two institutions in the Netherlands and only to people less than 25 years old, whereas it was fully covered by the social health insurance scheme in Austria. The patient's specialist requested reimbursement for the cost of the treatment but was refused on the grounds that appropriate care could have been obtained from a contracted provider in the Netherlands.

The ECJ was faced with three main questions (Nickless 2002):

- did the EC Treaty provisions on the free movement of services apply to health care provided in hospitals;
- the requirement of prior authorization for hospital treatment abroad violated these Treaty provisions;
- if so, whether the Dutch system of authorization could be justified.

In summary, the ECJ confirmed that Community law does not prevent Member States from organizing their health care systems but in doing so they must comply with Community law. It confirmed that health care is covered by rules on the freedom to provide services, and that there is "no need to distinguish in that regard between care provided in a hospital environment and care provided outside such an environment". It had been argued that as in the Netherlands, patients did not pay directly for hospital care, with sickness funds doing so on their behalf, the relationship between the patient and the hospital should not be considered a "service" (defined as an economic activity provided for remuneration) under the meaning of the Treaty. However, the ECJ ruled that a service did not necessarily have to be paid for by the person receiving it in order for it to be classified as a service. Thus the ECJ confirmed that the *Kohll* and *Decker* mechanism applies to all health care systems, regardless of whether they involve reimbursement or in kind benefits, and to both in-patient and outpatient care.

Turning to the requirement for prior authorization under the mechanisms set out in Regulation 1408/71, the ECJ held that a need to apply for prior authorization for treatment abroad would deter, or even prevent, people from applying to health care providers in another Member State. As such it constituted a barrier to the freedom to provide services. It did, however, accept that Member States could enact legislation restricting such freedom on "grounds of public policy, public security and public health". However, to do so they must demonstrate the existence of "overriding reasons relating to the public interest". It further clarified this position, indicating that such reasons would include:

- where there is a risk of seriously undermining a social security system's financial balance;
- where the objective of maintaining a balanced medical and hospital service open to all is jeopardized;
- where the maintenance of treatment capacity or medical competence on national territory is essential for the public health, and even the survival of, the population.

The ECJ accepted that the provision of hospital services were subject to planning and contracting in such a way that a balanced supply of facilities was ensured in a geographical area, providing a defined level of access. Complete freedom to provide services could interfere with the ability to maintain this provision. However, it also stated that constraints on free movement of services could only be justified if they were proven to be necessary and proportional and based on objective criteria that did not discriminate against providers established in another Member State. Unfortunately it did not define necessary or proportional.

Finally, the ECJ's decisions with regard to the Dutch system of authorization also raised an important new principle. The Dutch sickness funds based their decision on what was "usual" treatment. The ECJ accepted that a Member State can define the scope of its health care system and so can exclude provision or reimbursement of certain products or services. However, its decisions must be based on "objective criteria, without reference to the origin of the products". Similarly, prior authorization must be based on "objective, non discriminatory criteria that are known in advance, in such a way as to circumscribe the exercise of the national authorities' discretion, so that it is not used arbitrarily" and a decision must be made within a "reasonable time" and "be capable of being challenged in judicial or quasi-judicial proceedings". Consequently, the ECJ ruled that what is considered "usual" within professional circles must be based on what is "sufficiently tried and tested by international medical science" rather than just what is considered usual in Dutch professional circles. It continued that "to allow only treatment habitually carried out on national territory and scientific views prevailing in national medical circles to determine what is or is not normal will not offer those guarantees and will make it likely that Dutch providers will always be preferred in practice".

Additional clarification was provided by the 2003 ruling in the *Müller-Fauré and Van Riet* case (European Court of Justice, 2003). It examined two cases involving Dutch citizens who had obtained treatment abroad without prior authorization, in one case as an in-patient and in the other as an outpatient. In the case of outpatient care it ruled that the principle of freedom to provide services precludes legislation requiring prior authorization, even under a benefits-in-kind scheme, in the case of non-hospital care provided in another Member State by a non-contracted provider. In the case of hospital treatment, national authorities retained the right to authorize treatment but in doing so they had to ensure that treatment could be provided by a contracted provider without undue delay and when deciding they must take account not only of the patient's actual medical condition but also, where appropriate, the degree of pain or the nature of his or her disability, which might, for example, make it impossible or extremely difficult for him or her to work.

Free movement in practice

Given the considerable uncertainty that has surrounded the more recent ECJ rulings, it is believed that most patients seeking to travel abroad for care have done so using the E112 procedures. In practice, and with a few exceptions, most Member States have been reluctant to authorize care in another Member State using this mechanism if it can be provided on their own territory. In a study published in 2000, Palm reported that the United Kingdom had issued only about 600 E112 forms each year, although more recent figures are higher, at around 1000, with about 200 issued in France but only about 20 in Sweden. Numbers were, however, rather higher in Belgium and Luxembourg, with about 2000 and 7000 authorizations respectively (Palm et al. 2000). Differences in willingness to authorize treatment become even greater when population size is taken into account. Unfortunately, further analysis is not possible because of the fragmentary nature of available data from many countries.

The low volume of cross-border movement by patients cannot, however, be attributed entirely to a reluctance by funding organizations to pay for treatment abroad. Other factors also contribute, including distance (with its associated travel time and costs, which the funding body is not obliged to pay for), language difficulties (Starmans et al. 1997), lack of information about the type of health care provided, unfamiliarity with other health care systems, an unwillingness of local doctors to refer patients to other countries and the administrative costs of the procedures involved (Mountford 2000).

What movement does take place is concentrated in certain border areas where particular geographical factors come into play (as is the case with Luxembourg, or the area around the province of Limburg in the south of the Netherlands) or where specific referral pathways have been developed, and it often involves high technology care. In some areas entities called Euregios have been established to facilitate such linkages. Examples include Meuse-Rhine (involving Belgium, Germany and the Netherlands), Schleswig/Sudjutland (Denmark and Germany), Scheldemond (Belgium and the Netherlands) and Hainaut/Nord-Pas-de-Calais (Belgium and France) (Palm et al. 2000). The Euregios have made it possible to develop simplified procedures based on the E112 scheme, with a special form "E112+" being used in Euregio Meuse-Rhine, with an adaptation of it used in Hainaut/Nord-Pas-de-Calais, where individuals have a special E112 form ("E112TF") that is linked to their health insurance card. Requests for payment are sent directly from the treating health facility to the insurance company.

Yet with the exception of Scheldemond, the numbers of patients involved in these schemes is fairly small, not usually exceeding a few hundred (Busse 2002). Even in these situations, it seems most commonly to benefit those with access to sufficient information (Hermesse 1999) and who are able to overcome what are often considerable practical and legal obstacles (Coheur 2001).

A study of frontier worker's use of cross-border health care between France and Belgium found a lack of knowledge about entitlements to and reimbursement mechanisms for accessing cross-border care to be an important disincentive to seeking such care. In the same study, a lack of appropriate treatment facilities in the home country, close proximity of facilities to the workplace and a good reputation of providers in the non-home country were all important motivations for seeking cross-border care (Calnan et al. 1997).

The situation is, however, changing rapidly, with growing awareness of new opportunities to obtain care abroad, in part as a consequence of media coverage of the recent ECJ cases. Several factors are likely to stimulate this demand further, including increased movement in general, less willingness to accept waiting lists, implementation of new and experimental treatments in some Member States and not in others, greater integration in border areas, and increased scope to compare prices due to monetary union. An issue of particular importance for health services is the increase in numbers of pensioners from northern Europe moving to southern Europe on retirement, and one that may create particular challenges for Malta and Cyprus following accession.

Encouragement for patients to become more active participants in a European health care market is likely to come first from health care providers, who are seeking to safeguard their own positions in an emerging European market; second, by health insurers seeking the best health services for their clients at the lowest cost; and third, by politicians and the media, seeking to raise awareness of differences in levels of provision as a means of exerting pressure on some countries to increase expenditure on health care.

Benefits and risks

While some commentators have interpreted the current situation as opening the way to an unregulated European market for patients, others have argued that it offers potential to improve access to health care while maintaining control over the cost and quality of care (Pieters 1999). Such developments need not only be confined to border areas, where contracting across the frontier could make it easier to provide a comprehensive range of health services, especially as many border areas are relatively sparsely populated. The variety of initiatives developed in the Euregios with the aim of improving access to care across borders, promote complementarity among existing health services. In addition, with rapid technological development leading towards greater concentration of certain types of diagnosis and treatment, Europe-wide planning based on centres of excellence may offer a more cost-effective way of ensuring highly technical care in a few specialized areas.

Unfortunately, the existing legal framework is far from satisfactory, as it has evolved in a piecemeal fashion through a series of often quite atypical cases. This shifting and often ambiguous context makes it very difficult for health policy-makers to ensure that the principle of free movement leads to benefits and not problems. One area requiring more immediate attention relates to standards of care provided in different countries. As has already been noted, the ECJ's decision that existing provisions ensured an acceptable quality of care within the existing Member States has been questioned (Nickless 2001), and concerns are also likely to exist in relation to those candidate countries that have experienced long-term underinvestment in the resources (human and physical) required to provide effective modern health care.

It seems likely that the pace of developments in this area will accelerate in the coming years, with important, but as yet uncertain implications for health care systems. One area where caution will be required is to ensure that increasing mobility does not increase social inequalities in access to care. Wealthier and better-informed citizens are the most likely to benefit from greater access to health care abroad so national health policy-makers must ensure that developments do not undermine their commitment to solidarity.

Cross-border healthcare provision and enlargement

Preparations for integrating the candidate countries into the EU's arrangements for coordination of social security arrangements began some years ago. In 1999 the Commission presented proposals for Council Decisions on the participation of candidate countries into the EU schemes. The initial discussion on cross-border care was based largely on Regulation 1408/71 and so has rather been overtaken by events.

Given the relatively small number of patients moving under the mechanisms of Regulation 1408/71, in the future it is likely that attention will focus on alternative provisions, based either on recent ECJ rulings or on separate bilateral arrangements with other Member States. Enhanced mobility can be seen as bringing both benefits and risks. On the positive side, accession may offer increased opportunities to offer health services to other countries and make use of spare capacity. On the negative side, candidate countries may have concerns that their national health plans may be disrupted if EU social security arrangements are changed to allow easier access to more expensive cross-border care so that large numbers of their citizens seek to travel to other EU

Member States for health care. In the remainder of this chapter we examine some of these possible consequences of greater patient movement in an enlarged EU.

Will candidate countries become treatment centres for Europe?

Most candidate countries are able to provide health care at relatively low cost to patients from other countries, a policy that health care providers in some countries are hoping to take advantage of. Some candidate countries, such as Hungary, are already experiencing increasing inflows of patients from neighbouring EU Member States such as Austria. Others, such as Slovenia, are looking at how they might attract increasing numbers of patients from current Member States.

The cost of health care in a country is the sum of the costs of a large number of individual inputs. Some, such as pharmaceuticals, are internationally traded and so tend to reflect (imperfectly) world market prices. Others, such as staff costs, are in general not internationally traded and so reflect local costs.

As salaries make up between 65% and 80% of recurrent health expenditure (Saltman and von Otter 1995; Kolehamainen-Aiken 1997), international differences in cost of care reflect, to a considerable extent, the cost of salaries. Given the gap between the magnitude of salaries in health systems in current Member States and in most candidate countries, it is unsurprising that health care costs are much lower in candidate countries.

Comparison of costs in different countries is inevitably complex because of differences in costing methodologies, such as definitions of system boundaries and allocation of shared costs, but Table 11.1 does give some indication of the variety that can be found within Europe.

Table 11.1   Charges for hip replacement service in private hospitals in various European countries (November 2002)

Country	Cost of a hip replacement (specialist fee, stay, surgery, prosthesis)
Belgium	€6587 (European HealthNet)
Czech Republic	€1754
France	€4620 (European HealthNet), €20000 (American Hospital, Paris)
Germany	€7000 (through Medibroker)
Hungary	€6600 (Budapest's only private hospital)
Ireland	€5605 (through European HealthNet)
Slovenia	€5675 (results of a survey performed by the MoH of Slovenia in 2002 and of the outputs of the Health Sector Management Project in Slovenia 2002
Spain	€4340 (European HealthNet)
UK	€10640–14840 (BUPA Hospitals – range depends on type of prosthesis)

Source: Calls to hospitals in November 2002, European HealthNet (*www.surgeryabroad.net/prices.htm*)

Candidate countries may therefore be able to offer health care to patients from other EU Member States at very competitive prices, even taking into account travel costs. Even more competitive prices would probably be available for bulk purchases by insurers. However, as the table also shows, there is considerable variation among existing Member States, some of which may be more accessible to countries facing the greatest capacity problems. Thus, a hip replacement can be obtained in Spain for about half the price charged in London. Similarly, knee replacement in France is offered by private medical brokers at about 55% of the cost of that in Belgium (www.surgeryabroad.net/prices.htm) and around 40% of the private cost in the United Kingdom.

Looking ahead, increasing labour costs in some candidate countries may undermine their current competitiveness. In Slovenia, for example, labour costs rose, on average, fourfold, from 1997 to 2002 (Bitenc 2002). Prices for orthopaedic care in one leading Slovene hospital serving international patients were almost comparable to those across the border in Italy in 2002. Numbers of patients coming from Italy to Slovenia for pre-arranged care have steadily decreased throughout the latter half of the 1990s and early 2000s. Salaries are likely to increase further as candidate countries face pressures to improve working conditions for health professionals to reduce the scale of migration to richer Member States.

The cost of care is, however, only one factor determining whether patients will travel to candidate countries, not least because, in most cases, it is borne by the insurer and not the patient. Furthermore, travelling abroad to obtain health care is only ever going to be an option for certain conditions, in particular non-urgent surgery for conditions that do not require lengthy follow-up. Except for frontier workers and those living for prolonged periods in another country, such as pensioners, it is irrelevant for the majority of health care that now involves the management of long-term chronic disorders. Furthermore, as experience in border areas within existing Member States shows, there are many disincentives to obtaining care abroad, including differences in language and poor understanding of or incompatibility of administrative arrangements.

It is certainly true that there is an imbalance between supply and demand for health care within Europe, with some countries experiencing waiting lists because of inadequate supply, but these countries are, in general, not the closest to the candidate countries. Thus, in the case of Slovenia, which borders Italy, any competitive advantage it may have is undermined by the relatively high unemployment among physicians in Italy (WHO 2002). Waiting lists are virtually unknown in Germany (Busse 2000) so there is unlikely to be much demand to obtain more rapid treatment in the Czech Republic or Poland from German patients. However, an important question is whether candidate countries actually have sufficient capacity to make this a reality.

To assess the scope for redressing the supply/demand imbalance it is necessary to look at the capacity available in candidate countries, here focusing on the countries of central and eastern Europe that have land borders with the existing Member States. Although most have undergone a process of reform which includes strengthening primary care, their health care systems remain heavily weighted in favour of hospitals. Superficial analyses have previously engendered a widespread perception that these countries have considerable excess capacity in their health care systems. Yet even a brief look at the numbers of doctors and beds per head of population, in comparison with the current EU average, appears to show the opposite.

Looking within the overall figures, it can be seen that the numbers of general practitioners in all candidate countries in which data are available are lower than the EU average. In contrast, larger numbers are working in a hospital sector that, at least on paper, is much larger than in the west, at least in terms of the conventional measure of hospital beds.

Inevitably these statistics do not convey the complete picture. Modern health care requires a balanced combination of people with the right skills, appropriate facilities to work in, and access to appropriate technology. In many cases the pattern of care that these statistics describe is one that is based on a model in which labour was cheap but capital (which for many years had to be paid for with hard currency and, in some cases, was blocked by western export controls) was expensive. As a consequence, many patients that would elsewhere have been treated in ambulatory care were managed inefficiently in hospitals which had suffered from many years of underinvestment. Consequently, the apparent excess capacity may be somewhat illusory when the quality of facilities is taken into account.

A further problem is that, as in some current Member States, there are important geographical inequalities in provision. In Hungary, for example, while it is widely accepted that there is excess hospital capacity in Budapest there are considerable shortages of medical staff in some rural areas (Gaal et al. 1999).

Table 11.2   Indicators of health service provision in candidate countries

	No. doctors/ 100000 population	No. doctors in primary care/100 000 population	No. hospital beds/100 000 (2000)	Average LOS
Malta	263	n/a	542	4.63
Slovenia	215*	46	555*	7.6*
Czech Republic	337	72	855	8.8
Cyprus	260***	n/a	476***	–
Slovakia	323	45	797	9.4
Poland	226*	n/a	581*	–
Bulgaria	337	75	741	–
Hungary	361*	67	841	6.7
Lithuania	380	63	924	8.3
Estonia	322	58	718	7.3
Latvia	320	41	873	–
Romania	189	81	744	–
Turkey	127*	70	264	5.4*
EU average	387	103	596	8.2**

* 1999   ** 1998   *** 1997   LOS = length of stay in days
Ref: All data apart from Cyprus HFA 2002. Cyprus data source website: http://www.emro.who.int/emrinfo/CountryProfiles-cyp.htm/)

So what is the scope for offering health care to patients from other countries? Certainly there are places, especially in major cities, where such capacity exists and is of appropriate quality, but the scale of provision may be much less that the crude figures suggest. Provision of care to patients from other countries in such facilities may provide a lucrative source of income. However, this may introduce a distortion into the market that would have consequences for a more equitable development of health care provision in other parts of the country. It may also introduce an incentive for medical professionals to choose the more marketable specialities, such as cardiology and elective surgery, at the expense of primary care.

An example of a country actively exploring the scope to attract patients is Slovenia (Albreht 2002). Albreht argues that while Slovenia does not have spare capacity at present, there is scope for expansion in a number of areas such as orthopaedics, spa treatment and cardiac, plastic and gynaecological surgery that would respond to demand from other countries. However, as already noted, increasing labour costs may undermine price competitiveness. Providers in other candidate countries are exploring similar options but such arrangements are not conditional on EU membership, as shown by the small stream of patients already coming to countries such as Slovenia, Hungary and the Czech Republic for non-urgent surgery, paying for themselves.

Finally, greater cross-border mobility must take account of the degree of comparability of quality of care. As noted above, in the *Kohll* and *Decker* cases, the ECJ held that existing provisions on mutual recognition of health professionals provided sufficient safeguards to patients obtaining treatment elsewhere.

Given the requirement, set out in Article 152 of the Amsterdam Treaty, that health care is a responsibility for Member States, the EU has been hesitant about becoming involved in health care quality, except in respect of those elements that are internationally traded, such as blood products and pharmaceuticals. There are no EU-wide standards for health care or common agreement on quality assurance, increasingly a problem as Member States incorporate ever more quality measures into ever more selective contracts. While these changes are being undertaken to enhance standards of care, the existence of potentially incompatible national systems could ultimately fall foul of European competition law if a requirement to comply with a particular system was seen as indirectly discriminatory.

This issue is likely to become more important with growing recognition of the degree of variation in outcomes achieved in different health care systems. For example, the Eurocare study has found substantial differences in cancer survival across Europe, with poorest results in some of the candidate countries and in the United Kingdom.

In summary, it is likely that providers in some candidate countries will be able to use their competitive advantages of localized spare capacity and lower prices to attract from abroad some patients requiring a limited range of treatments, in particular non-urgent surgery. However, such patients are likely to be self-payers and there is no reason why they cannot do so already – EU membership will not change anything. They may also experience some increased demand from growing numbers of frontier workers, but given that such individuals have very low requirements for health care, the demand is likely to be relatively small, as it is in the existing Member States. One group of people who may place a more substantial demand on health care facilities is pensioners who move from northern Europe. This is likely to be of greatest importance in Malta and Cyprus.

Will patients from candidate countries seek treatment abroad?

The second question related to patient mobility is even more difficult to answer. As the earlier part of this chapter showed, the current legal basis for patient mobility is not only confusing but also evolving. On accession, there will legally be nothing to stop a patient in a candidate country seeking outpatient care in another country. The health insurer in the home country will have to contribute to the cost of treatment. However, whether the insurer should pay according to the cost in the country of treatment or what it would have cost in the home country will depend on the mechanism used. If the provisions of Regulation 1408/71 are used, then the home insurer must pay in the same way as if it was established in the country where the patient was treated, which in the case of patients from candidate countries going to current Member States is likely to be considerably more than being treated at home. If the patient invokes the *Kohll* and *Decker* mechanism, travelling without prior authorization, then the insurer will only be required to pay what the treatment would have cost in the country of residence. However, in deciding what those costs would be, the mechanism used must be transparent and non-discriminatory. In such a case there would be no additional cost to the home insurer, except what might arise indirectly from increased volumes of treatment if substantial numbers of patients were able to circumvent cost-containment measures in the country of residence that are based on limiting supply, as illustrated by waiting lists for example.

The situation is, however, changing rapidly. The procession of cases, often involving quite specific issues, have left many areas of uncertainty. One that is likely to attract increasing attention is where hospitals in one country, as in the Netherlands, are required to recover the cost of capital investment through their charges for treatment, while in others, as in Germany, the capital costs are largely paid by government. Is this a form of subsidy and so an indirect distortion of competition? This question has yet to be resolved.

Conclusions

Free movement of patients has been a reality in the EU for over 30 years. Yet the numbers of patients moving across borders to receive care has never been great. In a few border areas, where geographical and linguistic factors make it a sensible option, health care providers have developed solutions that bring mutual benefits. Yet even in these situations many disincentives to travel remain.

References

Albreht, T. (2002) Opportunities and challenges in the provision of cross-border care: View from Slovenia, *Eurohealth*, 8(4):8–10.

Bitenc, M. (2002) Report of the President of the Medical Chamber of Slovenia dr. 37th Assembly of the Medical Chamber of Slovenia, 20 March.

Bosco, A. (2000) *Are national social Protection Systems under threat? Observations on the recent Case Law of the Court of Justice.* Paris: Notre Europe.

Busse, R. (2000) *Health Care Systems in Transition: Germany.* Copenhagen: European observatory on Health Care Systems.

Busse, R. (2002) Border-crossing patients in the EU, *Eurohealth*, 8(4 special issue):19–21.

Busse, R., Drews, M. and Wismar, M. (2002) Consumer choice of healthcare services across borders, in R. Busse, M. Wismar and P. Berman (eds) *The European Union and Health Services – The Impact of the Single European Market on Member States.* IOS Press.

Calnan, M., Palm, W., Sohy, F. and Quaghebeur, D.N.A. (1997) Cross-border use of health care: A survey of frontier workers' knowledge, attitudes and use, *European Journal of Public Health*, 7(Supplement 3):26–32.

Coheur, A. (2001) Cross-border care: New Prospects for Convergence. Paper presented at the conference organized during the Belgian Presidence of the European Union. "European Integration and Health Care Systems: A Challenge for Social Policy." Ghent.

Cornellisen, R. (1996) The Principle of Territoriality and the Community Regulations on Social Security, *Common Market Law Review No. 3.*

Council of the European Communities (1981) Council Regulation 2793/81/EEC of 17 September 1981 amending Regulation (EEC) 1408/71 on the application of social security schemes to employed persons and their families moving within the Community and Regulation (EEC) 574/72 fixing the procedure for implementing Regulation (EEC) 1408/71. Official Journal of the European Union L275.

Council of the European Communities (1993) Council Directive 93/16/EEC of 5 April 1993 to facilitate the free movement of doctors and the mutual recognition of their diplomas, certificates and other evidence of formal qualifications. Official Journal of the European Union L165/1–24.

Department for Work and Pensions (2002) A summary of the European community Regulations on social security for migrant workers, http://www.dwp.gov.uk/publications/dss/1997/ie/annexa.htm.

European Commission (2002) Decision No. 183. Official Journal of the European Communities.

European Commission (2003) Communication from the Commission concerning the introduction of a European health insurance card. 73 final. 17 February 2003. Brussels: European Commission.

European Court of Justice (2003) *Müller-Fauré v Onderlinge Waarborgmaatschappij OZ Zorgverzekeringen and Van Riet v Onderlinge Waarborgmaatschappij ZAO Zorgverzekeringen.* C-385/99 13 May 2003.

Fillon, J.C. (1999) La Citoyennete de l'Union europeenne et la coordination de regimes de securite, *Journal des Tribunaux du Travail*, 747:393–403.

Gaal, P., Rekassy, B. and Healy, J. (1999) *Health Care Systems in Transition: Hungary.* Copenhagen: WHO Regional Office for Europe.

Hermesse, J. (1999) The opening of Frontiers to Patients: What Economic Consequences? AIM International Symposium Health Care without Frontiers within the European Union. Brussels, AIM.

Jamison, J., Butler, M., Clarke, P., McKee, M. and Oneill, C. (2001) *Cross-border Co-operation in Health Services in Ireland.* Armagh: Centre for Cross-Border Studies.

Kesteloot, K., Pocceschi, S. and van der Schueren, E. (1995) The Reimbursement of the Expenses for Medical Treatment Received by "transnational" patients in EU-countries, *Health Policy*, 43–57.

Kolehamainen-Aiken, R.L. (1997) Decentralisation and human resources: implications and impact, *Human Resource Development Journal*, 2(1):1–14.

Mossialos, E. and McKee, M. (2002) *EU Law and the Social Character of Health Care*. Brussels: Peter Lang.

Mountford, L. (2000) *Healthcare without frontiers? The development of a European market in health services?* London: Office of Health Economics.

Nickless, J. (2001) A Guarantee of Similar Medical Standards Right Across Europe: Were the European Court of Justice Decisions in Kohll and Decker Right?, *Eurohealth*, 7(1):16–18.

Nickless, J. (2002) A Guarantee of Similar Standards of Medical Treatment across the EU: Were the European Court of Justice Decisions in Kohll and Decker Right?, *Eurohealth*, 7(1):16–18.

Palm, W., Nickless, J., Lewalle, H. and Coheur, A. (2000) Implications of Recent Jurisprudence on the Co-ordination of Health Care Protection Systems – General report produced for the Directorate General for Employment and Social Affairs of the European Commission. Brussels: Association International de la Mutualité.

Pieters, D. (1999) De Nederlandse zorgverzekering in het licht van het recht van de EG, Achtergrondstudie in opdracht van de Raad voor de volksgezondheid en Zorg bij het RVZ-advies Europea en genondheidszorg. Zoetermeer.

Saltman, R.B. and von Otter, C. (1995) *Implementing planned markets in healthcare: balancing social and economic responsibility*. Buckingham: Open University Press.

Starmans, B., Leidl, R. and Rhodes, G. (1997) A comparative study on cross-border hospital care in the Euregio Meuse-Rhine, *European Journal of Public Health*, 7(3):33–41.

Van der Mei, A.P. (2001) Free Movement of persons within the European Community, Cross-border Access to Public Benefits. Maastricht: Hart Publishing.

Van Raepenbusch, S. (1997) Le champ d'application personnel du reglement no 1408/71 et la cioyennete europeenne: du travailleur migran au citoyen europeen, *Journal des Tribunaux du Travail*, 665:1–7.

WHO (2002) European Health for all Database. WHO Regional Office for Europe. www.surgeryabroad.net/prices.htm.

twelve

Closing the gap: Health and safety

Alison Wright-Reid, Martin McKee and Laura MacLehose

The EU and public health

To understand the role of the EU in the area of public health it is necessary to look back at the historical development of European integration. The EU arose from the 1950 Schuman Plan, which sought to ensure that the war in Europe that had ended only five years previously, which was the third between France and Germany in under a century, never happened again. The immediate goal was to pool coal and steel production in France and Germany, so limiting the ability of either to act militarily against the other, placing it under a supranational authority. This concept was formalized in the 1951 European Coal and Steel Community (ECSC), one of the precursors of the European Economic Community and subsequently the EU. Thus, while the EU is a political entity, its roots are firmly based in economic cooperation and the promotion of free trade.

As in all arrangements to promote free trade, considerations of public health cannot be ignored. Historically, there has always been a tension between the urge to ease the flow of goods across borders while preventing the simultaneous movement of infectious agents, most notably in the institution of quarantine by the Venetian Republic, which was especially vulnerable to plague and cholera due to its trading links with the Black Sea and the Arabian peninsula respectively.

Consequently, protection of health was included within the 1957 European Economic Community (EEC) Treaty, although only to the extent of providing a basis for action to restrict trade where health is threatened. Specifically, it permitted restrictions on imports and exports between Members States to protect the "health and life of humans, animals or plants". The rather general nature of this provision was subsequently qualified following the *Cassis de Dijon* case in the European Court of Justice (ECJ), which established the principle of proportionality. In other words, any action taken to restrict trade should be proportionate to the objective being pursued and not achievable in another way, such as enhanced labelling. Any action must also be part of a "seriously considered health policy" and be necessary to protect health while going no further than is necessary.

The unsatisfactory nature of these provisions was exposed by the BSE scandal in the 1990s, which was ultimately addressed under provisions relating to safeguarding agricultural markets rather than concern for human health. The lessons from this episode had a major impact on how public health was handled in the European Commission, including the creation of a new Directorate-General for Health and Consumer Protection.

The perennial challenge facing those working at the interface between health and trade policies is when to act, given that sufficient evidence of harm is often unavailable until it is too late. This dilemma has given rise to the concept of the "Precautionary Principle", which in essence means that where there are potential serious or irreversible threats to health a lack of scientific evidence should not be used as a reason for failing to put in place effective measures to counter this possible threat. The principle was set out in a non-binding Communication from the Commission in 2000 (Commission of the European Communities 2000). However, it is not yet enshrined in any binding EU legislation in relation to human health,[1] although the EU (and individual Member States) are bound by it in the context of actions governed by World Trade Organization (WTO) rules.

Health did, however, appear in some other places in the original treaties. The Treaty establishing the European Atomic Energy Community included provisions pertaining to radiation safety and research and the ECSC included provisions relating to the working conditions of coal and steel workers, including assessment of threats to their health. Of course, as noted elsewhere in this book, many aspects of the Treaties have implications for health systems (such as legislation relating to the free movement of personnel) but an explicit consideration of public health had to wait for the 1992 Maastricht Treaty, which contained a specific Article (Article 129) on public health, subsequently amended as Article 152 in the 1997 Treaty of Amsterdam.

It should also be noted that the Member States did feel able to take action on public health prior to the Maastricht Treaty, in particular by establishing the Europe against Cancer programme, which in turn set a precedent for the Europe against AIDS programme. These programmes were justified on the basis that the European Community has established an objective of promoting "an accelerated raising of the standard of living", illustrating that action is possible even on rather dubious legal grounds when the political will exists.

Article 129 and beyond

Article 129 of the Maastricht Treaty required that "the Community shall contribute towards ensuring a high level of human health protection by encouraging cooperation between the Member States and, if necessary, lending support to their actions". It continued "Community action shall be directed towards the prevention of diseases, in particular the major health scourges, including drug dependence, by promoting research into their causes and their transmission, as well as health information and education". To achieve these goals, it permitted adoption of "incentive measures, excluding any harmonisation of the laws and regulations of the Member States".

At Amsterdam, Article 152 went further in promoting a broad view of public health through calling for consideration of health in all EU activities, stating that "A high level of health protection shall be ensured in the definition and implementation of all Community policies and activities". It then goes on to reinforce the priorities outlined in the Maastricht Treaty stating:

> Community action, which shall complement national policies, shall be directed towards improving public health, preventing human illness and diseases, and obviating sources of danger to human health. Such action shall cover the fights against major health scourges, by promoting research into their causes, their transmission and their prevention, as well as health information and education.

Prevention of drug related health damage is again mentioned specifically, essentially as this was a means to ensure that it was treated as a public health issue and not, as some wished, as simply a criminal justice matter. In addition, safety related to blood and blood products and organs is mentioned for the first time.

The Maastricht and Amsterdam Treaty provisions for public health recognize, for the first time, that while health care remains the preserve of national authorities, there are public health benefits to be gained by means of cooperation through the institutions of the EU. In reality, cooperation between governments in areas of public health had always taken place, either on a government to government basis or through the World Health Organization. This at last recognized the importance of tackling some of the major threats to human health, such as the spread of communicable disease or promotion of tobacco at the level of the EU.

However, while the inclusion in the Treaty of a European competence in public health was widely welcomed, at least by those with an interest in promoting health, the Articles have been criticized, in particular because of the ambiguities and uncertainties in their wording. For example, the term "scourges", used to indicate threats to health, is nowhere defined, although this vagueness has also allowed the Commission to support a variety of public health related activities requiring coordinated action at the EU level. In particular, as will be described in more detail in the next chapter, it has supported a range of initiatives in communicable disease surveillance.

Yet the scope for action on public health is heavily circumscribed. Article 152 only permits adoption of "incentive measures designed to protect and improve human health, excluding any harmonisation of the laws and regulations of the Member States". Even in an area where it is widely agreed that action was needed, in the wake of scandals in which blood products were contaminated with HIV and Hepatitis C, the Article specifies that "measures . . . shall not affect national provisions on the donation or medical use of organs and blood".

While the Article requires that health considerations should be taken into account in all EU policies, unlike the situation with environmental protection where the precautionary principle is endorsed, the means of taking health concerns into account is unclear, with commentators frequently drawing attention to the incompatibility of this goal with the provision of subsidies for tobacco production.

One area where Article 152 is especially problematic is its specific statement that health systems are exclusively a matter for national governments. Elsewhere in this book it has been noted how, given that most of the inputs into health systems are subject to EU law, this effectively subjects health systems to arguments based on competition law without a possibility to take considerations of health into account. It also has the paradoxical effect of excluding the one sector that is arguably most closely related to promotion of health from consideration in health policy discussions. In summary, therefore, the present wording seems to permit action where there is consensus, but obstruct it where there are strong vested interests opposing health promoting activities (see also Chapter 14).

As this brief review shows, a competency in public health at the EU level is a relatively new concept and the measures available to achieve its somewhat undefined goals are themselves unclear. Yet, as will be described below, progress has been made in a number of key areas, building on the provisions in the EU treaties, with implications for enlargement. Yet several questions arise. How easy will it be for candidate countries to raise standards where necessary to EU levels? On the other hand, given that some candidate countries have already gone beyond what is required in the EU, will they have to dilute their policies? Are existing EU level initiatives in the field of public health sufficiently robust to respond to the needs of an additional 15 countries, many with very different health needs from the existing Member States? And what preparations are being made for enlargement?

To consider some of these questions this chapter and the next one will look at four key areas: health and safety, communicable disease surveillance and control, and, in Chapter 14, policies on tobacco and alcohol.

Health and safety legislation is selected as it exemplifies what is commonly, but falsely, seen as a tension between economic performance and health. Health and safety legislation, as noted earlier, was the first health related area in which the European Communities had competence. As the EU expands, it is important to assess how current requirements will impact on the candidate countries. Communicable disease control invokes the original tension between free trade and public health and represents an area where concerted European action has long been needed, if slow to develop, simply because micro-organisms have always enjoyed free movement, being completely unconstrained by national frontiers.

Health and safety at work: The case for a level playing field

Health and safety legislation is an essential response to market failure. In an ideal world, employers would invest in safety to reduce damage to their human and other resources, and workers would shun highly paid but dangerous work to maximize their working life. In reality, the short-termism that dominates unregulated free markets creates incentives for employers and workers to go for immediate gains at the expense of longer-term costs, many of which are borne by others.

Poor employers can flourish for quite some time, profiting while competitors spend time and money eradicating or minimizing safety problems. The poor employers simply consume people, discarding those too ill or injured to continue in employment, so transferring costs to the state, to insurance schemes and to their workers and their families.

The costs of poor safety are considerable: even in the current 15 Member States breaches of safety cost between 2.6% and 3.8% of GNP, or from 1% to 5% of operating profits in most sectors. Each year almost 5500 lives are ended in industrial accidents. A similar number are permanently disabled and 4.8 million people are unable to work for at least 4 days – many of these people will be badly injured or maimed. The United Kingdom has low rates of industrial injury, but even there an individual is twice as likely to be killed at work than to be murdered, and ten times as likely to die from asbestos exposure. If the United Kingdom's experience is typical, then 140 000 EU workers are, each year, disabled as a consequence of their work. One single health risk, asbestos, may claim as many as half a million European lives (Murray and Lopez 1996). The personal costs of inadequate health and safety are considerable. Of people sufficiently injured to claim workers' compensation [or the equivalent] nearly a quarter become dependent on state welfare, making this the third most common route into welfare dependency (Quinlan and Mayhew 1999). A study of people who have suffered from work related upper limb disorders showed that their promotion prospects fell by more than half, and that compared with uninjured colleagues they were twice as likely to become divorced and three and a half times as likely to lose their home (Morse et al. 1998). In the long term, reducing risks to health and safety increases productivity and profitability. The World Bank has estimated that two-thirds of occupationally determined loss of healthy life years could be prevented by occupational health and safety programmes. But, in the short term the strong externalities associated with health and safety policies allow some firms to make profits at the expense of more conscientious competitors. Likewise, firms in a country with poor safety standards can operate with a lower cost base than in safer states. To ensure a level playing field, the EU has imposed minimum health and safety standards. No Member State can ignore them but each, as the ECJ has ruled, has "full powers to adopt or maintain national measures which guarantee workers a higher standard of protection".

European legislation on health and safety

As noted previously, Europe's role in health and safety stretches back to 1951 when the European Coal and Steel Community established a programme of research and standard setting, and created special commissions for the steel and mining industries [including offshore oil wells]. In addition, the original six countries agreed the Euratom Treaty, creating a requirement to establish standards of protection in the nuclear industry. In 1957, the Treaty of Rome allowed for the introduction of provisions on health and safety if they were agreed unanimously by the Council of Ministers. Article 100 of the Treaty concerned maximum standards, while Article 118 allowed for minimum standards, but for employed people. Thus, even now, the more than 20 million workers who are themselves employers or are self-employed are only protected to the extent that governments have chosen to exceed the EU minimum. Some Directives were made under these provisions, but there was little progress until, in 1974, the Council initiated a social action programme that included specific reference to health and safety and led to new Directives on safety signs and vinyl chloride monomer. That programme also produced the Advisory Committee on Safety Hygiene and Health Protection at Work, which became the main forum for employers, trade unions and representatives of national authorities to debate the development of a detailed European health and safety policy.

The first Action Programme on health and safety, announced in 1978, led to more legislation, most significantly the "harmful agents Directive" (80/610/ EEC, later amended by 88/642/EEC) and the asbestos, lead and noise Directives. Six years later, the second Action Programme was more extensive but little faster, since the need for a unanimous decision by Council effectively gave any nation the power of veto. The need for unanimity not only prevented legislation from being agreed but it also produced distortions in Directives that are being not just perpetuated but exaggerated in next-generation Directives. This obstacle was removed in 1986 by the Single European Act which introduced qualified majority voting for health and safety Directives, and permitted a very ambitious third Action Programme in 1987 (to prepare for the single market in 1992). This third programme was spearheaded by the Framework Directive 89/391 on the introduction of measures to encourage improvements in the safety and health of workers at work. That Directive and its successors have become the dominant source of new health and safety law in Member States. In establishing these minimum standards, the EU's aim is to achieve harmonization, a more ambitious goal than simple convergence of national law. Harmonization has several aims. One is to give workers similar protection in different Member States. Another is to ensure that health and safety does not become marginalized as a consequence of competition. A third is to ensure that goods that move freely within the EU are safe. The safety of goods was addressed in the Single European Act with changes to Article 100A of the Treaty of Rome, resulting in the "new approach" product Directives, supported by the European standards organizations CEN and CENELEC. Article 100A Directives have included the machinery Directive (89/392/EEC) and the personal protective equipment Directive (89/686 EEC). Essentially, these laws set maximum standards, such that, where an item has been approved as meeting the appropriate standard by a qualified body in one Member State, another Member State cannot require that the testing be repeated, or that more stringent standards be met.

In the mid-1990s EU momentum on health and safety diminished as deregulatory pressures (including pressure from the Anglo-German Deregulation Group and from the Molitor Group) increased. Qualified majority voting had unleashed a considerable quantity of legislation, so to some extent a breathing space was welcomed. However, the consequences have been fewer Directives, less penetrating Directives and, allegedly, a tendency for Member States to treat the minimum requirements in Directives rather as though they were desirable targets. For example, in the United Kingdom there is constant pressure to avoid "gold-plating" Directives during transposition into national law.

Article 118a states that Directives should avoid imposing administrative, financial and legal constraints in a way which might hold back the creation and development of small and medium-sized enterprises (SMEs). SMEs are an increasingly important source of new employment, particularly in the candidate countries, and are a key element in the EU's employment strategy. Unfortunately it is becoming clear that SMEs are often significantly more dangerous employers than large enterprises.

How much detail should health and safety legislation go into? A fanatical level of detail in rules on safety has a certain appeal. But it also has considerable drawbacks. The scale of regulation can easily exceed the scope of any individual's memory or comprehension. In addition, there is often a long delay between the emergence of a risk and the development of an appropriate rule (five years or more for most legislatures). The Framework Directive escapes these problems by adopting the approach developed by many Member States. Under this approach, what must be achieved is stated (rather than how); certain processes must be undertaken (risk assessment, consultation); updating mechanisms are incorporated (practicability, and the review of assessments); and a link is created between economic goals and health and safety (proportionality or reasonable practicability).

Health and safety in the candidate countries

Ten years ago, many candidate countries had surprisingly effective health and safety systems, but cuts in resources during the transition period frequently inflicted lasting damage. While Malta and Cyprus have systems not dissimilar to those in the Member States, central and eastern European (CEE) states typically had "top-down" systems with trade unions functioning as inspectors (officials ensuring implementation of health and safety legislation). Often different ministries, with negligible cooperation, managed occupational safety and occupational health; managers were relatively powerless and employees were frequently conditioned to take neither initiative nor responsibility. This situation was not, however, uniformly good. In many cases, protection of the environment came a poor second to promoting employment. Results from monitoring of the working environment were sometimes manipulated to prove either that the safe standard was observed or that hazard pay was due; high levels of unemployment in some regions lead to acceptance of risk, with very poor working conditions in sectors such as mining and industries handling hazardous substances. Long-established practices have persisted in many places and an International Labour Office study found that the proportion of workplaces offering hazard pay ranged from 89% in Bulgaria to 25% in Hungary (Rice and Repo 2000). Such payments create an incentive for some trade unionists to promote, rather than prevent, dangerous working conditions as a means of improving salaries. Now new foreign owned enterprises typically offer safer working conditions, but tend to recruit a non-unionized workforce. Thus, in spite of support through European Commission financed twinning arrangements, tripartite relationships between government, employers associations and trade unions are extremely weak in some candidate countries.

Enlargement and health and safety

The EU's preference for tripartite relationships between governments, employers and workers is not simply political ideology: effective input from employers and workers makes for better law, greater commitment to that law and more effective implementation. In addition, effective trade union input to safety significantly lowers accident rates (Reilly et al. 1995). Most candidate countries have, however, adopted the *acquis* without worker or employer input, and many have changed their law without changing their systems.

There is often an assumption that EU law is better than existing national legislation, but pressure from new members, as well as from small and medium-sized enterprises, may provoke a reappraisal of the existing (low detail, high collaboration) model of legislation. Apart from stylistic arguments, is it adequate? The exclusion of the self-employed is perhaps the most important deficiency in EU law. With enlargement there will be increasing need to remedy this as, overall, about 22% of people working in candidate countries (33% in Poland) are self-employed, compared with 17% in the Member States. This is doubly important as the self-employed are more likely to be injured at work. Member States occupational accident statistics exclude the self-employed; their inclusion would increase the annual death toll from 6000 to 9000.

The Framework Directive makes no mention of enforcement. Yet without policing, the law has little value and workers obtain no protection. It is hard to determine whether this is a problem as EU monitoring addresses only transposition and accident statistics reveal more about reporting rates than compliance. Here, data on safety of equipment provides a useful example. A study of CE marked machines (marked to indicate conformity to EU safety standards) found that, in the Member States, less than one-sixth were properly marked or even safe (Raafat and Nicholas 1999). Criticisms have been made that some Member States fail to comply with the *acquis* that candidate countries are required to adopt upon accession. The EU intends to address compliance (European Commission 2002), but it is unclear how the small number of Commission staff will cope. Furthermore, the lead role is given to the Senior Labour Inspectors Committee – the only EU health and safety body which is not tripartite.

EU law necessitates a more participative style of inspection than the prescriptive model that has been in place in many candidate countries; employers and workers need detailed guidance and inspectors must consult and listen to workers, employers and experts. For the inspectors this will demand new attitudes, knowledge, skills and structures. The retraining demand is considerable and, notwithstanding the support provided by twinning arrangements, "reformed" inspectors often have few suitably experienced colleagues from whom to seek advice.

Providing adequate resources for enforcement is also a challenge, even in some current Member States. Romania has one inspector per 80 000 workers compared to 1 per 47 500 in Spain, about 1 per 10 000 in the United Kingdom, Denmark and Sweden, and 1 per 6000 in Finland (European Commission 2002). While Commission employees are not inspectors, their numbers are clearly relevant to any discussion of EU legislation or compliance. It is, therefore, startling to discover that the Commission's Health and Safety Unit has dwindled to just 24 people. After enlargement there will be only one Commission professional for every 10 million workers.

In summary, while some candidate countries begin with effective, compatible safety systems, most must compress 30 or more years of change into as many months, with few resources. The task is far from insignificant.

Note

1 The precautionary principle is not defined in any of the EU Treaties for health specifically. However, in Article 174 of the 1992 Maastricht Treaty the treaty legislates for the use of the precautionary principle for environmental protection. It states "Community policy on the environment shall aim at a high level of protection taking into account the diversity of situations in the various regions of the Community. It shall be based on the precautionary principle and on the principles that preventive action should be taken . . ."

References

Commission of the European Communities (2000) Communication From the Commission to the Council, The European Parliament, The Economic and Social Committee and the Committee of the Regions on the Health Strategy of the European Community. Brussels: Commission of the European Communities.

European Commission (2002) Adapting to change in work and society: a new community strategy on health and safety at work 2002–2006. COM 2002 118 final European Health and Safety Agency. The State of Occupational Safety and Health in the European Union – Pilot Study. Bilbao: European Union Commission.

Morse, T.F., Dillon, C., Warren, N., Levenstein, C. and Warren, A. (1998) The economic and social consequences of work-related musculoskeletal disorders: the Connecticut Upper-Extremity Surveillance Project (CUSP), *International Journal of Occupational and Environmental Health*, 4:209–16.

Murray, C.J.L. and Lopez, A.D. (1996) *The global burden of disease: A comprehensive assessment of mortality and disability from diseases, injuries and risk factors in 1990 and projected to 2020.* Boston, MA: Harvard University Press.

Quinlan, M. and Mayhew, C. (1999) Precarious employment and workers' compensation, *International Journal of Law and Psychiatry*, 22:491–520.

Raafat, H. and Nicholas, R. (1999) Analysis of the degree of machinery suppliers' compliance with relevant EU requirements. Birmingham: Health and Safety Unit, Aston University.

Reilly, B., Paci, P. and Holl, P. (1995) Unions, Safety Committees and Workplace Injuries, *British Journal of Industrial Relations*, 33(2):275–88.

Rice, A. and Repo, P. (2000) Health and Safety at the Workplace – Trade Union Experiences in Central and Eastern Europe. Budapest: ILO SRO-Budapest.

thirteen

Communicable disease control: Detecting and managing communicable disease outbreaks across borders

Laura MacLehose, Richard Coker and Martin McKee

Policies to detect and control the spread of communicable disease have long been a necessary corollary to policies on free trade. However, effective policies at an international level depend crucially on the quality of national surveillance and control systems.

The current wave of enlargement will create important challenges for these systems. First, the degree of development of these networks is already uneven in the existing Member States and will be even more so in an enlarged EU. Second, many of the candidate countries in central and eastern Europe have levels of communicable disease that are higher than in the current EU. Rates of HIV infection remain low compared to other parts of the world but are rising extremely quickly in some countries (Dobson 2001). Rates of tuberculosis have also increased markedly, in particular in the Baltic states, and especially among prison populations (Stern 1999), where there are growing rates of drug resistant disease (Farmer et al. 1999). Some animal borne infections, such as leptospirosis in Bulgaria (Stoilova and Popivanova 1999) and tick-borne encephalitis in the Baltic states (Randolph 2001) have increased as a consequence of changes in land use. Third, and perhaps most importantly, the expanded EU will have borders with several countries (Belarus, Ukraine, Republic of Moldova, Georgia, Armenia, Iran, Iraq and Syria) where levels of communicable disease are very much higher than in those on the borders of the current Member States. In this respect, the spread of multi-resistant tuberculosis from Russia to Finland highlights the need for concern (Loytonen and Maasilta 1998).

The development of communicable disease control in the EU

The roots of modern communicable disease control in Europe can be traced at least as far back as the fifteenth century. The relative lack of geographical barriers in the Eurasian land mass did much to foster international trade and increase prosperity but brought in its wake the threat of infectious disease and, especially, plague (McNeill 1976) and cholera. The Venetians introduced quarantine (from the Italian "quarante die" meaning "forty days") at their ports, a strategy subsequently adopted throughout western Europe to control the spread of disease. The quarantine policy, while initially effective, faced two major challenges in the mid-1800s. The first was the increasing volume and, especially, the speed of trade due to the introduction of the railway and the steamship. Delays caused by quarantine became increasingly costly and conflicted with calls for "free trade". The second was the appearance in the cities of Europe of cholera, which had circumvented the existing controls.

In an attempt to balance the interests of health and international trade, the first International Sanitary Conference convened in Paris in 1851, attended by representatives of 11 European countries. This initiated a process that was to lead to a series of International Conferences, giving rise to a permanent International Committee on Epidemics (1874), the adoption of the International Sanitary Convention (ISC), and ultimately paving the way for the current international system for control of infectious disease. By 1903 the International Sanitary Conference agreed that states would "immediately notify the other governments of the first appearance in its territory of authentic cases of plague or cholera" (Fidler 1999). This eventually led to the formulation of the International Health Regulations (IHR), which were adopted by the 22nd World Health Assembly in July 1969. The IHR, with which all EU Member States have agreed to comply, are currently being revised. The major changes are a new real time event management system, in which information will be drawn from a much wider range of sources than at present, so avoiding the problems that arise when an outbreak is reported in the international media but apparently remains unknown to the national authorities involved, strengthening of national surveillance capacities and inclusion of a much broader range of "public health emergencies of international concern" (the old regulations covered only smallpox, cholera, plague and yellow fever).

The complex relationship between trade and health made it inevitable that health would be taken account of in the Treaties establishing the European Communities. The Treaty of Rome created four freedoms of movement among Member States, covering persons, services, goods and capital, the first three of which have implications for communicable disease control. These freedoms have been progressively extended to the candidate countries through current Association Agreements. The four freedoms were, however, qualified, with Member States permitted to restrict movement for a variety of grounds, including the protection of health.

By the 1980s, however, as noted previously, it became clear that EU safeguards to health were unsatisfactory, eroding public confidence in the safety of certain goods, in particular foodstuffs. Furthermore, there was growing evidence that existing surveillance and control systems, based on national structures, were inadequate in the face of outbreaks that crossed borders. An evaluation of the response to five outbreaks affecting more than one country identified major weaknesses (Brand et al. 2000).

Development of common surveillance arrangements were, initially, slow to take off as enthusiasm for involvement of the European Commission in health matters was weak. Although Article 129 of the Maastricht Treaty provided a legal basis for action, EU efforts in the field of communicable disease were mainly focused on HIV/AIDS surveillance and prevention (European Parliament and Council 1996), under the Europe against AIDS programme that predated the Maastricht Treaty. However, it did lead to a programme of action in the field of public health that provided short-term project funding to support a range of networks assembled largely by groups of enthusiasts in national surveillance centres and academic departments who had identified a need for coordinated action that seemed to have been overlooked by governments of the Member States. The successes achieved by those networks made the case for further, more sustained action, identifying outbreaks that would otherwise have been missed. An example was an outbreak of legionnaires' disease where it was possible to link occurrences of disease in holidaymakers who had stayed in a hotel outside the EU but had since dispersed to several different countries (Joseph and Lee 1996). Indeed, of the travel associated legionnaires' disease clusters reported to the European Working Group on Legionella Infections in 1999 (EWGLI), 41% of these were detected by pooling international data and would have been missed by national surveillance systems alone (Lever and Joseph 2001).

More recently, communicable disease control has been given a much higher priority by political concerns about a potential threat from bioterrorism as it has been recognized that an effective response is critically dependent on the speed of initial detection of an outbreak. In this way, it is no different from occurrences of more conventional threats from communicable disease.

Current EU surveillance and control initiatives

From a somewhat hesitant beginning, collaboration at the level of the EU in the field of communicable disease control is now well established. It is based on two fora: the "Charter Group" and the "Network Committee", the former being made up of heads of national surveillance institutes and the latter, two experts on surveillance from each Member State. In 2002, the status of the Charter Group was formalized as the "Council for European State Epidemiologists for Communicable Disease" (CESE) (Hoile 2002). The pace with which these developments have taken place contrasts with the drawn out nature of policy-making in other health related areas in the EU, highlighting the possibility for rapid action where there is a relatively high degree of consensus.

The precise mechanisms for cooperation have, however, been controversial, in particular generating extensive debate about whether to base arrangements of dispersed networks or to develop a supra-national European centre (Tibayrenc 1997; Bradbury 1998; Editorial 1998; Giesecke and Weinberg 1998). The debate seemed to have been resolved in 1998 when agreement was reached on a "network approach" but as communicable disease has risen higher on the political agenda it has now been decided to create a European Centre on Communicable Disease, which is scheduled to be in place by 2005 (Byrne 2002). The new organization will, however, be very much smaller than its equivalent in the USA, with an initial staff of only 15, and will act primarily as a coordinating hub for the existing networks.

Until then, formal Europe-wide cooperation will continue to be based solely on the various networks in which interested centres can choose to participate. The legal framework for the networks was set out in Decision 2119/98/EC (European Parliament 1998), and reinforced in the November 1998 Council Conclusions on the Future Framework for Community Action in Public Health (European Commission 1998). Decision 2119/98/EC was complemented, in 1999, by Decision 2000/57/EC which established a European early warning and response system aimed at certain types of communicable disease events (European Commission 1999) and Decision 2000/96/EC outlined a list of communicable diseases to be progressively covered by the new EU networks (together known as "the Community Network") (European Parliament 1999). Two other major European programmes also began in the 1990s, a European intervention epidemiology training programme and two online EU surveillance journals, *EuroSurveillance Weekly* and *EuroSurveillance Monthly*.

The networks enable cases to be pooled, allowing detection of outbreaks involving more than one country that might previously have been missed and providing countries with information about outbreaks that may originate in their manufacturing processes but lead to cases elsewhere, so enabling rapid product withdrawal. Yet despite its many successes, the EU "Community Network" has yet to resolve a range of important issues, in particular security of funding, definition of organizational responsibilities, common preparedness planning and a lack of common control measures (MacLehose et al. 2001). Links with the new structures to combat any threat from bioterrorism remain unclear (Tegnell et al. 2002).

Because EU legislation in communicable disease control extends largely to coordination of efforts rather than harmonization of activities, weaknesses are increasingly apparent in relation to border health control. For example, a recently conducted survey of WHO European Region countries showed that screening policies and practices to detect tuberculosis infection among new entrants across Europe are extremely varied. Many countries have no formal policies and those that do differ in their formal arrangements. No two countries take the same regulatory, institutional or clinical approaches (Coker et al. in press). As in the past, in recent years control of communicable diseases associated with migration has provoked popular anxiety (Kraudt 1994). Proposed responses have often included separate, but linked, emotive issues such as immigration policy, "health tourism", migrant health workers, and mandatory screening of different populations. Evidence-based communicable disease control policy is likely to be a victim when the emotional temperature is fired by popular unease.

So while most effort in recent years has focused upon improving surveillance, coherent approaches to control that go beyond this have received considerably less attention. As the EU enlarges, the importance of resolving the organizational and funding issues facing the Community Network becomes more pressing, as does the need to ensure that the candidate countries are adequately prepared to participate in this process.

Communicable disease control in candidate countries

All the candidate countries have national communicable disease control systems, are members of WHO, and participate in WHO disease control initiatives. Several also participate in regional activities, such as the Task Force on Communicable Disease Control in the Baltic Sea Region [http://www.baltichealth.org/]. Yet as in existing Member States, systems for surveillance and control of communicable diseases differ and, in cases, are severely under-resourced. In a situation characterized by free movement, a weakness in surveillance anywhere undermines the integrity of the entire system.

To assess progress made by candidate countries in engaging with existing European mechanisms a questionnaire was circulated to key informants in each country, supplemented with a review of available information on the various networks. Although some countries were participating in many of the networks (Table 13.1), there were important gaps. In particular, Cyprus, perhaps because it only became a member of the European Region of WHO in May 2003, did not participate in any of them.

Respondents were also asked about the strengths and weaknesses of existing systems. The findings were, inevitably, dominated by the views from the countries of central and eastern Europe. Strengths included having strong legal frameworks for surveillance and control, a long tradition of reporting, high levels of attainment, for example in terms of immunization coverage, and the comprehensiveness of national reporting. Emergency preparedness was reported as strong with just over half of the countries responding having a written epidemic preparedness plan, while all had a rapid response team in place for epidemics. Four main areas of weakness were identified: the need for the introduction or enhancement of modern information technology; greater participation in international initiatives; enhancement of laboratory facilities; and better training in modern epidemiological methods.

These views largely reflect the strengths and weaknesses of the Soviet system of communicable disease control. Communicable disease control was given a strong emphasis under the Soviet system reflecting Lenin's remark that "If communism does not defeat the louse, the louse will defeat communism" (MacLehose et al. 2002). However, although surveillance systems were extensive and well organized, resource constraints and a focus on other priorities meant that the systems have often failed to keep pace with developments elsewhere.

Although efforts are now being made to include candidate countries in the EU surveillance systems, these have been somewhat limited to date as illustrated by the somewhat uneven participation in networks. Respondents to the survey indicated an enthusiasm for greater participation but many identified cost as a

Table 13.1 Participation in EU Networks by candidate countries, June 2003

Network	BUL	CYP	CZE	EST	HUN	LIT	LTV	MTA	POL	ROM	SLO	SVK	TUR
European Working Group on Legionella Infection (EWGLI)	X		X	X	X	X	X	X	X	X	X	X	X
European Network on Human Gastrointestinal Infections (Enter-net)			X		X		X		X				
European Influenza Surveillance Scheme (EISS)									X	X	X	X	
Euro-IBIS (Meningococci)			X					X					
Euro-IBIS (Haemophilus Influenzae)			X										
European Anti-microbial Resistance Surveillance System (EARSS)	X		X	X	X			X	X	X	X	X	
European Network for Diagnostics of "Imported" Viral Diseases (ENIVD)			X		X	X			X		X	X	
Euro HIV	X		X	X	X	X	X	X	X	X	X	X	X
Helics (nosocomial infections) EuroTB	X		X	X	X	X	X	X	X	X	X	X	X

Source: Survey undertaken by authors

barrier to participation. Few reported receiving any assistance from the EU to support their involvement. Other reasons given for not participating included structural factors (such as the absence of a national reference laboratory for the particular disease covered in the network), "network issues" (such as a lack of information on the networks, not yet being accepted by the network, language difficulties and not being invited to participate) and insufficient staff to participate. The reported lack of information about networks is a cause for concern as uptake of the freely available journal *EuroSurveillance* is low in the candidate countries. None of the respondents reported that *Eurosurveillance Weekly* was read widely in their country and only one said that *Eurosurveillance Monthly* was widely read. However, the key informants, while admittedly a highly selected group, were well aware of the relevant EU legislation relating to communicable disease.

The new programme of Community action in the field of public health offers scope to address concerns about lack of involvement in networks as it states that "applicant countries should be actively involved in the development and implementation of the programme and consideration should be given to a strategic approach to health in those countries, and especially to their specific problems" (2002). International collaboration is improving and some countries reported that they had instituted changes that would improve national surveillance systems, including improvements in information systems and laboratory facilities, expanding national surveillance networks, enhancing training in epidemiology and participating in EU network meetings.

Beyond an enlarged Europe: New neighbours – a need for wider cooperation for health

While the countries in central and eastern Europe experienced a transient worsening in economic conditions following transition, this was much less than in most of the countries that emerged from the Soviet Union (Bloom and Malaney 1998; UNICEF 2001). Some of the worst outcomes have been in Belarus, the Republic of Moldova, the Russian Federation and Ukraine, countries that will be neighbours of an enlarged EU. Thus, while by 1999, economic recovery meant that Poland and Slovenia had Gross Domestic Products (GDP) in excess of 1989 levels, in Russia and Ukraine GDP fell to 57% and 36% of their 1989 levels respectively (World Bank).

Economic decline during the past decade has been accompanied by substantial increases in poverty, with an estimated 50 million people in this region living on less than $2.15 per day in the late 1990s (Klugman et al. 2002). The health consequences of economic decline have been exacerbated by weaknesses in systems of social support, both formal and informal. In the Russian Federation, for example, increases in mortality in the early 1990s were greatest in regions experiencing the most rapid pace of transition and where measures of social cohesion are weakest (Kennedy et al. 1998). A wide range of health indicators of diminished social wellbeing, such as suicide among teenagers, alcohol-related deaths, sexually transmitted diseases and tuberculosis, have all deteriorated over the past decade (Shkolnikov et al. 2001; UNICEF 2001).

Major social change has had consequences for the prison sector, with profound consequences for communicable disease control, especially for tuberculosis and HIV. Overcrowded prisons in the former Soviet Union have been described as the "epidemiological pump" for multi-drug resistant tuberculosis (Farmer et al. 1999) but there is now evidence that they are also contributing to a potential explosion of HIV. The Russian Federation has the second highest incarceration rate in the world after the USA and rates are only slightly lower in Belarus and Ukraine.

The challenge facing an enlarged EU is that communicable diseases are not contained by national frontiers while the scope to implement surveillance and control systems often is. The countries that will border the EU's eastern boundary in 2004 are very different from those it currently borders, which can be illustrated by considering two infectious diseases, tuberculosis and HIV.

Tuberculosis

Even on the basis of official Russian Federation statistics, which are likely to underestimate the scale of the problem because of weaknesses in case detection, diagnosis and reporting, the incidence of tuberculosis has increased markedly during the 1990s, from 34 in 100 000 in 1991 to 95 in 100 000 in 2000. Reported death rates from tuberculosis have also risen, from 7.7 in 100000 in 1989 to 20.4 in 100000 in 2000 (Shilova and Dye 2001). Similar trends have been observed in Ukraine and Belarus.

The reasons for the worsening situation are complex. They include a deterioration in socioeconomic conditions, with increasing rates of unemployment, poverty, homelessness and migration. This situation was compounded by a hierarchical health system that was unable to respond to changing circumstances, retention of inefficient national tuberculosis screening programmes and professional bodies that were largely unexposed to modern concepts of public health control and clinical management. Further factors included high incarceration rates in often appallingly overcrowded conditions, not only in prisons but often in even worse pre-detention trial centres. These institutions have played a central role in the spread of tuberculosis (Stern 1999). On release from prison most infected ex-prisoners have been unable to access care in the civilian sector. Anti-tuberculosis drugs have often been supplied erratically which, along with individualized approaches to clinical management and poorly developed mechanisms to support treatment adherence, has led to high rates of drug resistance and multi-drug resistance (Drobniewski et al. 1996; Farmer et al. 1999; Kimmerling et al. 1999; Coker et al. 2003). Yet many of these factors applied, initially, to the Baltic states, which, unlike their ex-Soviet neighbours, have now adopted internationally advocated tuberculosis control approaches. The Russian Federation, Ukraine and Belarus have struggled to do so (Perelman 2000; Wolfheze Workshop 2003). Although the World Health Organization (WHO) has been extremely active in promoting Directly Observed Therapy-Short Course (DOTS) in the Russian Federation in particular, successful pilot regions have depended extensively upon external assistance and it seems likely that changes already adopted may not been sustained in the absence of such external financial support.

HIV

Until the early 1990s the Russian Federation, Belarus and Ukraine were relatively untouched by the HIV epidemics that were afflicting much of the rest of the world. Since then, rates of increase have become the highest in the world (UNAIDS 2002), with explosive outbreaks especially among injecting drug users (Rhodes et al. 2002). This epidemic now seems to be moving into a second stage, leaking out from the drug-using population via heterosexual spread fuelled by commercial sex work, exacerbated by high rates of other sexually transmitted diseases (Borisenko et al. 1999; Barnett et al. 2000; Hamers and Downs 2002). This is in marked contrast to the situation in countries of central and western Europe (EuroHIV; Federal AIDS Centre; AIDS infoshare; UNAIDS; World Bank) From a situation in which only a few cases of HIV infection had been reported by the mid-1990s (Rhodes et al. 1999a; Rhodes et al. 1999b), the number of HIV infected individuals notified in the Russian Federation had risen to 197 497 by June 2002, corresponding to a prevalence of 136 in 100 000. Yet this is still likely to be a substantial underestimate (Borisenko et al. 1999) as surveillance mechanisms are likely to have missed many people in high risk, marginalized populations. Thus UNAIDS has estimated that, by the end of 2001, 700 000 people in the Russian Federation were living with HIV, while Vadim Pokrovsky, a noted Russian expert, has suggested the figure might be as high as 1.4 million (Badkhen 2002; UNAIDS 2002). Ukraine and Belarus have both witnessed similar increases in numbers of reported cases to those in the Russian Federation although the rate of increase has been slightly slower than in the Russian Federation (Hamers and Downs 2002). The impact is also being felt elsewhere, with recorded rates of syphilis doubling in Finland in 1995, with most cases traced to Finnish men who had travelled to the Russian Federation (Hiltunen-Back et al. 2002).

As with tuberculosis the epidemic growth and the failure of prevention are multi-factorial (Rhodes et al. 1999a; Rhodes et al. 1999b). The causes include the growth in commercial sex work, changing cultural values stressing greater sexual freedom and sexual expression through partner change, a widespread feeling of hopelessness and fatalism that promotes risk-taking behaviour, and deteriorating public health systems (Borisenko et al. 1999; Rhodes et al. 1999a; Rivkin-Fish 1999; Atlanti et al. 2000; Barnett et al. 2000; Kalichman et al. 2000; Parker et al. 2000).

Public health responses have, in most cases, been slow, poorly focused and inadequately funded. Where changes have taken place they have often been driven by the international donor community. In the Russian Federation, concern about HIV/AIDS led to the passage, in 1995, of a federal law "On the prevention and spread in the Russian Federation of disease caused by the Human Immunodeficiency Virus". While the aims were laudable, including provision of anonymous medical examinations to detect HIV infection, pre- and post-test counselling, health promotion, improved epidemiological surveillance, free medical care and social support for those infected, and anti-discrimination measures. In practice, however, implementation has been patchy. A further factor is that efforts to control HIV have failed to reach populations most at risk of acquiring the infection, especially injecting drug users, commercial sex workers, homosexual men, and prisoners.

There is little evidence of coherent strategies within the countries to link the three principle agents of AIDS prevention: medical institutions, voluntary organizations and educational institutions. Furthermore, some promising initiatives have been threatened by active opposition from Russian Federation Pro-Life organizations, conservative political parties and the church (Chervyakov and Kon 1998).

Policy-makers have failed to adapt to major shifts in cultural values and behaviour among young populations in the Russian Federation and Ukraine (and to a lesser degree in Belarus) at a time when they should have been embracing novel, innovative approaches to prevention. Action remains constrained by outmoded thinking and often ineffective practices.

Conclusions

Public health does not feature prominently in the *acquis communautaire* and has not had a high profile in the enlargement process to date. Yet, as this chapter has shown, joining the EU brings with it a wide range of obligations which impact on public health.

Under the principle of subsidiarity, the EU should only undertake activities where the benefits of action bring benefits that are greater than that which can be achieved by Member States acting alone. This principle is perhaps most clearly demonstrated in communicable disease control. The expanding role of the EU in communicable disease surveillance and control offers the potential for more effective public health action, with the inclusion of the candidate countries bringing benefits to all. Yet, to date, opportunities to help the candidate countries prepare for more active participation in these networks appear to have been squandered, to a considerable extent reflecting the reactive nature of European initiatives. Few contain any mechanism to help those where capacity is negligible to get onto the first rung of the ladder. Indeed, the penalties for failure within many EU programmes actively discourage the risk-taking that is needed to initiate activities in the candidate countries that are in the greatest need. This is clearly an area where greater efforts are urgently needed.

Implementing public health measures is not without cost. Upgrading working practices to meet European health and safety standards will be time consuming and may require considerable additional investment. Securing the resources to upgrade laboratory facilities and staff skills to ensure effective communicable disease surveillance will pose challenges for some countries. These investments will ultimately reap benefits, not only in terms of better health but also by facilitating trade between the candidate countries and the rest of the EU. Yet there are also risks, not least that some of the problems will be displaced beyond the new borders of the EU. Will European companies emulate their American counterparts, which relocate production in Mexico, where working conditions are much less intensively regulated? Will products, and in particular foodstuffs and pharmaceuticals, that fall below EU manufacturing standards leak into the European market from less regulated countries? These are certainly risks, and they indicate the need for effective systems of surveillance throughout the enlarged EU and beyond its new borders as a means of protection for everyone. Enlargement of the EU will have important consequences for the surveillance and control of communicable disease, not only because of the greater volume of travel not only within the expanded Union but also across its new frontiers. These changes make it essential that the systems that are in place to detect and manage communicable disease are functioning effectively, with access to communication systems that, like microorganisms, transcend national borders. In many candidate countries, as in some existing Member States, there is still some way to go.

References

(2002) Stability Pact, http://www.stabilitypact.org. Accessed 10 February.

Atlanti, L., Carael, M., Brunet, J.B., Frasca, T. and Chaika, N. (2000) Social change and HIV in the former USSR: the making of a new epidemic, *Social Science & Medicine*, 50:1547–56.

Badkhen, A. (2002) Global pandemic: Russia on the brink of AIDS explosion. San Francisco: San Francisco Chronicle.

Barnett, T., Whiteside, A., Khodakevich, L., Kruglov, Y. and Steshenko, V. (2000) The HIV/AIDS epidemic in Ukraine: its potential social and economic impact, *Social Science & Medicine*, 51:1387–403.

Bloom, D.E. and Malaney, P.N. (1998) Macroeconomic consequences of the Russian mortality crisis, *World Development*, 26:2073–85.

Borisenko, K.K., Tichonova, L.I. and Renton, A. (1999) Syphilis and other sexually transmitted infections in the Russian Federation, *International Journal of STD & AIDS*, 10:665–8.

Bradbury, J. (1998) European infectious diseases centre takes shape, *Lancet*, 352:969.

Brand, H., Camaroni, I., Gill, N. et al. (2000) *An evaluation of the arrangements for managing an epidemiological emergency involving more than one EU member state*. Bielefeld: LOGD.

Byrne, D. (2002) speech 02/152, 15 April.

Chervyakov, V. and Kon, I. (1998) Sex education and HIV prevention in the context of Russian politics, in R. Rosenbrock (ed.) *Politics behind AIDS policies: case studies from India, Russia and South Africa*. Berlin: Wissenschaftszentrum Berlin fur Sozialforschung.

Coker, R.J., Dimitrova, B., Drobniewski, F. et al. (2003) Tuberculosis control in Samara Oblast, Russia: institutional and regulatory environment, *The International Journal of Tuberculosis and Lung Disease*, 10: 920–32.

Coker, R.J., Bell, A., Pitman, R., Hayward, A. and Watson, J. (In press) Screening programmes for tuberculosis in new entrants across Europe, *The International Journal of Tuberculosis and Lung Disease*.

Dobson, R. (2001) AIDS-dramatic surge in ex-Soviet Union, no respite worldwide, new data show, *Bulletin of the World Health Organization*, 79:78.

Drobniewski, F., Tayler, E., Ignatenko, N. et al. (1996) Tuberculosis in Siberia 2. Diagnosis, chemoprophylaxis and treatment, *Tubercle and Lung Disease*, 77:297–301.

Editorial (1998) Not another European Institution, *Lancet*, 352:1237.

European Commission (1998) Council Conclusions of 26 November 1998 on the future framework for Community action in the field for public health. European Commission.

European Commission (1999) Commission Decision of 22 December 1999 on the early warning and response system for the prevention and control of communicable diseases under Decision No 2119/98/EC of the European Parliament and of the Council (2000/57/EC). Official Journal of the European Commission 26 January 2000 L21/32–35.

European Parliament (1998) Decision No 2119/98/EC of the European Parliament and of the Council of 24 September 1998 setting up a network for the epidemiological surveillance and control of communicable diseases in the Community.

European Parliament (1999) Community Decision of 22 December 1999 on the Communicable diseases to be progressively covered by the Community network under Decision No 2119/98/EC of the European Parliament and of the Council. (2000/96/EC). Official Journal of the European Commission 3 February 2000 L28/51–53.

European Parliament and Council (1996) Decision 647/96/EC adopting a programme of Community action on the prevention of AIDS and certain other communicable diseases.

Farmer, P.E., Kononets, A., Borisov, S.E. et al. (1999) Recrudescent tuberculosis in the Russian Federation, in P.E. Farmer, L.B. Reichman and M.D. Iseman (eds) *The global impact of drug resistant tuberculosis*. Boston, MA: Harvard Medical School/ Open Society Institute.

Fidler, D. (1999) *International Law on Infectious Diseases*. Oxford: Clarendon Press.

Giesecke, J. and Weinberg, J. (1998) A European Centre for Infectious Disease?, *Lancet*, 352:1308.

Hamers, F.F. and Downs, A.M. (2002) HIV in central and eastern Europe, *Lancet*, 361:1035–44.

Hiltunen-Back, E., Haikala, O., Koskela, P. et al. (2002) Epidemics due to imported syphilis in Finland, *Sexually Transmitted Diseases*, 29:746–51.

Hoile, E. (2002) New chair of the Council for European State Epidemiologists outlines some immediate changes, *Eurosurveillance*, 6(42).

Joseph, C. and Lee, J. (1996) Outbreak of Legionnaires Disease Associated with the Hotel Imbat, Kusadasi, Turkey. Final Report and Recommendations from the Epidemiological, Environmental and Microbiological Investigations carried out by the PHLS in conjunction with the Turkish Representative of the European Working Group for Legionella Infections. PHLS.

Kalichman, S.C., Kelly, J.A., Sikkema, K.J. et al. (2000) The emerging AIDS crisis in Russia: review of enabling factors and prevention needs, *International Journal of STD & AIDS*, 11:71–5.

Kennedy, B.P., Kawachi, I. and Brainerd, E. (1998) The role of social capital in the Russian mortality crisis, *World Development*, 26:2029–43.

Kimmerling, M.E., Kluge, H., Vezhina, N. et al. (1999) Inadequacy of the current WHO re-treatment egimen in a central Siberian prison: treatment failure and MDR-TB, *The International Journal of Tuberculosis and Lung Disease*, 3:451–3.

Klugman, J., Micklewright, J. and Redmond, G. (2002) Poverty in transition: social expenditures and the working-age poor. Innocenti Working Paper No. 91. Florence: UNICEF Innocenti Research Centre.

Kraudt, A.M. (1994) *Silent Travellers: germs, genes, and the "immigrant menace"*. Baltimore, MD: The Johns Hopkins University Press.

Lever, F. and Joseph, C. (2001) On behalf of the European Working Group for Legionella Infections (EWGLI) Travel associated Legionnaires Disease in Europe in 1999, *Eurosurveillance*, 6:53–61.

Loytonen, M. and Maasilta, P. (1998) Multi-drug resistant tuberculosis in Finland – a forecast, *Social Science & Medicine*, 46:695–702.

MacLehose, L., Brand, H., Camaroni, I. et al. (2001) Communicable disease outbreaks involving more than one country: systems approach to evaluating the response, *British Medical Journal*, 323:861–3.

MacLehose, L., McKee, M. and Weinberg, J. (2002) Responding to the challenge of communicable disease in Europe, *Science*, 295:2047–50.

McNeill, W.H. (1976) *Plagues and People*. Harmondsworth: Penguin.

Parker, R.G., Easton, D. and Klein, C.H. (2000) Structural barriers and facilitators in HIV prevention: a review of international research, *AIDS*, 14(Suppl. 1):S22–32.

Perelman, M.I. (2000) Tuberculosis in Russia, *The International Journal of Tuberculosis and Lung Disease*, 4:1097–103.

Randolph, S.E. (2001) The shifting landscape of tick-borne zoonoses: tick-borne encephalitis and Lyme borreliosis in Europe, *Philosophical Transactions of the Royal Society of London. Series B, Biological Sciences*, 356:1045–56.

Rhodes, T., Ball, A., Stimson, G.V. et al. (1999a) HIV infection associated with drug injecting in the Newly Independent States, eastern Europe: the social and economic context of epidemics, *Addiction*, 94:1323–36.

Rhodes, T., Lowndes, C., Judd, A. et al. (2002) Explosive spread and high prevalence of HIV infection among injecting drug users in Togliatti City, Russian Federation: Implications for HIV prevention, *AIDS*, 16:F25–31.

Rhodes, T., Stimson, G.V., Crofts, N. et al. (1999b) Drug injecting, rapid HIV spread, and the "risk environment": implications for assessment and response, *AIDS*, 13 (Suppl. A):S259–69.

Rivkin-Fish, M. (1999) Sexuality education in Russia: defining pleasure and danger for a fledgling democratic society, *Social Science & Medicine*, 49:801–14.

Shilova, M.V. and Dye, C. (2001) The resurgence of tuberculosis in Russia, *Philosophical Transactions of the Royal Society of London. Series B, Biological Sciences*, 356:1069–75.

Shkolnikov, V., McKee, M. and Leon, D.A. (2001) Changes in life expectancy in Russia in the mid-1990s, *Lancet*, 357:917–21.

Stern, V. (1999) *Sentenced to die. The problem of TB in prisons in Eastern Europe and central Asia*. London: International Centre for Prison Studies, King's College London.

Stoilova, N. and Popivanova, N. (1999) Epidemiologic studies of leptospiroses in the Plovdiv region of Bulgaria, *Folia Medica (Plovdiv)*, 41(4):73–9.

Tegnell, A., van Loock, F., Hendricks, J., Baka, A. and Vitozzi, L. (2002) BICHAT: an EU initiative to improve – and response to bioterrorism, *Eurosurveillance Weekly*, 6.

Tibayrenc, M. (1997) European Centres for disease control, *Nature*, 389:433.

UNAIDS (2002) Report on the global HIV/AIDS epidemic.

UNICEF (2001) A Decade of Transition, Regional Monitoring Report No 8. Florence: UNICEF, Innocenti Research Centre.

Wolkfheze Workshop (2003) Eighth Wolkfheze Workshop on TB Control in Europe, Wolfheze, Netherlands 7–12 June.

World Bank http://www.worldbank.org/data/databytopic/class.htm.

fourteen

Free Trade versus the protection of health: The examples of alcohol and tobacco

Anna B. Gilmore, Esa Österberg, Antero Heloma, Witold Zatonski, Evgenia Delcheva and Martin McKee

EU accession: Raising or lowering standards?

The European Union (EU) is above all an economic entity concerned with free trade and in particular the free movement of goods, capital, people and services, the cornerstones of its internal market. Some of these goods (the best examples being cigarettes and alcohol) and the services used to promote them (advertising) may, however, be detrimental to health (Box 14.1 and Box 14.2). A potential conflict could therefore arise between desire to promote the internal market and the need to protect health. For similar reasons, joining the EU is often seen as a process that will raise health standards in the candidate countries, as the opening of borders brings faster economic growth and consequently a rise in living standards. Yet the removal of borders also brings potential threats to health, in particular where trade in products detrimental to health is promoted.

Given the important role that tobacco and alcohol play in determining patterns of health in Europe, they will serve as the focus for this chapter. We start by examining the implications for tobacco control, considering issues under three main domains. First are the broad trade issues that arise when the internal market expands to accommodate new Member States. Second are the specific legislative issues that fall under the rubric of the *acquis communautaire* and the requirement that acceding states align their legislation with that of the EU, with the latter taking precedence in areas where it exists. Finally, we address issues

Box 14.1 Tobacco as a health issue in the EU and accession states

Tobacco is the single largest cause of preventable disease and premature death in the European Union, accounting for over half a million deaths each year and over a million deaths in Europe as a whole (Peto et al. 1994). While male deaths from tobacco are now steady, the number of female deaths continues to increase. This is largely because of the rapid increase in tobacco-related mortality in the southern European countries where, due to the later start of their epidemic, female deaths from tobacco have yet to be realized to any great extent.

The health impacts in the accession states, excluding Malta, are even more devastating. Smoking prevalence in central and eastern Europe has traditionally been high, particularly among men, but the entry of the tobacco transnationals with their aggressive marketing campaigns has pushed rates upwards (Connolly 1995). Male smoking rates in the region remain among the highest in the world (Corrao et al. 2000) and rates among women and young people are rising rapidly.

As a result, lung cancer rates, which provide the best indication of the health impact of tobacco, have reached higher levels in eastern Europe than ever observed in the west (Pajak 1996). Indeed the risk of tobacco-related premature mortality has been found to be approximately twice as high in former socialist states than in EU countries (Peto et al. 1994) and it is suggested that tobacco may explain 50% of the male mortality gap between these two regions (Pajak 1996). In 1990, it is estimated that men in the former socialist states had a 19% chance of premature death from tobacco compared with 10% in the EU and women a 2% chance compared with 1% in the EU (Peto et al. 1994).

Box 14.2 Alcohol as a health issue in the EU and accession states

Alcohol presents a more complex challenge to health than tobacco, as there is evidence that moderate consumption by older people may be beneficial to health by protecting against heart disease. However, when drunk to excess, or in ways and settings that are hazardous, it is an important cause of disease and premature death in Europe. The threat it poses to health is especially great in central and eastern Europe, although the precise nature of this threat varies reflecting national differences in consumption.

The candidate countries of central and eastern Europe can be divided into those where consumption has traditionally been predominantly wine, beer or spirit based, reflecting differences in local agricultural patterns. Where spirit drinking is common, as in Poland and the three Baltic states, the main health effects are those associated with acute intoxication, including injuries and violence and, especially, sudden cardiac death. In the southern part of this region, in Slovenia, Hungary and Romania, where wine (and brandies of various sorts) are consumed, liver cirrhosis is a more common manifestation.

However, in all of these countries, patterns and levels of consumption are changing, with some degree of homogenization, reflecting active marketing of new products by the alcohol industry as well as higher disposable incomes and changes in traditional gender differences. Thus, as with tobacco, the health effects of alcohol on young women are growing and are likely to continue to do so.

that arise from the expansion of the Common Agricultural Policy (CAP). We will focus, particularly when exploring the legislative issues, on two accession states, Poland and Bulgaria, chosen for their very different initial positions on this issue. Poland is considered by many to be a European leader in its stance on tobacco control while Bulgaria has so far been unable effectively to address the challenges posed by tobacco.

Having identified potential issues facing the candidate states, we will then examine the precedents set when a current EU Member State, Finland, acceded in 1995. At the time of its accession Finnish legislation on alcohol and tobacco control was among the strongest in Europe and we explore how disparities between the stronger Finnish and weaker European legislation were resolved in this instance.

First, however, it is necessary to understand something about the EU treaty provisions for public health.

Free trade versus the protection of health: The limitations of the EU treaties

The potential conflicts between trade and health outlined above are ones that the EU treaties inadequately address. Although the EU's competence in the field of public health has gradually expanded culminating in Article 152 of the Treaty of Amsterdam, which requires that a high level of health protection be "ensured in the definition and implementation of all Community policies and activities", it remains effectively impossible to implement harmonizing legislation purely for public health purposes (Gilmore and McKee 2002). This presents a major challenge to those wishing to protect the health of European citizens and one which the European Convention's first draft treaty for Europe, does not adequately address (Belcher et al. 2003). This means, for example, that most tobacco and alcohol control laws have been enacted as internal market measures under Article 100a (now Article 95) using the argument that differing national legislations must be synchronized to enable the smooth running of, and facilitate the free movement of goods and services within, the internal market.

The limitations of this approach are perhaps best illustrated by the annulment of the EU's first comprehensive ban on direct and indirect tobacco advertising and sponsorship (98/43/EC) in the European Court of Justice (ECJ) in October 2000 following a challenge by the German Government and four British tobacco companies (Gilmore and McKee 2002). The Advocate General's opinion (Opinion of Advocate General Fennelly 2000) and the subsequent ECJ ruling (European Court of Justice 2000) concluded that the Directive had exceeded its legal base as an internal market measure: it did not facilitate the movement of goods but regulated it and did not equalize the conditions of competition in the tobacco advertising market but essentially eradicated that market (Hervey 2001). The restrictions the Directive placed on trade in tobacco were seen as disproportionate to those needed to ensure the proper functioning of the internal market (European Court of Justice 2000), highlighting the underlying problem that, as long as treaty provisions prevent the passage of harmonizing legislation for public health purposes alone, the EU will always be faced with the dilemma that what is needed to protect public health may be considered disproportionate to that needed to protect the internal market (Gilmore and McKee 2002). This clear subordination of public health to trade in the European treaties led some, at the time, to question whether all consumer protection laws were potentially under threat in this way. Certainly, where major corporate interests are threatened, such challenges are most likely, although as the example of the unsuccessful tobacco industry's challenge to the 2001 tobacco products Directive (2001/37/EC) showed (Gilmore and McKee 2002), the ECJ does at least take account of public health concerns.

Expanding the internal market: What are the health concerns?

The addition of ten new countries in 2004 will increase the population of the EU by 20% to more than 450 million. The further addition of Bulgaria, Romania and Turkey would make the EU the largest single market in the world (Euromonitor 2003). This represents a major opportunity for any industry selling its products within the internal market just as the formal creation of the single market did at the end of 1992.[1] Indeed much can be learnt about the potential impacts of accession from the tobacco industry's attitudes and approach to the creation of the single European market as illuminated through previously secret internal tobacco industry documents released through litigation (Bero 2003).

These documents indicate that although the creation of the market brought potential threats to the tobacco industry in the form of tax harmonization and abolition of duty-free sales, overall the multinational companies recognized the benefits that would accrue from the shift towards their high-priced international brands and the greater economies of scale (British American Tobacco 1988; British American Tobacco 1989). Although competition would increase pushing prices down, pricing could be used "as a key marketing weapon to take advantage of the new market environments" (Bingham 1992). By contrast, smaller national companies and state owned monopolies would be more vulnerable (British American Tobacco 1989). British American Tobacco (BAT) recognized the particular opportunities in southern Europe where state owned monopolies still dominated the tobacco trade and BAT had only tiny market shares. In a document titled "Secret. The European Community: the Single market 1992" BAT outlined its 1992 marketing and business strategy:

> BATco. market strategy is to defend and develop its position in existing Operating Company markets, whilst aggressively taking up the opportunities created in the markets of Southern Europe. These priority opportunity markets will be Italy, Spain, France and Greece where there is growth potential for our strategic international brands. . . .
> . . . .
> BATCO. Policy towards State Monopolies is, with the co-operation of the other free enterprise companies, to press for an end to discriminatory practices and to secure freedom to determine prices. (Bingham 1992)

No longer able to protect their markets through tariff and non-tariff barriers as such monopolies have traditionally done, the French, Spanish and more recently the Italian monopolies bowed to the increased competition that arose. In October 1999, following their individual privatizations, Spanish Tabacalera and French Seita merged to form Altadis (Altadis) and in July 2003 BAT acquired Ente Tabacchi Italiano (ETI) of Italy (Anon 2003a).

Although trade has been liberalized between the Members States and candidate countries since the early 1990s, Bulgaria still has its state owned tobacco monopoly and thus a significant degree of protectionism.[2] Should this monopoly still be in place by the time these countries accede (which is unlikely given current pressure from the International Monetary Fund and others) (Weissman and White 2002) these protectionist measures could not be retained. This would have major implications for tobacco control. First, as in southern Europe, it would almost certainly herald the demise of state monopolies whose inefficiencies are generally seen as beneficial to tobacco control (Campaign for Tobacco-Free Kids 2002). It is also suggested that transnational tobacco companies (TTCs) behave differently to state owned monopolies – they market their products more heavily, introduce new, more attractive products that are sold through a larger number of outlets and are more likely to challenge attempts to control tobacco use (Mackay 1992; Campaign for Tobacco-Free Kids 2002). They also favour the production of international filter brands over products using locally produced tobacco leaf, with consequences for local leaf growing. Second, both economic theory and empirical evidence show that removing barriers to trade in tobacco products leads to increased consumption (Taylor et al. 2000; Bettcher et al. 2001). This occurs through an increase in both supply and demand, the latter driven by and through competition, which reduces prices and increases advertising (Bettcher et al. 2001). Although these issues are most pertinent to Bulgaria, which presents a particular opportunity to the TTCs, increased competitiveness is likely to occur throughout the newly enlarged internal market and may push down prices and increase advertising (where it is permitted). The presence of effective tobacco control policies, particularly tax and advertising controls, will therefore be essential to safeguarding tobacco control in the region.

In addition to easier access to markets, accession will bring other benefits for the tobacco industry, most notably considerable economies of scale both in terms of manufacturing and marketing, a more stable business environment in central and eastern Europe, and greater demand for their products by those whose incomes grow (Anon 2002b; Globan 2002; Euromonitor 2003). The global tobacco industry clearly hopes to encourage smokers to use their increased earnings to switch to more expensive brands, thereby increasing profits (Globan 2002). Their interest has been summed up in one trade journal:

> major players are greedily eyeing up the 130 million new upwardly mobile consumers in a geographical area which will be far better regulated than before and an improved environment for doing profitable business. (Globan 2002)

Finally, expansion of the internal market will bring countries with far lower cigarette prices into the EU, thereby increasing price differentials and hence the incentive to bootleg cigarettes (Box 14.3). It will also create new EU borders with countries to the south and east, where prices are lower still and smuggling is widespread.[3] Maintaining high cigarette prices is one of the most effective weapons in the struggle to control tobacco use. It seems certain that bootlegging and smuggling will increase with enlargement, which, when combined with the downward pressure on prices through greater competition described above, will pose a major challenge for tobacco control, particularly as a significant proportion of cigarettes consumed throughout Europe is already contraband (Joossens and Raw 2000) (see Box 14.3).

The response to this challenge could have taken two forms – the high tax/ tobacco control response or the low tax/tobacco industry response. The first would have ensured rapid tax increases in accession states so that price differentials within the EU could be narrowed as quickly as possible while simultaneously looking beyond the new EU borders to work with other former Soviet and ex-Yugoslav states to encourage tax increases and collaborative action to control smuggling. Unfortunately the second response triumphed. The European Commission and candidate countries caved in to industry pressure, which was easily wielded within finance and agricultural ministries (Szilagyi and Chapman 2003). As a result, the candidate countries have been granted inordinately long delays before having to implement the full EU cigarette excise rates, as will be explored further below.

This is already having negative impacts. The Finnish Minister of Health for example announced at the 2003 World Conference on Tobacco or Health in Helsinki that Finland would be lowering its cigarette excise rates when Estonia joins in an attempt to pre-empt an increase in bootlegging. However, in December 2003 Finland did not decrease its excise rates on cigarettes when it decided to decrease its excise duty rates on alcoholic beverages from the beginning of March 2004.

Finland faces a similar problem with alcohol. It is estimated that the accession of Estonia, in tandem with the abolishment of duty free allowances that have occurred since 1995 (see below), will increase total alcohol consumption in that country by some 20–30%. Although difficult to estimate, these figures do not seem excessive considering that alcohol prices in Estonia, to which Finns have easy access, are on average about half, and for vodka only about one-fifth of the Finnish prices. Finland has thus far maintained high taxation rates on alcohol to limit consumption (Österberg and Karlsson 2002). However, on 3 December 2003 the Finnish parliament decided to decrease, from 1 March 2004, the excise duties on distilled spirits by 44%, the excise duties on intermediate products by 40%, the excise duties on wine by 10% and the excise duties on beer by 32%. This was done in order to combat the increase of travellers alcohol imports from Estonia, which is becoming a full member of the EU on 1 May 2004. Similarly, Denmark decreased its excise duty on distilled spirits by 45 per cent on 1 October 2003 before it was forced to give up its travellers import quota for distilled spirits on 1 January 2004.

Signing the acquis: Complement or compromise?

As indicated above, all acceding countries have to align their legislation with that of the EU and where conflict exists, EU law takes precedence. The question arises therefore, will accession to the EU complement or compromise tobacco

Box 14.3 Cigarette smuggling and bootlegging in the EU

Bootlegging is the smaller scale illegal cross-border trade of tobacco products that are not intended for personal use, and smuggling, the large-scale organized smuggling of tobacco on which no duty has been paid. Bootlegging is related to price differentials while smuggling is not (Joossens and Raw 1998). Instead it appears to be associated with the presence of organized crime, a culture of street selling and the complicity of the industry (Joossens 1999). The industry benefits in a number of ways: it stimulates consumption by ensuring a supply of cheap cigarettes (the industry gains its normal profit regardless of whether cigarettes enter the legal or illegal market) and enables the industry to penetrate markets that would otherwise block its products. In addition the industry uses the presence of smuggled cigarettes to argue for a reduction in tobacco taxation, despite growing evidence of its own direct involvement in smuggling (Campbell and Maguire 2001; The International Consortium of Investigative Journalists 2001). Duncan Campbell of the Centre for Public Integrity, in submitting evidence to the United Kingdom House of Commons Health Committee has written:

> smuggling . . . has been BAT [British American Tobacco] company policy since the late 1960s. Smuggling of BAT products evolved from an ad hoc activity into an organised and centrally managed system of law breaking. The company directors and managers who were involved, were, on evidence that is plentifully available, fully aware that what they organised was unlawful in those countries where they placed smuggled products (Health Committee Session 1999–2000 2000).

Further information on the tobacco industry's role in smuggling is available on a number of websites, for example the Guardian (*http://www.guardian.co.uk/bat*) and Centre for Public Integrity websites (*http://www.publici.org/story_01_030301.htm#newsstories*). There have now been several official investigations in different parts of the world and a series of court cases accusing the industry of smuggling cigarettes (Dickey and Nordland 2000) in which a number of senior tobacco industry executives or affiliates have been convicted (Associated Press 1997; Dow Jones Newswires 1998). Following a two-year investigation by the EU's anti-fraud unit, the Commission and Member States have brought a series of legal actions against the tobacco industry in the US courts in an attempt to recover billions of Euros of customs revenues lost through smuggling (Anon 2000; Black and Martinson 2000). The most recent lawsuit, launched in October 2002 against US-based company RJ Reynolds, goes further than any previous case by accusing the company of direct complicity in facilitating money laundering schemes and other criminal enterprises (*European Community et al. v. RJR Nabisco* 2003).

Smuggling has been made easier by the European customs and transit arrangements designed to promote international trade by road (Joossens 1999), again highlighting the potential conflict between trade liberalization and public health. International action, including controls on cigarette transport, holds the key to controlling smuggling (Joossens and Raw 2000). Spain is one of the few countries to have successfully tackled this problem and its example shows that with concerted action at both national and international levels, involving collaboration with the European Anti-Fraud Office, and political pressure by the EU, smuggling can be reduced, contrary to the claims of the industry which uses the evidence of smuggling, in which it is itself complicit, to argue that the only solution is to reduce tobacco taxes and thus price differentials.

control? To answer this question, we first need to examine the current status of tobacco control legislation in the EU and the accession states, for which Poland and Bulgaria serve as examples. We can then turn to consider the potential impacts of accession on each of the key tobacco control policies currently covered by EU law.[4] Despite the focus on Poland and Bulgaria, the issues that arise will be germane to all candidate countries.

The European Union's role in tobacco control

The Union's first major foray into public health was the 1987 adoption of the "Europe against Cancer" programme; a programme that has underpinned the development of a European tobacco control policy (Gilmore and McKee in press). The establishment of the Europe against Cancer programme led to major advances in the field of tobacco control with seven Directives and one non-binding Resolution agreed between 1989 and 1992 (Gilmore and McKee in press). From the mid-1990s, however, progress stalled, largely due to the growing influence of the tobacco industry lobby within Europe but also to the obstructive role played by certain Member States, most notably Germany (Neuman et al. 2002; Gilmore and McKee in press). More recently, progress has been hampered by legal challenges as noted above. These have been initiated by the industry and the German Government (occasionally in association with other Member States). The latest challenge, again from the German Government, concerns the decision in the 2003 advertising Directive to advance the ban on Formula 1 advertising by one year from that anticipated in the annulled 1998 Directive (Bloomberg.com 2003). Despite challenges and constraints, current EU laws cover a number of areas (Table 14.1) including advertising, taxation and labelling.

Poland

Poland is the largest of the accession countries with a population of 38.5 million (WHO 2002) and one of the largest tobacco markets in Europe. Its tobacco industry was privatized between 1995 and 1996 and, encouraged by Poland's very high tobacco consumption rates, most of the major tobacco transnationals moved into the country, leaving only one domestic manufacturer (European Bank of Reconstruction and Development 2001). With 20 000 hectares under tobacco plantation, Poland is also one of the largest tobacco leaf producers in central and eastern Europe. Although some locally grown tobacco is used in manufacturing, a shift in consumer preferences to international cigarette brands has led to a growth in tobacco leaf imports (Anon 1997a) and a decline in local production (Anon 1997b). Despite pressure from the tobacco transnationals, the Polish Government was the first in the region to enact comprehensive tobacco control legislation and, since 1995, has developed a set of tobacco control policies that are more comprehensive than those currently in force in the EU.

A 1995 law included bans on television, radio, cinema and some print

Table 14.1 Major EU tobacco control Directives (please note that some of the earlier Directives have been replaced by later Directives as indicated in the table)

Labelling and product regulation

Labelling Directives (& Smokeless Tobacco), 1989, 1992	89/622/EEC	Tar and nicotine yield to be printed on the side of each pack and health warnings on the front of each pack. Each warning to cover 4% of the appropriate surface, 6% for countries with two official languages and 8% for countries with three official languages.
	92/41/EEC	Amended Directive 89/662 by introducing warnings for packaging of tobacco products other than cigarettes and banning the marketing of certain tobacco products for oral use.
Tar yield Directive, 1990	90/239/EEC	Sets a maximum tar yield of 15mg per cigarette by 31 December 1992 and 12mg per cigarette from 3 December 1997.
Tobacco Products Directive, 2001 (Replaces Directives 89/662/EEC, 92/41/EEC and 90/239/EEC)	2001/37/EC	Specifies a reduction in tar yield from 12mg to 10mg, nicotine and carbon monoxide limits, health warnings to cover 30% of the pack front, additive and ingredient disclosure, a ban on misleading product descriptors such as "light" and "mild".

Taxation

Tax Directives, 1992, 1995, 1999 and 2002 (1999 and 2002 Directives amend earlier Directives)	92/78/EEC 92/79/EEC 92/80/EEC 95/59/EEC	Set minimum levels of duty on cigarettes and tobacco.
	99/81/EC	Requires an overall excise duty (specific and *ad valorem* combined) of at least 57% of the final retail selling price of the price category most in demand, plus a VAT rate of 13.04%.
	2002/10/EC	Introduces a fixed minimum amount of taxation expressed in Euros by requiring that the minimum excise rates outlined above shall be at least €60 per 1000 cigarettes for the price category most in demand.

Advertising and sponsorship

Television Broadcasting Directive, 1989 (Minor amendments made by Directive 97/36/EC)	89/552/EEC	Bans all forms of TV advertising for tobacco products.
Tobacco advertising and sponsorship Directive, 1998. Annulled October 2000	98/43/EC	A comprehensive ban on tobacco advertising and sponsorship.
Directive on advertising of tobacco products	2003/33/EC	Bans cross-border sponsorship, advertising in printed publications, on the internet and radio.

advertising; permitted adverts had to carry a warning covering 20% of the advertisement (Zatonski and Harville 2000). It outlawed the production and sale of smokeless tobacco, sales to minors, the use of vending machines and prohibited smoking in schools, health care facilities and enclosed workplaces (except in designated areas). It also required health warnings to cover 30% of the cigarette pack, making these warnings the largest in the world at that time. In 1999, the regulations were strengthened, most notably with a comprehensive ban on advertising, including indirect advertising and sponsorship. Officially only point of sale advertising is now permitted.

Smoking rates are now declining and health indicators are improving as a result (Zatonski et al. 1998). Through the 1990s male smoking rates fell from 60% to approximately 40% and female smoking rates from 30% to 20%. Life expectancy rose rapidly by about four years in men and three years in women after a 30 year period of stagnation and it is estimated that approximately one-third of this change is due to the reduced incidence of smoking (Zatonski et al. 1998). For the first time since the Second World War the steady increase in lung cancer mortality rates has ceased and even reversed in men aged under 65 (Zatonski and Tyczynski 1997). Such improvements stand in contrast to other eastern European countries that were slower to implement effective anti-tobacco measures.

Bulgaria

Bulgaria has traditionally been a major producer of cigarettes, with large export markets in eastern Europe and the former Soviet Union countries during the Soviet era. Since transition however, cigarette production and exports have declined markedly. The domestic tobacco company Bulgartabac, established by the Government in 1947, dominates the Bulgarian market and attempts to privatize it have so far been unsuccessful – a deal to sell the company to a Deutsche Bank backed consortium was cancelled in October 2002 when the Bulgarian Supreme Administrative Court overruled the Government privatization agency (Anon 2003b). Although the situation remains uncertain, tobacco farmers have registered their resistance to privatization through protests in Sofia.

As in Poland, smoking is a major contributor to ill health in Bulgaria. Bulgaria has recorded a 20% increase in lung cancer incidence since 1980 and smoking is estimated to be responsible, directly or indirectly, for about 22% of current mortality (National Statistical Institute Bulletin 2001). Although cigarette consumption in Bulgaria is currently lower than in Poland, smoking rates are higher in both men and women and consumption has been increasing over the last decade at a time of decreases in Poland.

Tobacco production has a long history in Bulgaria and is an important contributor to the national economy, accounting for 5% of all Bulgarian exports, somewhat more than in Poland, and between 0.5 and 0.7% of the world tobacco leaf supply. Between 2 and 3% of the population in a country with unemployment rates of 16–18% work in tobacco production (National Statistical Institute Publishing 2001) and many tobacco farmers belong to the Turkish minority party, whose leader, Mehmet Dikme, is Minister of Agriculture. This makes tobacco farmers a powerful group (as demonstrated in the protests over privatization) and any threat to their employment and to tobacco exports is politically very sensitive.

Bulgaria's public health authorities have attempted to implement antismoking campaigns and tobacco control legislation throughout the 1990s, including the 1997 amendments to the 1973 Public Health Act, the 1998 Radio and Television Act and the October 2000 Tobacco Products Act which prohibit tobacco advertising and introduce labelling, albeit only to cover 4% of the pack (Delcheva 2002). As will be seen below, much of this legislation was prompted by the accession process. To date, however, these measures have met with little success in reducing smoking levels, prompting the Ministry of Health to conclude in 2001 that such measures had not delivered the anticipated results (Ministry of Health 2001). This failure appears to be due to problems of enforcement and the need to support these measures with a broader approach to tobacco control and an effective communications strategy.

A comparison

From the brief descriptions above it is apparent that EU tobacco control legislation is less comprehensive than the existing Polish legislation but more comprehensive than the Bulgarian. Moreover, as Poland has served as a role model for its neighbours, many of whom have since enacted similar measures, European legislation is also weaker than that of many other candidate countries particularly in the area of tobacco advertising. We turn then to examine the impact accession will have on key tobacco control policies.

Tobacco advertising

The annulment of the 1998 advertising ban in the ECJ led the Commission to draft a new Directive (Table 14.1). The usual safeguard clause[5] was initially omitted and we have previously highlighted concerns that this could have left Member and accession states such as Poland vulnerable to challenge for having or attempting to introduce more stringent advertising bans (Gilmore and Zatonski 2002). Fortunately however, a last minute amendment introduced a safeguard clause, foreclosing this scenario.

As a result of the ECJ's narrow interpretation of EU competence, the new Directive is, however, considerably weaker than the 1998 Directive it replaces (Commission of the European Communities 2000). Thus it only bans direct advertising that crosses borders, namely advertising via print media (other than trade journals), radio and internet, sponsorship of cross-border events and the free distribution of tobacco products. Indirect advertising (for example via the use of clothing with cigarette brand logos), a key component of modern advertising strategies which focus on brand rather than product promotions, is specifically excluded from the Directive. Thus while it should help protect Poland and other accession states with comprehensive bans on tobacco advertising from the unwanted entry of direct advertising materials from other

EU members with less comprehensive advertising restrictions, such states will be powerless to prevent the entry of indirect advertising materials.

In Bulgaria, the EU advertising Directives have had a more direct and positive impact. Transposition of Directives 89/552/EEC and 98/43/EC (the annulled Directive) has formed the basis of Bulgarian tobacco advertising bans. Thus Bulgaria and other accession states, such as Estonia, where the 1998 advertising ban also served as a basis for new advertising legislation, ironically have benefited from the overturned advertising Directive and now have more effective controls on indirect advertising than some existing EU Member States.

Tobacco regulation: Cigarette content and labelling

The 2001 EU Tobacco Products Directive includes maximum tar yields; greatly enlarged warnings covering 30% of the front surface and 40% of the back surface of each pack; the disclosure of ingredients and additives and a ban on misleading product descriptions such as "light" or "mild". The size of the health warnings specified in the 2001 Directive was based on the Polish warnings so these would not be jeopardized when Poland accedes. The challenge to the Directive, once again brought by the German Government and the tobacco industry (Gilmore and Zatonski 2002) raised temporary concerns that this threat might be realized, as happened on Finland's accession (see below) and that, even if Poland had succeeded in keeping its warnings, the import of cigarettes with smaller health warnings would have indirectly threatened Polish tobacco control by enabling local manufacturers to argue that the size of the warnings should be reduced to allow fair competition (Gilmore and Zatonski 2002). The challenge was, however, overturned and as a result, other measures in the Directive, in particular the ban on product descriptors, will strengthen Polish tobacco control.

In Bulgaria the Products Directive, particularly its restriction on tar and nicotine yields, has faced considerable resistance from local producers who have called for delays in its transposition in order to adapt their own production procedures. The issue is particularly sensitive as it has implications for local leaf requirements. It is likely that Bulgaria will refer to Greece's accession in relation to this matter as Greece was allowed delays like those requested by Bulgaria for similar reasons. Nevertheless, the Directive offers major benefits to Bulgarian tobacco control particularly in respect of its health warnings, which are considerably larger than the 4% warnings currently in place, and its ban on misleading descriptors.

Taxation

EU Directives specify a minimum taxation rate of 70%. This comprises an overall excise duty of at least 57% which should include a combination of specific (a fixed amount per 1000 pieces) and *ad valorem* (proportional to the retail price) tax, plus 13.04% VAT. The Polish Government has steadily been increasing taxation, partly in anticipation of accession, and in 2000, moved from a specific to a mixed system of taxation, the *ad valorem* component introduced to allow for inflation. The Polish Government estimates that total excise taxes currently constitute 46% of cigarette price (25% of this *ad valorem* tax) and VAT stands at 22% (Polish Statistical Office). Thus while accession would require at least an 11% rise in excise tax, it would allow a drop in VAT of 9%. With income increasing in Poland, the 2% overall increase in taxation required could pass largely unnoticed. Nevertheless, as a result of industry pressure, a temporary delay in tax harmonization has been granted until 2009 (Anon 2002a).

While Bulgaria's taxation arrangements are in line with European Union requirements for most tobacco products, this is not yet the case for cigarettes, which are taxed well below the levels required and include differential rates for filter and non-filter cigarettes (Commission of the European Communities 2001a). Bulgaria, along with all the candidate states other than Malta, has agreed a long derogation in implementing the required rates. As indicated above, the delays in tax harmonization are a major cause for concern and it is unfortunate that one of the major potential benefits that accession offered for tobacco control – increases in tobacco taxation – has not been adequately harnessed.

The Framework Convention on Tobacco Control

Although not formally part of EU legislation at the time of writing, no discussion on international tobacco control is complete without mention of the Framework Convention on Tobacco Control (FCTC), the world's first international health Treaty. This legally binding Treaty will establish guidelines for international governance on tobacco in recognition of the fact that individual states can no longer effectively control the global factors that drive the tobacco epidemic (Health Committee Session 1999–2000 2000; Joossens and Raw 2000). On 21 May 2003 the World Health Assembly adopted the Framework Convention despite the obstructive stance taken throughout the preceding four years of negotiations by a few key states, most notably the United States, Japan and Germany (Gilmore and Collin 2002; Waxman 2002; World Health Organization 2002).

It is now beholden on states to sign and ratify the treaty; ratification by 40 countries is needed for the treaty to enter into force in those countries and any others that sign thereafter. The FCTC includes areas covered by EU legislation as well as others that are not. It is therefore described as a mixed convention, which requires ratification both by the Community and individual Member States. On the day the treaty opened for signature Commissioner Byrne and the Greek presidency signed on behalf of the EU (European Commission 2003). Ten of the 15 EU Member States – Denmark, Finland, France, Greece, Italy, Luxembourg, the Netherlands, Spain, Sweden and the United Kingdom, and three of the candidate countries – Czech Republic, Hungary and Malta, were also among the first signatories. Concerted efforts will be required on behalf of all current and accession states and the European Commission to ensure the Treaty is successfully ratified despite intense industry opposition.

The common agricultural policy

Tobacco subsidies

Approximately €1000 million, 2.3% of the European Commission's agricultural subsidies budget, is spent directly on tobacco subsidies each year. This compares with a paltry €2 million spent on smoking prevention. Soil and climate conditions in Europe support the growth of leaf varieties for which there is little commercial market and tobacco subsidies have therefore led to the dumping of this high tar leaf in countries with no effective restrictions on tar levels (Townsend 1991). Unsurprisingly the tobacco subsidies have been widely criticized and described by the European Court of Auditors as "a misuse of public funds" (Townsend 1991; Court of Auditors 1994).

Nevertheless, not only were EU tobacco subsidies renewed in April 2002, but Polish tobacco farmers have used their existence to argue their own need for funding, despite the falling demand for home-grown tobacco leaf. The Polish Government, keen to gain the farmers' support for accession, obliged. Tobacco subsidies, previously unknown in Poland, were introduced two years ago and already account for a greater proportion of the state budget than the tobacco control programme.

In Bulgaria where tobacco cultivation is a more important source of revenue, tobacco subsidies are a sensitive issue. Although Bulgarian tobacco farmers receive greater state subsidies than farmers in most other central and eastern European states, these subsidies are still far below levels of EU support, which will make it increasingly difficult for the Bulgarian farmers to compete. In addition, a further shift in consumption from local cigarettes to international brands will undoubtedly follow accession and the almost inevitable privatization of Bulgartabak, and lead to a fall in requirements for locally produced leaf as has occurred in Poland and the former Soviet Union (Gilmore and McKee submitted). Indeed Turkey's experience to date is a lesson in point. Following liberalization of the tobacco market under IMF pressure in the 1980s, Tekel lost a substantial portion of its market share to the tobacco transnationals and use of local leaf declined to such an extent that excess leaf had to be burnt (Daghli 2003). Life for the tobacco farmers became harder still when in 2000, under IMF and World Bank pressure, tobacco subsidies, which were first introduced in 1961, ended (Daghli 2003).

It is still unclear what will happen to the Common Agricultural Policy (CAP) with enlargement (see also Chapter 15) but the option of extending current subsidies to the more agriculturally-oriented candidate countries is clearly unaffordable and it seems inevitable that the policy will be reformed. The Commission produced a Communication on sustainable development in preparation for the 2002 Johannesburg World Summit. Along with a reorientation of the CAP, this recommended a phasing out of tobacco subsidies and the identification of alternate sources of income and economic activity for tobacco workers and growers (Commission of the European Communities 2001b). The CAP is being reviewed in 2003 and while certain Member States – particularly France, which gains most from agricultural subsidies – are hugely resistant to change, others will use enlargement and pressure from the World Trade Organization to argue for reform. Within these changing contexts an end to tobacco subsidies, albeit some years down the line, may finally be possible. The Turkish experience, where tobacco farmers are far poorer and tobacco a more important contributor to the economy, shows it is achievable. However, the timing and nature of any reform in relation to enlargement remain uncertain and the addition of further groups of farmers with powerful political links prepared to lobby for the status quo could make progress that much more difficult.

Previous accession: Lessons from Finland

It is clear from the earlier parts of this chapter that accession poses potential threats to tobacco control. Although many of the direct threats have been resolved through recent legislative changes, including the introduction of a safeguard clause and agreement (although not yet ratification) of the Framework Convention, indirect threats through the entry of advertising materials still exist. One way to assess whether these potential threats might be realized in practice is to examine a previous accession of a country with strong public health policies, that of Finland.

Following its initial application for membership in 1992, Finland became a member of the European Economic Area (EEA) on 1 January 1994 and a full member of the EU in 1995. The EEA agreement was in many respects the same as the Treaty establishing the European Communities, and Finnish legislation therefore had to be harmonized with that of the EU on joining the EEA (Alavaikko 2000). Until this point Finnish laws on alcohol and tobacco were among the strongest in Europe and considerably stricter than those required by the EU. They were seen by many in Finland as being necessary to limit alcohol-related social problems, ill health and premature death. They were, however, found to restrict free movement of goods and, as shall be seen, Finland was required to bring its policies into line with the weaker EU position.

Alcohol

Finland, like geographically similar places including Iceland, Norway, Sweden and the Russian Federation had a long experience of adverse health consequences of heavy drinking, in particular of spirits. Consequently, as in two other Nordic countries, Norway and Sweden, it had implemented strict controls on access to alcohol. The organized response to the problems posed by alcohol dates from the middle of the twentieth century when the temperance

movement successfully tackled the "control" exerted by alcohol on the population. Alcohol consumption fell but increased again in the 1920s despite the
prohibition that was introduced in 1917. Prohibition remained in place until
1932 when it was replaced with a new system of alcohol control which
provided the foundations for Finnish alcohol policies until EU accession
(Österberg 1985).

The Finnish alcohol control system was based on a comprehensive state
alcohol monopoly ("Alko") which maintained a strict control of all aspects of
alcohol production, sales and marketing. Advertising of alcohol was either
very heavily controlled or totally banned (except in a few business journals)
and alcohol was heavily taxed. Alko was empowered to grant licences for
manufacturing other alcoholic beverages than distilled spirits and for sale
for on-premise consumption in restaurants. It also set the on-premise prices for
alcoholic beverages, thereby heavily controlling the earnings of private restaurant owners, and also set off-premise prices and taxation levels for all alcoholic
beverages. The taxation system was guided by public health goals and aimed
both to discourage heavy drinking and to promote low-alcohol beverages (such
as wine or beer) rather than high-alcohol drinks (such as spirits). Alcohol consumption in rural areas was especially heavily restricted, with a ban on purchase
for off-site consumption, although this legislation was abandoned in 1968. In
addition, the 1932 Alcohol Act permitted restaurants in rural areas to serve
alcoholic beverages only to travellers to the area and not to local residents.
Additionally, until 1969, in all parts of the country, the minimum age for purchase of alcoholic beverages for off-site consumption was 21. After 1969, this
was lowered to 20 for strong alcoholic beverages and 18 for alcoholic beverages
up to 22% alcohol by volume, the same age at which alcohol could be consumed legally in restaurants and other places where drinking took place on the
premises (Makela et al. 1981). The importation of duty free alcohol was also
highly restricted until 1995.

Alcohol policy in Finland began to change prior to EU accession, largely as a
consequence of consumer pressure. By the late 1980s and early 1990s therefore
practically all Alko stores had converted from assistant-service to self-service,
Saturday closures during the summer months were abandoned, opening hours
extended and the stores relocated from inaccessible locations into shopping
malls. Thus, by the time Finland began to negotiate its entry to the EEA its
laws were viewed as quite liberal within the country, although from an EU
perspective they were considered highly restrictive (Karlsson and Osterberg
2001).

The consequences of accession

EU accession combined with continuing national pressure for relaxation of
alcohol legislation led to major changes to Finnish alcohol control. On 1
January 1995 the 1994 Alcohol Act repealed the alcohol monopolies on
production, import, export and wholesale (Holder et al. 1998) prompting many
changes in alcohol marketing and availability. Those with relevance to public
health are outlined in Box 14.4.

Box 14.4 Changes in alcohol legislation as part of EU accession preparations

Licensing of production was relaxed allowing more private alcohol producers to operate. For example, production licences were granted to domestic manufacturers of distilled spirits.

Alcohol advertising became legal. Between 1977 and 1994, all alcohol advertising was banned in Finland, except in some business magazines. Taking as a basis the EU Council Directive 89/552 ("Television without Frontiers"), the 1994 Alcohol Act legalized the advertising of alcoholic beverages with an alcohol content up to 22% alcohol by volume (Alavaikko 2000) requiring only minor restrictions on the format that the advertising took, for example, banning advertising aimed at minors.

Duty-free alcohol purchases were liberalized. Minimum periods that travellers must spend abroad to qualify for duty-free imports were abandoned on 15 February 1995. Until then, travellers returning to Finland could bring alcoholic beverages duty-free only if staying outside Finland for 24 hours. In May 1996, however, a shorter 20 hour limit was reintroduced for Finnish travellers from non-EU countries (Paaso and Österberg 1996).

At the same time the requirement that non-EU or non-Nordic citizens entering Finland could only bring alcoholic beverages duty-free if staying in Finland at least 72 hours (with the exception of air travel, where no time limits were required) was also reintroduced.

Duty-free allowances have been increased. As a result of EU membership duty-free allowances of alcoholic beverages have increased progressively since 1994 (Table 14.2), leading to increases in the amounts imported to Finland (Österberg and Pehkonen 1996; Österberg 2000).

Changes in pricing and taxation. Until 1994, pricing and taxation of alcoholic beverages had been the responsibility of Alko. One aim of this system had been to use the pricing mechanism to discourage excessive drinking and the consumption of harmful beverages (defined generally as distilled spirits) in favour of the consumption of less harmful beverages (mostly defined as wines and beer). Before 1994 taxes on alcoholic beverages inside each beverage category (distilled spirits, intermediate products, wine and beer) were based on the value of the beverages rather than on the amount of alcohol they contained. This favoured domestic products and cheap beverages and worked against imported and expensive beverages. It was, therefore, in conflict with European competition law (Horverak and Österberg 1992). In 1994 and 1995, Finland introduced new tax systems where excise duties on alcoholic beverages were based on volume of pure alcohol. In this respect, the new taxing system is both non-discriminatory and transparent. In addition, from 1995, restaurants have been free to set prices of beverages at will.

Table 14.2 Travellers' duty-free allowances of alcoholic beverages from other EU Member States from 1995, litres

From	Distilled spirits	Intermediate products	Wine	Beer
1 January 1995	1 distilled spirits or	3 intermediate products	5	15
1 January 1998	1	3	5	15
1 November 2000	1	3	5	32
1 January 2003	1	3	5	64
1 January 2004*	10	20	90	110

* Figures for guidance as to amount reasonable for personal use

The consequences for public health

In 1994, total alcohol consumption in Finland (recorded and unrecorded) was estimated at about 8 litres per head. In 1995 it increased to 8.8 litres, mainly due to increases in alcohol imports by travellers. Since then unrecorded alcohol consumption is believed to have decreased somewhat while recorded alcohol consumption has increased to 7.6 litres (Figure 14.1) giving an estimated total consumption figure of 9.3 litres of alcohol per head in 2002. Given the close connection between total alcohol consumption and alcohol related problems, it is likely that the increase of about 15 per cent in total alcohol consumption between 1994 and 2001 has contributed to the growth in alcohol-related problems in Finland. The number of violent crimes increased from 401 per 100 000 inhabitants in 1994 to 548 in 2000. Between 1994 and 1999 deaths due to alcoholic liver cirrhosis increased from 8.1 to 9.9 per 100 000 inhabitants and the total number of deaths from alcohol related illnesses increased from 14.5 to 20.3 per 100 000 inhabitants.

Figure 14.1   Reported consumption of alcoholic beverages in Finland 1950–2000 (litres of 100% alcohol equivalent per head)

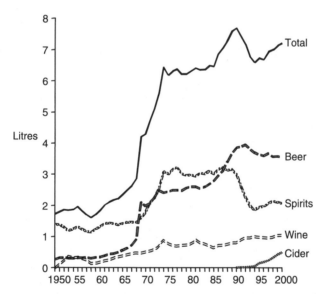

Sources: Alcohol Statistical Yearbook 1950–2000; Stakes Unit for Statistics and Registers

Tobacco

Finland was one of the first countries in Europe to take comprehensive action on tobacco control (Heloma 2003). The Finnish Tobacco Act dates back to 1976. It comprised a wide variety of tobacco control measures including a total ban on advertising and statutes on cigarette product control and labelling (Leppo

1978). A health warning became mandatory for all tobacco product packages and in the case of cigarettes was required to cover 33% of the largest surface on the pack. In addition, new tobacco products could not enter the market without receiving prior approval and an inspection certificate from the National Board of Health. Approval was based on package design and yields of tar, nicotine and carbon monoxide as tested by a government laboratory for compliance with tar and nicotine limits set by the Council of State. A certified label based on this inspection and including information on the concentrations of tar, nicotine and carbon monoxide of the cigarette had to be printed on cigarette packages.

On Finland's entry to the EEA, it had to harmonize its tobacco control legislation to comply with the European Union Directives on labelling and tar yield. This led to a considerable weakening of Finnish legislation. The most significant change was that the large 33% health warning had to be reduced to only 6% of the package surface, a European Union requirement for countries with two official languages. The advance product approval also had to be cancelled; the European Union permitted the control of tobacco products only after they had already appeared in the market.

When Finland eventually entered the EU in 1995, no specific European legislation on tobacco advertising existed except for a ban on tobacco advertising on television that had been included in the 1989 Television Broadcasting Directive. The absence of comprehensive European legislation on tobacco advertising enabled Finland to keep its stricter national legislation in force. However, import of tobacco advertising through media from other parts of Europe could not be prevented. For example, although the current Finnish national law bans both direct and indirect tobacco advertising, indirect advertising on television from Formula 1 races is still abundant. Thus tobacco control was weakened both directly through joining the EU and indirectly as a result of joining an internal market where the free movement of advertising products could not be blocked.

Public health impact

These negative changes were to some extent counterbalanced by further national legislation on smoke-free workplaces (other than restaurants) introduced in 1994. Nevertheless, the downwards decline in tobacco consumption ceased in 1995 and plateaued thereafter (Figure 14.2). The impacts on smoking prevalence are less clear cut although EU entry once again coincided with a levelling out in the earlier decline in smoking prevalence in both genders (Figure 14.3).

Summary

It is clear that although pressure from Finnish consumers led to some relaxation of alcohol regulations in the 1980s and 1990s, the major changes to Finnish alcohol and tobacco legislation arose as a result of joining the EEA and subsequently the EU and were to address conflicts with European competition law. Although a causal relationship is difficult to prove, the observed trends in

Figure 14.2   Tobacco consumption in Finland per person aged 15 or over, 1980–2002

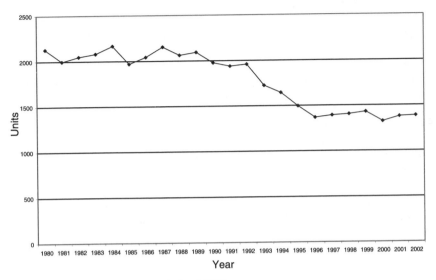

Source: Statistics Finland. (Statistics Finland 2002)

Figure 14.3   Proportion of daily smokers, 1980–2002

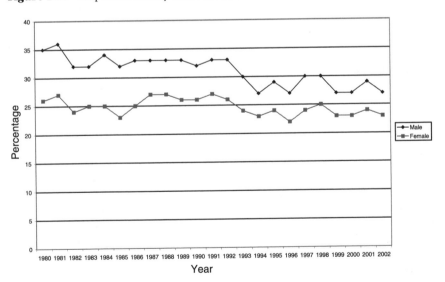

Source: Statistics Finland. (Statistics Finland 2002)

health since 1995 at least suggest that there is a relationship between increased alcohol consumption and alcohol related ill health. The impact on smoking has been less marked although earlier declines in consumption and smoking prevalence have slowed. However, in part reflecting long-standing policies, Finland, along with Sweden, still has the lowest smoking prevalence rates of all EU Member States (Heloma 2003).

It is worth noting however, that although it is widely believed that the changes in Finland's alcohol policy were a necessary alignment with European legislation, other countries have successfully challenged interference in policies on alcohol that seek to protect public health. For example, Sweden maintained its total ban on alcohol advertising when it joined the EU. The ban on alcohol advertising was, however, challenged and after the decision of the ECJ and later a Swedish Court, advertising for alcoholic beverages up to 15 per cent alcohol by volume was allowed in Sweden in 2003. A case arising in Spain has confirmed that local bans on alcohol advertising on grounds of public health are consistent with European Union legislation. The legality of Catalan legislation banning advertising of alcoholic beverages over 23% by volume in certain places such as cinemas and public transport was upheld by the ECJ (1991). In its ruling the ECJ observed on the one hand that such a law could constitute an obstacle to imports, and on the other hand the law contributes to the protection of public health. As the Catalan law did not involve a *total* prohibition on alcohol advertising, the law was not found by the ECJ to be disproportionate to its objective and it was thus granted a derogation under Article 30 (ex Article 36) of the EC Treaty.

Conclusions

This chapter illustrates how the current round of enlargement, as with previous rounds, presents both opportunities and threats to public health. Although the chapter focuses on tobacco and alcohol, the findings could equally apply to any other consumer good that has potential health impacts.

The threats emerge from a number of areas. The expansion of the internal market represents a major opportunity to any industry trading its goods within the EU – it brings greater economies of scale and adds millions of new consumers with increasing disposable incomes. Simultaneously it presents challenges to public health.

Using the example of tobacco, the removal of barriers to trade within the expanded internal market, the widening of price differentials within the EU and between the EU and its new neighbours and the shift of the EU borders will tend to promote competition, stimulate bootlegging and smuggling, and in turn push down prices and push up consumption. Many of these changes, in particular the liberalization of trade, had already occurred in the early 1990s, partly as a result of transition rather than the accession process per se and have resulted in increasing smoking prevalence rates in many countries, particularly among women who had traditionally smoked little (Forey et al. 2002; Szilagyi and Chapman 2003).

The ability to mitigate these threats is limited by the EU treaties that treat tobacco, despite its appalling impacts on health, almost like any other consumer good while at the same time precluding the enactment of binding EU legislation for public health purposes. However, even within the constraints set by the Treaties, further action could have been taken to limit these threats particularly by ensuring adequate taxation rates in the candidate countries. Although accession will lead to some increases in cigarette excise, the ease with which long derogations were apparently agreed is a real missed opportunity for public health that will have ramifications across the expanded EU.

In other legislative areas the impact of accession has been both positive and negative, depending on the starting point of the country concerned and the state of EU legislation at the time. Candidate countries such as Poland, that have comprehensive tobacco control legislation, stand to gain least (in terms of tobacco control) from accession, while those with weaker laws, such as Bulgaria, stand to gain more. The advent of European tobacco control legislation in the late 1980s and early 1990s had a similar impact – the most notable gains were made in countries such as Greece and the Netherlands that had weak legislation while those with more comprehensive policies were less affected (Gilmore and McKee in press).

Until recently, accession looked set to threaten Polish tobacco control (Gilmore and Zatonski 2002). Although the capricious state of EU tobacco legislation made it impossible to be certain whether such risks would be realized, the Finnish experience with tobacco, as with alcohol, demonstrates that threats to countries with strong public health legislation must be taken seriously. Fortunately, however, most of the potential threats to Polish tobacco control disappeared in 2003 as EU legislation was clarified – a safeguard clause was inserted in the new advertising Directive, the Products Directive was ruled as valid and the FCTC agreed.

Overall therefore there will be some benefits to tobacco control in Poland – most notably in the ban on misleading descriptors such as "light" and "mild" that form part of the Products Directive, protection from the entry of direct advertising products from other Member States, and increases, albeit slow, in tobacco taxation. In other areas – the introduction of tobacco subsidies under European Union influence – the accession process has been detrimental. As the Bulgarian experience demonstrates, in other candidate countries anticipation of accession has had a greater and more positive influence on tobacco control. Although some aspects of EU public health legislation, such as tobacco control, have been criticized as being weak, for candidate countries with even less stringent controls accession does present opportunities to improve health. Bulgaria is an example of where the national public health authorities can gain support for their smoking prevention efforts by referring to the *acquis communautaire*.

On a broader note it is worth highlighting that although the EU began discussions on a comprehensive tobacco advertising ban in 1989, it has still only succeeded in introducing a ban on direct advertising. In contrast, the majority of candidate countries have, in the last few years, implemented fairly comprehensive bans that cover both direct and indirect advertising. The relative ease with which the candidate countries have achieved this is perhaps an indication of the barriers to enacting public health law at a European level where there are strong vested interests opposing it, and should serve as a warning to the candidate states of the potential difficulties to come.

Three main lessons emerge from this chapter. The first is the need for effective supranational public health policies, illustrated here through the inability of a national tobacco advertising ban in Finland to control the entry of advertising from elsewhere and the potential threats to the Polish warning labels had the products Directive been overturned. The need for supranational measures is of course not limited to free trade areas such as the EU although it may be particularly acute in such areas. It is rather a broader reflection of the way in which the tobacco industry has harnessed the processes of globalization to its advantage in undermining national tobacco control policies. The second is that the EU is above all an economic entity where trade appears to trump public health at all turns. As the negative Finnish experience illustrates with regard to both alcohol and tobacco, real reassurance to Poland and those other candidate countries that value their public health legislation and wish to balance the benefits of accession against the threats to health may only be obtained by giving public health a greater status in the European Union treaties. The opportunities for ensuring the necessary Treaty changes are fast running out. The third is that the public health community must learn to engage more readily and in a more timely manner in these trade debates so that in future, potential benefits can be harnessed and harms mitigated. Meanwhile, collaborative action will be needed to encourage candidate countries to increase cigarette excise rates more rapidly than is officially required and to control the likely increases in smuggling.

Notes

1 The 1986 Single European Act signed in Luxembourg and The Hague came into force on 1 July 1987. It paved the way for the progressive establishment of a common market over a period that would conclude on 31 December 1992.

2 Turkey also still has a state owned monopoly but due to International Monetary Fund recommendations on market reform the tobacco market was liberalized in the 1980s and the transnational tobacco companies have had a presence since that time. In Romania, the former tobacco monopoly was recently returned to state ownership following an unsuccessful privatization but the transnational tobacco companies have already gained a significant marketshare following market liberalization (Prislopeanu 2003).

3 The new border will for example include Belarus where approximately 40% of cigarettes are thought to be smuggled (ERC Statistics International plc 2001), Moldova with its breakaway Trans-Dniester region, seen as a hotbed of illegal activity including cigarette smuggling (Wines 2002; International Crisis Group 2003) and the Balkans where between 25% and 80% of cigarettes in the individual countries are believed to be smuggled (ERC Statistics International plc 2001) and where links between the mafia, the tobacco industry and governments have been alleged (Barnett and Ravina 2001; Forster et al. 2001; Traynor 2003).

4 Smoke-free environments, while an essential component of any comprehensive tobacco control strategy, are not effectively covered by binding EU legislation, and unlike goods such as tobacco or services such as cigarette advertising, are not affected by the principles of free trade that underpin the EU Treaties. They are not therefore considered here.

5 A safeguard clause allows Member States to introduce their own more stringent legislation thereby ensuring that EU legislation forms a minimum requirement rather than a ceiling.

6 Although other Treaty clauses confer almost the same protection on Member States as the safeguard clause, there are slight differences. Article 95(4) refers to the right to

maintain existing legislation (not *introduce* it) and Article 30 permits health protection measures which are not the subject of an existing Directive as long as they are proportionate.

References

(1991) Judgment of 25/07/1991, *Aragonesa de Publicidad Exterior and Publivia/Departamento de Sanidad y Seguridad Social de Cataluña* (Rec. 1991, p.I–4151).

Alavaikko, M. (2000) The influence of economic interests on alcohol control policy: a case study from Finland, *Addiction*, 95 (Supplement 4):S565–79.

Altadis: The birth of Altadis http://www.altadis.com/en/quienes/nuestrahistoria.html (last accessed 15 August 2003).

Anon (1997a) Statistics. Imports–exports of tobacco leaf, *Tobacco Journal International*, 2:72–5.

Anon (1997b) Statistics. Production of unmanufactured tobacco, *Tobacco Journal International*, 2:72–5.

Anon (2000) European Union: Plans to sue, *Tobacco Journal International*, 5(3).

Anon (2002a) EU grants tax harmonization delay to Poland, *Tobacco Reporter*, April:12.

Anon (2002b) EU enlargement: an unknown quantity (http//www.tobaccojournal.com/show_artikel.php3?id–2851 (last accessed 9 June 2003) *Tobacco Journal International*, 6 December.

Anon (2003a) British American Tobacco gets ETI. – United Kingdom, *Investors Chronicle*, 25 July.

Anon (2003b) Bulgaria – Deal cancelled, *Tobacco Journal International*, 1:6.

Associated Press (1997) Former B&W executive convicted of cigarette smuggling. Associated Press, 16 October.

Barnett, A. and Ravina, P. (2001) Clarke Tobacco Firm linked to Serb "smuggler", *The Observer*, 15 July.

Belcher, P., Mossialos, E. and McKee, M. (2003) Is health in the European Convention?, *Eurohealth*, 9:1–4.

Bero, L. (2003) Implications of the tobacco industry documents for public health and policy, *Annual Review of Public Health*, 24:267–88.

Bettcher, D., Subramaniam, C., Guindon, E. et al. (2001) *Confronting the tobacco epidemic in an era of trade liberalisation*. Geneva: WHO, TFI.

Bingham, P. (1992) Secret. The European Community: the Single market 1992. 03/02/1989. Guildford Depository. BAT. Bates No: 301527819-58. Guildford: British American Tobacco.

Black, I. and Martinson, J. (2000) Tobacco firms sued over EU smuggling, *The Guardian* 7 November.

Bloomberg.com (2003) Bloomberg.com. Germany to Take EU to Court Over Tobacco Ad Ban, 1 August 2003 http://quote.bloomberg.com/apps/news?pid=10000100&sid=a.PNQyMITB58&refer=germany (last accessed 17 August 2003).

British American Tobacco (1988) Common Market "1992 and all that". [Undated, circa January 1988]. Guildford Depository. BAT. Bates No: 300027445-61. Guildford: British American Tobacco.

British American Tobacco (1989) Report of the European Team June 1989 Volume 1. June. Guildford Depository. Bates No: 301529103-66. Guildford: British American Tobacco.

Campaign for Tobacco-Free Kids (2002) Public Health and International Trade Volume II: tariffs and privatisation. Washington, DC: Campaign for Tobacco-Free Kids.

Campbell, D. and Maguire, K. (2001) Clarke company faces new smuggling claims, Manchester: *The Guardian*, 22 August.

Commission of the European Communities (2000) Proposal for a Directive of the European Parliament and of the Council on the approximation of the laws, regulations and administrative provisions of the Member States relating to the advertising of tobacco products and related sponsorship. Brussels.

Commission of the European Communities (2001a) Regular report on Bulgaria's progress toward accession, *SEC*, 1744:3–109.

Commission of the European Communities (2001b) A sustainable Europe for a better world: A European Union strategy for sustainable development (Commission's proposal to the Gothenburg European Council) 15 May. Com (2001) 264 final. Brussels.

Connolly, G. N. (1995) Tobacco, trade and Eastern Europe, in K. Slama (ed.) *Tobacco and Health*. New York: Plenum Press.

Corrao, M.A., Guindon, G.E., Sharma, N. and Shokoohi, D.F. (2000) *Tobacco Control Country Profiles*. Atlanta, GA: American Cancer Society.

Court of Auditors (1994) Special Report No 8/93 concerning the common organisation of the market in raw tobacco together with the commission's replies. Official Journal of the European Communities, C65 volume 37, 2 March.

Daghli, E. (2003) Tobacco Control Policy in Turkey. 3–8 August. Abstract book p. 149. 12th World Conference on Tobacco or Health.

Delcheva, E. (2002) Implementing EU tobacco legislation in Bulgaria: challenges and opportunities, *Eurohealth*, 8(4):34–6.

Dickey, C. and Nordland, R. (2000) Big tobaccos next legal war, *Newsweek*, 31 July.

Dow Jones Newswires (1998) RJR affiliate to pay $15M for acting as smuggling front, 22 December.

ERC Statistics International plc (2001) *The World Cigarettes I and II: The 2001 survey.* Suffolk, UK: ERC Statistics International plc.

Euromonitor (2003) *The Enlarged European Union: a statistical handbook.* London: Euromonitor.

European Bank of Reconstruction and Development (2001) *Poland: Investment profile 2001.* London: EBRD.

European Commission (2003) European Commission Press Release, IP/03/847. EU among first to sign Convention on Tobacco Control. Brussels, 16 June 2003. http://www.europa.eu.int/rapid/start/cgi/guesten.ksh?p_action.gettxt=gt&doc=IP/03/847|0|RAPID&lg=EN (last accessed 17 August 2003) Brussels: European Commission.

European Community et al v. RJR Nabisco, I. e. a. (2003) United States District Court, Eastern District of New York, October 2002 (available on http://www.tobaccofreekids.org/pressoffice/rjrlawsuit.pdf, last accessed 16 August 2003).

European Court of Justice (2000) Judgement of the Court Case C-376/98 (*Federal Republic of Germany v European parliament and Council of the European Union*) 5 October.

Forey, B., Hamling, J., Lee, P. and Wald, N. (2002) *International Smoking Statistics*, 2nd edn. Oxford: Oxford University Press.

Forster, N., Husic, S. and Wagstyl, S. (2001) EU hits at BAT plan for Serbia plant, *Financial Times*, 13 August.

Gilmore, A. and Collin, J. (2002) A wake up call for global tobacco control: will leading nations thwart the world's first health treaty?, *British Medical Journal*, 325:846–7.

Gilmore, A. and McKee, M. (2002) Tobacco control policies: the European Dimension, *Clinical Medicine*, 2:335–42.

Gilmore, A. and McKee, M. (in press) Tobacco control in the European Union, in E. Feldman and R. Bayer, *Tobacco control and the liberal state: the legal ethical and policy debates*.

Gilmore, A. and McKee, M. (submitted) Exploring the impact of foreign direct investment on Tobacco Consumption in the Former Soviet Union, *Tobacco Control.*

Gilmore, A. and Zatonski, W. (2002) Free trade v. the protection of health: how will EU accession influence tobacco control in Poland, *Eurohealth*, 8(4):31–3.

Globan, T. (2002) EU enlargement: an unknown quantity, *Tobacco Journal International*, 6 (November/December).

Health Committee Session 1999–2000 (2000) Inquiry into the tobacco industry and the health risks of smoking. Memorandum by Duncan Campbell in respect of planning, organisation and management of cigarette smuggling by British American Tobacco plc and related issues (http://www.parliament.the-stationery-office.co.uk/pa/cm199900/cmselect/cmhealth/27/0021603.htm) House of Commons.

Heloma, A. (2003) Impact and implementation of the Finnish Tobacco Act in Workplaces. People and Work Research Reports 57. Helsinki: Finnish Institute of Occupational Health.

Hervey, T.K. (2001) Up in Smoke? – Community (Anti)-Tobacco Law and Policy, *European law review*, 26:101–25.

Holder, H.D., Kühlhorn, E., Nordlund, S., Österberg, E., Romelsojö, A. and Ugland, T. (1998) *European Integration and Nordic Alcohol Policies. Changes in Alcohol Controls and Consequences in Finland, Norway and Sweden, 1980–1997*. Aldershot: Ashgate.

Horverak, Ö. and Österberg, E. (1992) The prices of alcoholic beverages in the Nordic countries, *British Journal of Addiction*, 87:1393–408.

International Crisis Group (2003) Moldova no quick fix, IGC Europe Report no. 147, 12 August. ICG, Chisinau/Brussels.

Joossens, L. (1999) Smuggling and cross-border shopping of tobacco products in the European Union. A report for the Health Education Authority. December. Health Education Authority.

Joossens, L. and Raw, M. (1998) Cigarette smuggling in Europe: who really benefits?, *Tobacco Control*, 7:66–71.

Joossens, L. and Raw, M. (2000) How can cigarette smuggling be reduced?, *British Medical Journal*, 321:947–50.

Karlsson, T. and Osterberg, E. (2001) A scale of formal alcohol control policy in 15 European Countries, *Nordic Studies on Alcohol and Drugs*, 18 (English supplement):117–31.

Leppo, K. (1978) Smoking control policy and legislation, *British Medical Journal*, 1:345–7.

Mackay, J. (1992) US tobacco export to Third World: Third World War, *Journal of the National Cancer Institute*, (Monographs):25–8.

Mäkelä, K., Österberg, E. and Sulkunen, P. (1981) Drink in Finland: Increasing alcohol availability in a monopoly state, in E. Single, P. Morgan and J. de Lint *Alcohol, Society and the State. Vol 2 The Social History of Control Policy in Seven Countries*. Toronto: Addiction Research Foundation.

Ministry of Health (2001) National Health Care Strategy "Better health for a better future of Bulgaria" 2001–2010. Sofia: Ministry of Health.

National Statistical Institute Bulletin (2001) Main results from survey on health status of the Bulgarian population, *National Statistical Institute Bulletin*, 3.

National Statistical Institute Publishing (2001) Annual Statistics. National Statistical Institute Publishing.

Neuman, M., Bitton, A. and Glantz, S. (2002) Tobacco industry strategies for influencing European community tobacco advertising legislation, *Lancet*, 359:1323–30.

Opinion of Advocate General Fennelly (2000) Case C-376/98 (*Federal Republic of Germany v European parliament and Council of the European Union*), Case C-74/99 (*The Queen v Secretary of State for Health and Others, ex parte Imperial Tobacco Ltd. And Others*) 15 June.

Österberg, E. (1985) From home distillation to the state alcohol monopoly, *Contemporary Drug Problems*, 12:31–51.

Österberg, E. (2000) Unrecorded alcohol consumption in Finland in the 1990s, *Contemporary Drug Problems*, 27:271–99.

Österberg, E. and Karlsson, T. (2002) *Alcohol Policies in EU Member States and Norway. A collection of Country Reports*. Helsinki: Stakes.

Österberg, E. and Pehkonen, J. (1996) Travellers imports of alcoholic beverages into Finland before and after EU, *Nordic Alcohol Studies*, 13:22–32.

Paaso, K. and Osterberg, E. (1996) Regulations concerning alcohol imports by travellers in Finland and Sweden, *Alkoholipolitiikka*, 61:491–7.

Pajak, A. (1996) Contribution of smoking, in C. Hertzman, S. Kelly and M. Bobak (eds) *East-West life expectancy gap in Europe, environmental and non-environmental determinants*. Dortrecht: Kluwer Academic publishers.

Peto, R., Lopez, A.D., Boreham, J., Thun, M. and Clark, H. (1994) *Mortality from smoking in developed countries 1950–2000: Indirect Estimates from National Vital Statistics*. Oxford: Oxford University Press.

Prislopeanu, I. (2003) Into the next round, *Tobacco Journal International*, 3(May/June):107.

Statistics Finland (2002) Tobacco Statistics. Helsinki: Prima Oy.

Szilagyi, T. and Chapman, S. (2003) Hungry for Hungary: examples of tobacco industry's expansionism, *European Journal of Public Health*, 11:38–43.

Taylor, A., Chaloupka, F.J., Guindon, E. and Corbett, M. (2000) The impact of trade liberalisation on tobacco consumption, in P. Jha and F. Chaloupka *Tobacco control in developing countries*. Oxford: Oxford University Press.

The International Consortium of Investigative Journalists (2001) Tobacco companies linked to criminal organizations in lucrative cigarette smuggling. 3 March 2001 http://www.publici.org/story_01_030301.htm (last accessed 16 August 2003).

Townsend, J. (1991) Tobacco and the European common agricultural policy, *British Medical Journal*, 303:1008–9.

Traynor, I. (2003) Montenegrin PM accused of link with tobacco racket, *The Guardian*, 11 July.

Waxman, H. (2002) The Future of the Global Tobacco Treaty Negotiations, *New England Journal of Medicine*, 346:936–9.

Weissman, R. and White, A. (2002) Needless Harm, International Monetary fund support for tobacco privatisation and for tobacco tax and tariff reduction and the cost to public health. Washington, DC: Essential Action.

WHO (2002) European Health for all Database. WHO Regional Office for Europe.

Wines, M. (2002) Trans-Dniester "Nation" Resents Shady Reputation, *New York Times*, 5 March.

World Health Organization (2002) Fifth session of the Intergovernmental Negotiating Body, Framework Convention on Tobacco Control, 14–25 October (http://www.who.int/gb/fctc/E/E_Index) Geneva: World Health Organization.

Zatonski, W. and Tyczynski, J. (1997) *Epidemiologia nowotworów zlosliwych w Polsce w pietnastoleciu 1980–1994 [Epidemiology of cancer in Poland in 1980–1994]*. Warszawa: Centrum Onkologii – Instytut im. M. Sklodowskiej-Curie.

Zatonski, W. and Harville, E. (2000) Tobacco Control in Poland, *Eurohealth*, 6:13–15.

Zatonski, W., McMichael, A.J. and Powles, J.W. (1998) Ecological study of reasons for sharp decline in mortality from ischaemic heart disease in Poland since 1991, *British Medical Journal*, 316:1047–51.

chapter fifteen

Opportunities for inter-sectoral health improvement in new Member States – the case for health impact assessment

Karen Lock

Health impacts of non-health sector policies

Health is a theme that cuts across all policy sectors although awareness and acceptance of this by policy and decision-makers across Europe is not as high as it might be. While health care systems play a vital role in improving people's health, the need to prevent ill health in the first place is an essential requirement for successful sustainable development policy in any country. In most countries in Europe, the interface between the health and non-health sectors is still fairly limited, confined to links between health care and social care, and between public health and environmental health and communicable disease control. Health is not routinely on the agenda of other ministries or agencies even though the financial burden of negative health impacts of their policies usually fall on the health sector.

Although the importance of taking account of the health impact of policies in other sectors is acknowledged in the EU Treaty (Article 152, Amsterdam Treaty 1997), it has only infrequently been applied at a European or Member State level. The EU has previously been criticized for taking a disease-focused approach and ignoring the wider determinants of health, many of which are affected by its own policies. Similarly, although the accession process has required candidate countries to sign up to some specific provisions related to health and environment, public health has rarely been an important issue in negotiations on chapters of the *acquis*, even though many EU policies directly or indirectly affect population health. Chapter 14 discussed the negative effect of EU trade policies on national tobacco and alcohol control policies, and the consequent negative health implications. The health impacts of internal market policies are also covered in detail in Chapters 12, 13 and 16. However, many other EU policies also have potentially large population health impacts including agriculture, transport, energy and employment policies. In these sectors the direct health impacts are less obvious and public health is often not on the agenda.

The Common Agricultural Policy (CAP) is the EU's largest and arguably the most important policy issue. In 2002 approximately 45.2% of the EU budget was allocated to it (Schäfer Elinder 2003). This appears incongruous as the agricultural sector only contributes between 1% and 3% to the total Gross Domestic Product (GDP) in the majority of current Member States, with only Spain and Portugal (4%) and Greece (8%) having larger agricultural sectors (CIA 2002). The basic aim of any agricultural policy should be to provide adequate food for the population. In reality the situation in the EU is a much more complex combination of agriculture, environment, food and trade with no real consideration of health. The CAP comprises a set of laws and policy instruments which regulate the production, trade and processing of agricultural products in the EU. Currently about 90% of the agricultural budget is allocated to subsidies to farmers.

The objectives of the CAP as set out in Article 33 of the EC (Amsterdam) Treaty are:

- To increase agricultural productivity;
- To ensure a fair standard of living for the agricultural community, by increasing individual earnings of those employed in agriculture;
- To stabilize markets;
- To assure the availability of supplies;
- To ensure that supplies reach consumers at reasonable price.

The CAP provides certain benefits in terms of maintaining farm incomes and a level of food security, but at the expense of Europe's consumers. According to the UK National Consumer Council figures, in 1996 consumers paid an extra €39 billion through inflated food prices. By their calculations, for every €100 that farmers gain from the CAP, consumers and taxpayers pay out €142 (National Consumer Council 1999). The CAP fails to promote healthy products like fruit and vegetables but encourages overproduction and distribution of surplus foods such as meat, sugar and dairy products which current dietary advice recommends the European population should cut back on (Schäfer Elinder 2003). Intensive agricultural systems that the CAP encourages are also linked to a wide range of food safety problems (such as antibiotic use, pesticide residues and increased zoonoses and foodborne infections). Public health has never been considered an important factor in the CAP and does not feature in the most recent reforms agreed on 26 June 2003 (Council of the European Union 30 June 2003). The EU agricultural sector continues to ignore the negative health implications of the CAP through its promotion of poor nutrition and inequalities in access to food which are created through subsidies, trade barriers and other economic incentives in the CAP (Schäfer Elinder 2003).

Transport is another important European policy issue. There is pressure to create an integrated European transport network to facilitate the working of the internal market and enhance regional development (European Commission 2002). Large amounts of structural funds have been invested in road building in less developed areas in poorer member states such as Ireland. This investment in infrastructure improvements has had little or no assessment of health impacts despite the increasing public awareness and scientific evidence for the health effects of transport policy through traffic injuries, air pollution, noise and impact on levels of physical activity (Dora and Racioppi 2003), with several studies from different Member States showing that health impacts of transport policy have been poorly considered despite the requirement for environmental impact assessment (Dora and Racioppi 2003).

Despite the fact that several international policy instruments – the UNECE Espoo Convention and the European Directives on Environmental Impact Assessment, for example – cite emphasis on human health protection as a major reason to carry out environmental impact assessments (EIAs) (1985; 1987), in practice the consideration of health impacts has largely been neglected or has been inadequate.

Clearly considerable scope exists outside the health care sector to prevent ill health at a population level. Increasingly, governments and supranational institutions are starting to acknowledge the wider determinants of population health and thus, the relevance of health impacts of non-health policies. In some cases, awareness of health impacts has increased as a result of major public concern about health protection. For example, the discovery in the UK of Bovine Spongiform Encephalopathy (BSE) in cattle and the realization that poor agricultural practices and bad policy-making, which did not take public health into account, led to BSE being transmitted to humans as a new fatal disease (new variant Creutzveld-Jakob disease) (The BSE Inquiry 2000). Such high profile examples have highlighted the impact on human health of decisions made in other policy areas and the knock-on effects that such developments can have, including effects on people's perceptions of risks and on public confidence in policy-makers and scientists. A recent survey of 28 European governments (including current and new Member States of the EU) found that in all but four countries health was seen as a theme that cuts across other policy areas, and all but one stated that they thought health might be relevant when developing polices or programmes in other policy sectors (Welsh Assembly Government 2003). However, 15 out of 28 stated that health is only considered opportunistically and its inclusion is not systematically included in policy development.

How can we improve consideration of health in decision-making?

Health impact assessment (HIA) is one approach that is being increasingly perceived by policy-makers across Europe as a mechanism that could be used to increase awareness and consideration of public health at a policy and project level.

The health impact assessment (HIA) approach is grounded in the broad

---

Box 15.1 What is health impact assessment?

The most quoted definition of HIA was developed at a WHO consensus conference:

> HIA is combination of procedures, methods, and tools by which a policy, pro-
> gramme, or plan may be judged as to its potential effects on the health of popu-
> lation and the distribution of those effects within the population. (Gothenburg
> consensus paper, European Centre for Health Policy, WHO 1999)

HIA is a systematic, yet flexible and adaptable approach to help those developing
and delivering policies to consider the potential (and actual) impact of a proposal
on population health and wellbeing, and on the equity effects within the population (that is health inequalities, the impact on specific vulnerable groups). HIA
also identifies practical ways to improve and enhance the proposals, and its primary output is a set of evidence-based recommendations which feed into the
decision-making process. It enables a wide range of factors that can affect human
health – directly or indirectly – to be identified and taken into account at an early
stage in planning and decision-making (Lock 2000; Health Development Agency
2002).
  It can help by:

- making links between health and other policy areas thus helping to
  generate a better understanding of the interactions between policy areas;
- ensuring that the potential health consequences of political decisions –
  positive or negative – are not overlooked by raising awareness of the
  relevance of health in different policy sectors;
- facilitating greater integration and coordination between policies and
  action across all sectors by identifying new opportunities to protect and
  improve health and by informing discussions and decisions on
  appropriate action. (Breeze and Lock 2001)

---

determinants of human health. These include personal, social, cultural, economic, environmental and other factors that influence the health status of
individuals and populations (Table 15.1). Many health determinants are inter-
related and there are several cross-cutting issues that affect health such as poverty and education. The systematic nature of health impact assessment means
that health impacts are considered by way of a number of categories. The categories encompass a series of intermediate factors that are determinants of
health, through which changes due to a policy or project can impact on people's
health. The precise categories used and their component parts may vary according to the nature of the proposed policy, programme or other development thus
providing sufficient flexibility in the application of the health impact assessment concept in different circumstances. Table 15.1 illustrates one example of
such a classification. This broad model of health obviously means that the
greatest scope for improving population health often lies outside the control of
the health services, often within specific EU policy competencies.

Table 15.1 Classification of the broad determinants of health used in health impact assessment

Category of health determinants	Some examples
Pre-conceptual/in utero	Maternal health, health of foetus during pregnancy
Behavioural/lifestyle	Diet, smoking, physical activity, risk-taking behaviour (for example unsafe sex, illicit drugs)
Psycho-social environment	Community networks, culture, religion, social inclusion
Physical environment	Air, water, housing, noise, waste
Socioeconomic status	Employment, education, training, household income
Provision of and access to public services	Transport, shops, leisure, health and social services
Public policy	Economic, welfare, crime, agriculture, health policies
Global policy issues	International trade, European Union policy, multinational industries (for example tobacco, food, oil)

The European basis for health impact assessment of inter-sectoral policies

There is a long tradition of applying impact assessment methodologies in the EU and in individual Member States. The first European Directive on Environmental Impact Assessment was adopted in 1985 (1985). There is also experience with social impact assessment and, more recently, integrated forms of impact assessment such as sustainability assessment and integrated impact assessment. A legal basis for conducting HIA emerged in Article 129 of the Maastrict Treaty (1993) and remained in Article 152 of the Amsterdam Treaty (1997). Article 129 on public health stated that "health protection shall form a constituent part of the Community's other policies". However, as Article 129 precluded harmonizing legislation it had little influence on policy within Member States (McKee et al. 1996). It also did little to foster an intersectoral approach to policy at a European level (Mossialos and McKee 2000) as there was a discrepancy between the intentions of Article 129 and the lack of internal means to carry it out. Article 152 of the Amsterdam Treaty (ratified in 1999), stated "a high level of human health protection shall be ensured in the definition and implementation of all community policies and activities". This strengthened the Community obligation, and created an opportunity to develop HIA to ensure that this goal would be achieved. Yet while there has been much discussion about integrating public health into other policies, taking advantage of HIA, the only examples of progress so far have been pilot HIA projects funded through Directorate-General (DG) Sanco, as part of the EU Health Strategy 2000, with further examples expected to be funded in the new public health programme 2003–2008 (2002). An initial guide to taking health impacts into account when developing policy was published by DG Sanco (European Commission 2001). This is an untried and unevaluated HIA screening tool which has yet to be implemented at any level of EU decision-making. In the new public health programme HIA is supported as a cross-cutting theme, in which health impact assessment of proposals under other Community policies and activities, such as research, internal market, agriculture or environment will be used as a tool to ensure the consistency of the Community health strategy. However, while work on HIA continues there is still some scepticism about its future potential due to its currently unproven nature (Hubel and Hedin 2003).

Yet even if HIA were implemented within the EU it is not clear how it would be integrated into policy-making. Health is, of course, not the only consideration in policy-making and final decisions will be the result of a number of other considerations or factors. HIA does not mean that health considerations will take primacy over all others in policy-making. Decision-making may involve trade-offs between different objectives, of which health will only be one alongside economic, environmental, employment, social welfare, trade and other considerations. This is a major barrier to effective HIA implementation at a policy level, and has yet to be resolved. A realistic aim is to ensure that possible health consequences of actions are not overlooked. In this way, any negative impacts on people's health and wellbeing can be anticipated, removed or mitigated.

Integrating health into other impact assessments in the EU

Although the European Commission is starting to develop HIA methods as part of its public health programme, HIA is unlikely to become mandatory, in contrast to Environmental Impact Assessment (EIA) which, in the EU, has a statutory legal basis. This is mainly mandated by the terms of the EIA and Strategic Environmental Assessment (SEA) Directives of the EU (1985; 1987). HIA, EIA, SEA and other impact assessments have much in common. It has been argued that procedures for HIA could be most easily introduced with the inclusion of health in existing processes for EIA. While health effects are currently supposed to be dealt with within the EIA legislation, they are actually poorly assessed, either completely absent or restricted to an environmental health focus such as pollution levels of specific substances. Although health protection is always defined as a key issue in any environmental assessment, in practice, little has really been achieved in integrating health considerations into the process (Breeze and Lock 2001). The ownership of the EIA, SEA or other impact assessment process by agencies that have no direct stake in the health sector has been shown to be an obstacle to the effective integration of health concerns. Some recent European initiatives are attempting to strengthen the health elements of environmental impact assessments, including development of integrated impact assessment procedures and work between WHO and European governments towards integrating aspects of HIA in a new European legal protocol on SEA (Breeze and Lock 2001). On 21 May 2003 the UNECE Strategic Environmental Assessment (SEA) protocol was launched at the 5th Pan European Ministerial Conference European Environment for Europe held in Kiev (http://www.kyiv-2003.info/main/index.php). Thirty-five European countries and the EU have now agreed and signed the protocol, which should come into force in about 2005 once it has been ratified by each country. This legal protocol represents new opportunities of getting public health considerations into assessments of national and EU policies that require environmental assessments. Unlike the EIA Directive, the SEA protocol includes a clear definition of health and identifies the health determinants that should be considered. It also requires health authorities to be involved and hence could provide a mechanism to institutionalize HIA in European law (Breeze and Lock 2001).

This protocol may have implications for the health sector in candidate countries in the future. First, it may be an important means to enhance the position of public health in intersectional policy but it could also impact on scarce public health resources by placing additional legal demands on health systems to contribute to the SEA process. The other potential route of embedding health considerations in routine policy-making in the EU and Member States is through the development of so-called "integrated assessment tools". The EU is currently in the process of developing such an integrated approach for use in screening new Commission proposals (Hubel and Hedin 2003). Details of how health will be included and how the tool will be piloted and then applied are currently unavailable.

The use of Health Impact Assessment in current and new Member States

Although HIA is neither a mandatory requirement in the EU, nor part of the accession process, in the recent pan-European survey 12 governments recognize the HIA approach (Welsh Assembly Government 2003). Several current Member States already have considerable experience at applying HIA at local, regional and national level including Denmark, Finland, Germany, Ireland, the United Kingdom (England, Wales and Scotland), the Netherlands and Sweden. A brief overview of the applications of HIA in some Member States is given in Table 15.2.

Many candidate countries have begun to develop their ability to undertake HIA, identifying needs and conducting capacity building workshops. For example, a Hungarian policy paper looked at opportunities and barriers to using HIA as a tool for intersectoral policy-making (Ohr 2003), which has led to the initiation of a process of HIA development by the Hungarian Ministry of Health. Several others have been developing HIA methods and conducting pilot projects. Various approaches have been developed, including environmental health impact assessment as well as broader HIA. In the process of developing national Environmental Health Action Plans, the WHO Regional Office for Europe has worked with several national environmental health departments to develop an approach for integrating health into environmental impact assessment. Examples include Poland, Hungary, Lithuania, Czech Republic, Slovakia and Estonia, with HIA being applied to projects such as waste management and transport. Many central and eastern European countries have a strong tradition of environmental health protection and this approach to HIA has been developing in parallel with broader public health approaches, often simply termed health impact assessment. An overview of HIA activity in candidate countries is given in Table 15.3.

Table 15.2 Selected examples of how HIA has been applied in EU Member States

Country	Administrative level at which HIA conducted (national, regional, local)	Policy sectors to which HIA has been applied
Netherlands	Health impact screening of national policy	Housing policy, education budget, environmental energy tax, national budget
England	National	Regeneration (New Deal), fuel poverty, burglary reduction initiative
	Regional	London Mayoral strategies including transport, waste disposal, economic development
	Local	Housing schemes, regeneration projects, farmers markets
Wales	National	Home energy efficiency scheme, Objective 1 programme, tourism (national botanical garden)
	Local	Power station development, landfill sites, housing renewal scheme
Sweden	National	Agriculture, alcohol policy
	Local county council level	Various

Sources: Welsh Assembly Government (2003), Health Development Agency HIA gateway website (http://www.hiagateway.org.uk/).

National HIA case study: the health effect of the EU Common Agricultural Policy in Slovenia

The Slovenian Ministry of Health is one of the few countries in Europe to have actually conducted an HIA at a national level. This is an assessment of the health impacts of adopting the CAP following accession. This arose from the complex and bureaucratic accession negotiation process with the European Commission. Agricultural policy was a concern for all candidate countries and the agricultural chapter of the *acquis* was still being negotiated when the HIA was begun in Slovenia.

HIA was seen as a useful method to investigate health concerns arising from the varying effects of agriculture, food and nutrition policy. This was particularly important in relation to the agricultural sector, where public health effectively did not feature in the negotiations with the Commission. The process was in six stages: policy analysis; rapid appraisal workshops with stakeholders from a range of backgrounds; review of research evidence relevant to the policy; analysis of Slovenian data for key health-related indicators; a report on the findings to a cross-government group and evaluation.

The major difficulty in the initial stages was clarifying the policy options to be assessed. Although there were national proposals for new agricultural policy and a food and nutrition action plan, these were still at the stage of development

Table 15.3 Examples of HIA projects and development in new Member States

Country	HIA guidelines and/or training	HIA projects	Administrative level at which HIA conducted (national, regional, local)
Czech Republic	Health risk assessment (National Institute of Public Health, Prague) Health Impact Assessment in the Hygiene Service (Volf and Janout 2001)	Development regional plan-strategic health plan (planned)	Regional
Estonia	Guidelines for health impact assessment of municipality policies (Estonian Centre for Health Promotion 2002)	Pilot project: health impact assessment in Rapla municipality (in progress)	Local
Lithuania		Annual report of the National health Council health policy assessment (1998, 1999, 2000)	National
		Toxic substances health impact assessment (2003 planned)	National
		Environmental health impact assessment of waste management system, Siauliai region	Regional
Malta		Consideration of health issues in EIA for abattoir waste incinerator (preliminary HIA)	Local
Slovakia	HIA Workshop for nine central and eastern European countries (2002, 2003)		
Slovenia	Two day HIA training course run at National Institute of Public Health (2002)	Health effects of agriculture and food policies after accession (2002–2003) (Lock et al. 2003)	National

Source: Welsh Assembly Government (2003); Lock et al. (2003); Personal communication.

rather than being firm Government proposals. To complicate matters the HIA had to take into account the effect of adopting the CAP into Slovenian law. This could not be done with any degree of certainty as there were ongoing negotiations with the EU about the nature and amount of common agricultural policy subsidies that Slovenia would be allocated on accession, Furthermore, the date of accession had still not been confirmed. These issues were not resolved until December 2002, when the CAP subsidies were finally agreed between the EC and the Slovenian Government. The complexities of European agricultural policy and how it will be applied in Slovenia made conducting a detailed HIA very difficult. The CAP is an enormous and relatively inflexible body of legislation. The HIA project involved agricultural economists at the University of Ljubljana who modelled and interpreted potential policy scenarios that would be likely to occur in Slovenia when integrating the CAP requirements into Slovenian national policy. Obviously, the adoption of the CAP has an enormous influence on national policy, and it was decided that the main focus of the HIA should be the broad effects of the CAP adoption. Thus it looked at the effects of some of the specific commodity regimes including the fruit and vegetable, wine, and dairy sectors, and the policy instruments for rural development. The policy analysis also had to consider any impact on national proposals, which promoted rural development, including the development of rural diversification and environmentally friendly policies. Although these national proposals were based on the CAP, it was widely believed that the EU negotiations would prevent them being adopted in full.

The most important part of an HIA is identifying and collecting information on the health impacts that may arise from a policy. The HIA approach taken in Slovenia involved national and regional stakeholders. The first HIA workshops were held in March 2002 in the north-east region of Promurje. Sixty-six people participated, including representatives of local farmers, food processors, consumer organizations, schools, public health, non-governmental organizations, national and regional development agencies and officials from several government ministries, including Agriculture, Economic Development, Education, Tourism and Health, as well as a representative of the president of Slovenia (Lock et al. 2003). The participants were asked to identify potential positive and negative health impacts of the proposed agricultural policies. This was achieved by conducting a series of rapid appraisal workshops, which were facilitated by use of a semi-structured grid assessment framework. This prompted participants to consider the core policy issues and identify potential health impacts using the main determinants of health. As part of this process, participants were asked to identify which population groups would be most affected by each policy area.

The qualitative information gained from the workshops enabled construction of a picture of probable positive and negative health impacts, including areas of speculation and disagreement. The next step was to combine this information on potential health impacts with evidence from other sources in order to test the "hypotheses" proposed in relation to health impacts. For example, one theme from the workshops was the hypothesis that adoption of the CAP would result in larger farm sizes and intensified production methods, leading to loss of small family farms, increased rural unemployment, and a consequent increase in ill health, including depression. This was in regions that already had high rates of alcohol-related deaths and suicide. The next stage set out to clarify whether evidence supported the links between adopting the CAP and loss of small family farms, links between farm intensification and increased rural unemployment, and links between either of these and increased rates of ill health. This review produce recommendations aimed at identifying policy instruments in the CAP that could help to maintain small farms, such as conversion from grain to horticulture production more suited to smallholdings.

Unsurprisingly, evidence for the links between the policy issues identified in the workshops was found to be patchy or not available in an up-to-date, easily synthesizable form. For the HIA to proceed, the next stage was to map a more detailed evidence base for how agriculture and food policies affect health. Evidence reviews were provisionally commissioned by WHO that linked relevant agriculturally related health determinants and health outcomes for the six policy topics identified in the stakeholder workshops. These policy topics were environmentally friendly and organic farming methods, mental health and rural communities, socioeconomic factors and social capital, food safety, occupational exposure and issues of food policy, including price, availability, diet and nutrition.

The final aspect of the project collected health and social indicators in Slovenia. These indicators are determinants of health and were used in the HIA as measures of intermediate health outcomes. This allowed the interpretation of the literature review evidence for the Slovenian context. The Institute of Public Health, Ljubljana, coordinated the national and regional data collection. As with many HIAs, uncertainty about the extent of policy change after accession meant that for many indicators we were unable to quantify the health outcomes precisely and could only predict the direction of the effect.

The HIA report was presented to the Ministry of Health to inform the National Food and Nutrition Action Plan. This report presented the results and offered recommendations to the Government of Slovenia on a range of agricultural issues including the fruit and vegetable, grain and dairy sectors, and rural development funding, although it clearly could not advise on all aspects of the CAP.

This was the first project to attempt to estimate specific national health impacts of incorporating the CAP, and the first prospective HIA undertaken of national agricultural and food policy. Although a formal evaluation has not yet been undertaken, several important learning points have already arisen. The main problems encountered during the HIA were the complexity of the policies being assessed and the lack of evidence of health impacts. As the CAP is such a huge and difficult policy area it was essential to have effective cross-governmental working in place at a national and regional level to tackle the policy issues. Relatively good intersectoral relationships existed between the Ministry of Health and other ministries, including agriculture and economic development, before the HIA commenced. The HIA helped to develop new communication mechanisms between the ministries on these issues. In common with many HIAs elsewhere, this HIA was limited by pressures of time and human resources, as everyone involved had to work on the HIA in addition to carrying out their existing responsibilities. At the start of the work most people in Slovenia were unfamiliar with the methods or aims of HIA. The project initially failed to recognize the importance of the public health capacity building that was required, and found that some data or evidence from sources was not tailored to a form best suited for use in the HIA.

Even though this was planned as a pilot project feeding into national policy development, the political time frames created pressure to provide support for the Slovenian Government's position during the EU negotiations on the CAP subsidies. However, often this was not possible. In 2002 the goal of accession had been a moveable target, and the proposed nature of EU subsidies changed regularly. Consequently, it proved very difficult to quantify or assess some outcomes with any certainty. However, the process of conducting the HIA has achieved some important intermediate outcomes that were not initially foreseen. The HIA involved experts from the Ministry of Agriculture who were negotiating the Slovenian policy position on subsidies with the EC. This not only put wider health and social issues on the agricultural policy agenda, but resulted in agricultural experts arguing the case for "healthy" agricultural policy in the Slovenian national media. The end result was that the health and agricultural sectors have begun to have a better understanding of each others' objectives, and have begun to support each other in some of the agriculture and food policies that they want implemented in Slovenia after accession.

Conclusion: What are the opportunities and constraints of HIA for candidate countries?

There is a growing experience of HIA applied to non-health sector policies in Europe including employment, housing and transport policies and national budget allocations (IIUE 1999 (English translation 2001); NSPH 2000; Varela Put et al. 2001). Various methods and approaches have been used, all of which aim to assess the impact of a policy on public health. Despite this, there is still much uncertainty about what HIA can realistically do for policy-making and how it can be used by current and acceding Member States to improve health considerations in non-health policy-making.

In many respects the experience of HIA of agriculture and food policies in Slovenia is similar to that found in other policy contexts in current Member States. The major benefits seem to result in strengthening policy-makers' understanding of the interactions between health and other policy areas, and to create new opportunities for improving intersectoral relationships (Lock et al. 2003). For example, in Slovenia, the ability of HIA to involve a wide range of stakeholders was considered a very important part of the process. It broadened the perspective brought to bear on the issues. By engaging other ministries and sectors in public health issues, it created shared agendas and goals in the future policy negotiations. However, such wide-ranging stakeholder involvement may not always be necessary. Two health assessments of the EU CAP have been conducted by the Swedish Institute of Public Health (Dahlgren et al. 1996; Schäfer Elinder 2003). The most recent (Schäfer Elinder 2003) has contributed to improved intersectoral working but was limited to a desk-based expert-led study.

In terms of achieving more specific outcomes, the HIA process still faces many problems, especially in such complex policy environments as agriculture and environmental policy, exactly those that should be subject to health assessments at a European level. These include the often discussed issues of the correct timing of an HIA, the weak evidence-base for HIA, and how to embed HIA in governmental organizational culture.

Timing is a particularly problematic issue. The experience in Slovenia, as in earlier examples in the Netherlands and Wales, was that if an HIA is begun too early, policies may be still too vague or change too frequently to make a detailed assessment possible (Breeze and Hall 2001; Varela Put et al. 2001). Conversely, a HIA that feeds into the decision-making too late will also have little or no ability to effect change. This was the case in the health assessment of the carcass disposal policy in response to the foot and mouth disease outbreak that was conducted by the UK Department of Health. A rapid, early health assessment was crucial in influencing policy change and getting public health onto the agenda early in the foot and mouth disease outbreak (Department of Health 2001).

So far all the methods used to conduct HIAs at national policy level have been broadly similar, using assessment based on broad determinants of health. By maintaining the focus on health determinants in this way HIAs will always reveal large uncertainties in the evidence for potential health impacts. In many EU policies such as the CAP, the causal pathways are very complex, and the current evidence base is patchy and often not relevant for assessing specific policy options (Parry and Stevens 2001). Yet this does not mean that there is no evidence to assess health impacts of a policy. There is continuing discussion about how best to assemble relevant evidence that can enable HIA to contribute to policy-making (Mindell et al. 2001; Parry and Stevens 2001), which may require a trade-off between timeliness and depth.

The way HIA is applied by governments will affect its ultimate long-term influence on policy. Those countries that have effective HIA programmes have institutionalized HIA in various ways (Banken 2001; Breeze and Hall 2001; Varela Put et al. 2001). However, the Netherlands is the only European country that has institutionalized a national HIA programme. The HIA in Slovenia was conducted as a one-off project. However, in Slovenia there was at least a clear mechanism of how the HIA would feed into government strategy making. If HIA is not embedded in the organizational structure of decision-making bodies, benefits to intersectoral working may be lost. This was the case in British Columbia, Canada, where, owing to political changes, HIA fell off the policy agenda after previously having a central cabinet-level role (NSPH 2000).

The need for health involvement across policy sectors will become more important after accession to the EU. Any new Member State thinking of introducing HIA as a mechanism for improving intersectoral working needs to think more broadly about the most appropriate means of developing and embedding public health in current intersectoral practice, including the need for public health capacity building. In the wider context of policy-making, HIA should be seen as one, albeit useful, tool that can be used to embed public health across policy sectors including those where there are major EU competencies such as agriculture. It is clearly not the only way to support effective intersectoral working or "healthy" policy development.

Its strengths include a structured approach, the flexibility of methods and involvement of stakeholders in the process. However, the public health community has not yet reached a common understanding of HIA, and how it can be used in policy-making. This is confusing to decision-makers wishing to apply HIA. The experience gained in Slovenia shows that HIA has potential for candidate countries as a means of contributing to more integrated intersectoral policies, not only in agriculture but a range of policy areas. Further evaluation of the outcomes of such exercises should enable us to direct the development of HIA in the most practical way to support such governments who are already undergoing a rapid process of change make "healthier" policy choices.

References

(1985) Council Directive 85/337/EEC of 27 June 1985 on the assessment of the effects of certain public health and private projects on the environment.

(1987) Council Directive 97/11/EC of 3 March 1997 amending Directive 85/337/EEC on the assessment of the effects of certain public and private projects.

(2002) Decision No 1786/2002/EC of the European Parliament and of the Council of 23 September 2002 adopting a programme of Community action in the field of public health (2003–2008).

Banken, R. (2001) Strategies for institutionalising HIA. Brussels: WHO Europe, ECHP Policy Learning Curve no. 1.

Breeze, C. and Hall, R. (2001) Health Impact Assessment in government policymaking: developments in Wales. Brussels: WHO Europe, ECHP Policy Learning Curve.

Breeze, C. and Lock, K. (2001) Health Impact Assessment as part of Strategic Environment Assessment. Rome: WHO Regional Office for Europe.

CIA (2002) The world factbook 2002, http://www.cia.gov/cia/publications/factbook/ges/pl.html#Econ.

Council of the European Union (30 June 2003) CAP Reform – Presidency compromise (in agreement with the Commission). http://register.consilium.eu.int/pdf/en/03/st10/st10961en03.pdf, Brussels.

Dahlgren, G., Nordgren, P. and Whitehead, M. (1996) *Health Impact Assessment of the EU Common Agricultural Policy.* Stockholm, Sweden: National Institute of Public Health.

Department of Health (2001) A rapid qualitative assessment of possible risks to Public Health from current foot and mouth disposal options. London: Department of Health.

Dora, C. and Racioppi, F. (2003) Including health in transport policy agendas: the role of health impact assessment analyses and procedures in the European experience, *Bulletin of the World Health Organization,* 81(6):399–403.

European Commission (2001) Ensuring a high level of health protection. Luxembourg: EC Health and Consumer Protection Directorate General.

European Commisssion (2002) White paper. European transport policy for 2010; time to decide. Brussels, http://europa.eu.int/comm/energy_transport/en/lb_en.html.

Health Development Agency (2002) Introducing health impact assessment: informing the decision-making process. London: Health Development Agency.

Hubel, M. and Hedin, A. (2003) Developing health impact assessment in the European Union, *Bulletin of the World Health Organization,* 81(6):461–2.

IIUE (1999 (English translation 2001)) Preliminary study: Health Impact Assessment of Housing Policies in the Netherlands. NSPH.

Lock, K. (2000) Health Impact Assessment, *British Medical Journal*, (20 May): 1395–8.

Lock, K., Gabrijelcic, M., Martuzzi, M. et al. (2003) Health impact assessment of agriculture and food policies: lessons learnt from HIA development in the Republic of Slovenia, *Bulletin of the World Health Organization*, 81(6):391–8.

McKee, M., Mossialos, E. and Belcher, P. (1996) The influence of European law on national health policy, *Journal of European Social Policy*, 6:268–9.

Mindell, J., Hansell, A. and Morrison, D. (2001) What do we need for robust quantitative health impact assessment?, *Journal of Public Health Medicine*, 23(3):173–8.

Mossialos, E. and McKee, M. (2000) A new European health strategy, *British Medical Journal*, 321:6.

National Consumer Council (1999) CAP reform: cheap food and rural conservation?, *European Review*, 6:5.

NSPH (2000) Health Impact Screening National Budget 2000. Intersectoral Policy, Ministry of Health, Welfare and Sport, Netherlands.

Ohr, M. (2003) Getting health impact assessment into the policy process in Hungary. Conditions for developing healthy public policy. Budapest: Centre for Policy Studies, Central European University and Open Society Institute.

Parry, J. and Stevens A. (2001) Prospective health impact assessment: pitfalls, problems and possible ways forward, *British Medical Journal*, 323:1177–82.

Schäfer Elinder, L. (2003) Public Health aspects of the EU Common Agricultural Policy: Developments and recommendations for change in four sectors: fruit and vegetables, dairy, wine, tobacco. Stockholm, Sweden: National Institute of Public Health.

The BSE Inquiry (2000) The BSE Inquiry: The Report. 16 volumes. London: The Stationery Office.

Varela Put, G., den Broeder, L., Penris, M. and Roscam Abbing, E. (2001) Experience with HIA at national policy level in the Netherlands. Brussels: WHO Europe, ECHP Policy Learning Curve no 4.

Volf, J. and Janout, V. (2001) Health impact assessment in the Hygiene Service in the Millennium, *Hygiena*, 46(3):148–56.

Welsh Assembly Government (2003) Health impact assessment and government policy-making in European countries. Cardiff.

sixteen

European pharmaceutical policy and implications for current Member States and candidate countries

Panos Kanavos

Introduction

The issues

Before 1989, most pharmaceutical supplies in the then communist central and eastern European countries came from their domestic state-owned drug companies. Poland, the then Czechoslovakia, Hungary and Slovenia had strong domestic (mostly generic) pharmaceutical industries that also exported their surpluses to the Soviet Union. Transition forced these countries to consolidate their national pharmaceutical industries, as well as to accept changing patterns in pharmaceutical consumption, favouring imports of western-developed medicines. These changes had profound implications for the nature of intervention in pharmaceutical markets by the competent authorities established by national governments.

This can be seen across the spectrum of pharmaceutical business. In the regulatory field, despite progress in reform of practices and policies, there were (and still are) concerns about the process of approval and licensing of medicines, the length of time it takes to approve a medicine and the criteria applied. In the area of intellectual property rights protection, many countries in the region had to address important policy trade-offs, for instance, the granting of product (rather than process) patent rights and patent term extensions, which would limit the freedom of operation of their national generic industries. At the other end of the spectrum, full patent rights (compliance with the WTO – TRIPs (World Trade

Organization – Trade-Related Aspects of Intellectual Property Rights) Agreement, the introduction of Supplementary Protection Certificates (SPCs), and long periods of marketing exclusivity), are a necessary condition for inward investment in the pharmaceutical sector. In the pricing and reimbursement sphere, as the ratio of imported to locally produced pharmaceuticals gradually increased and countries in the region were faced increasingly with international prices charged by multinational pharmaceutical manufacturers, their statutory health insurance systems suffered deficits and had to review their initial policies of free pricing, introducing interventionist measures either for the pricing of medicines, or their reimbursement, or both, in order to contain the rate of growth of expenditure. The latter, in particular, has been growing as a proportion of total health care expenditure since transition started after 1989.

The process of striking a balance in these three areas (regulation, intellectual property rights protection, pharmaceutical pricing and reimbursement) has by no means been easy and straightforward. Accession has presented all countries in the region with further challenges. In the areas of regulation and intellectual property rights protection, eastward enlargement presents considerable opportunities to business and consumers over the medium to long term, but also challenges, particularly to regulators over the short term. In both policy areas, there have been considerable achievements so far in incorporating the *acquis communautaire* (see Table 16.1), but there is also unfinished business. Candidate countries certainly need to do more on improving transparency, reducing regulatory delays, and strengthening overall compliance with EU norms, among others, whereas the trade-off between introducing SPCs and maintaining Bolar provisions has generated much debate.

Supplementary Protection Certificates are a means of extending the validity of patents, by up to five years, to compensate for the often lengthy period between the patent application and obtaining marketing authorization. Bolar provisions refer to the right to undertake pre-patent expiry development and registration of generic medicines in order to ensure that these products can come on to the market immediately after patent expiry of the original product. In the field of pharmaceutical pricing and reimbursement, although the role of EU regulatory authorities is limited as this is a national issue, there are clearly areas of EU policy or EU jurisprudence that affect national policy. Two of these areas are parallel trade, where a product is sold in one Member State at a lower price than in another one, and then traded between the two, undercutting the higher price, and transparency, in relation to the method used to set prices of medicines, and in particular demonstration that it is non-discriminatory. There are particular concerns about the likelihood of parallel exports from candidate countries as a result of interventions by their governments to lower pharmaceutical prices, and, indeed, whether national procedures on reimbursement negotiation are in accordance with the EU Directive on transparency.

Data, methods and structure

Information on pharmaceutical regulation pertaining to central and eastern European economies is very scarce and up-to-date information is patchy (Gaal

Table 16.1 Status of regulatory and intellectual property issues in central and eastern European candidate countries, 2003

	Regulatory issues				Intellectual Property issues		
	Transparency	Delays	Fully EU compliant	Post-marketing surveillance	IPR[1] system compliant with Treaties	SPC in operation	Bolar provision in operation
Czech Republic	Yes	Yes	No	Yes	Yes	Yes	No
Estonia	Yes	No	Yes	Yes	–[2]	Yes	No
Hungary	No	Yes	No	Yes	Yes	Yes	No
Latvia	Yes	Yes	No	Yes	Yes	Yes	Yes
Lithuania	Yes	No	Yes	Yes	No	Yes	No
Poland	No	Yes	No	No	No	Yes[3]	Yes
Slovakia	No	Yes	No	Yes	No	Yes	Yes
Slovenia	Yes	No	No	Yes	No	Yes	Yes
Bulgaria	Yes	No	Yes	Yes	No	No	No
Romania	No	Yes	No	Yes	No	No	No

Notes: [1] IPR: Intellectual Property Rights
[2] – indicates not known or not available.
[3] But it will be valid from the time of accession and, as is the norm with other SPC systems in other enlargement countries, it will have no retro-active power.
Source: Author's own research.

et al. 1999; Hinkov et al. 1999; Busse 2000; Hlavacka and Sckackova 2000; Jesse 2000; Karski and Koronkiewicz 2000; Vladescu et al. 2000; Karaskevica and Tragakes 2001; Albreht et al. 2002). Very few studies exist analysing pharmaceutical policies in the region at the macroeconomic level, thereby examining national policies and comparing their likely outcomes (Kanavos 1999; Freemantle et al. 2001; Kanavos 2001; Petrova 2001; Mrazek 2002). Even fewer studies examine the (likely) impact of pharmaceutical policy changes in these countries (Eldridge et al. 2000; King and Kanavos 2002; Eicher 2003). In light of this, this chapter has relied on three distinct sources of material: first, a review of the relevant literature, comprising studies on pharmaceutical pricing and reimbursement, market research reports, and official publications of the EU and the European Medicines Evaluation Agency (EMEA). The second key source was a questionnaire survey of national senior decision-makers, comprising Directors of Pharmaceutical Regulation in Ministries of Health, Pharmacy Directors in National Health Insurance Funds and Directors of Drug Regulatory Agencies. The survey was conducted in mid-2002 and was administered by email to decision-makers previously identified by the WHO Regional Office for Europe. The survey covered the eight candidate countries (Czech Republic, Estonia, Hungary, Latvia, Lithuania, Poland, Slovakia and Slovenia) plus Bulgaria and Romania. It requested respondents to provide a detailed account of the systems of regulation and intellectual property rights protection for pharmaceuticals in their country and the extent to which they complied with international norms and treaties, the methods of financing health care, the stakeholders involved in the pricing and reimbursement of pharmaceutical products, and the methods for pricing pharmaceuticals and policies on pharmaceutical reimbursement. Finally, the third source of material was a questionnaire survey administered to national pharmaceutical industry associations requesting their view on whether national reimbursement systems fulfil the principle of transparency as envisaged by EU Directives. Individual responses to the questionnaire were accompanied by follow-up telephone interviews that sought to clarify certain issues and expand on others.

The next section reviews the challenges facing candidate countries in the areas of regulation and intellectual property rights, after which comes an overview of methods for pricing of pharmaceuticals and a discussion of cost-containment measures applying to pharmaceutical prices; the section concludes that current EU Member States and candidate countries present many similarities in their approaches to pharmaceutical pricing. The remaining sections analyse reimbursement policy in candidate countries and the type of policies that are in place, before examining policy options for the candidate countries and drawing together the conclusions.

Intellectual property rights protection and regulatory issues

Intellectual property rights protection

There are six areas of intellectual property rights protection that have been the subject of intense negotiations between the EU and the candidate countries.

The first is overall intellectual property standards, particularly the patent type and the patent protection term. Other important issues include the existence or not of Supplementary Protection Certificates (SPCs) and early experimental testing (Bolar provisions), regulatory data protection, compulsory licensing and parallel trade.

Intellectual property standards and their enforcement in the acceding countries must be similar to those in the EU and compatible with the provisions of TRIPs (Trade Related Aspects of Intellectual Property Rights). Significant progress has been made in upgrading national legislation and in individual negotiations with a number of candidate countries. Nevertheless, many of the pharmaceutical products that will be launched in several candidate countries over the next few years may have only process patents, despite product patent protection now having been introduced in all candidate countries. Process patents do not in principle allow the same degree of patent protection as product patents, thereby allowing unauthorized manufacturing of products patented in the current EU Member States to be produced and sold in candidate countries. However, parallel trade of products covered by process patents in candidate countries into "western" Europe is disallowed.

The second is the burning issue of SPCs, as, currently, only Slovenia allows for a patent term restoration along the lines of EU SPCs. Recently, the Czech Republic amended its patent legislation to include an SPC rule and Poland will introduce SPCs as soon as it becomes a full EU member in June 2004. There was also concern about Bolar provisions in several of the accession countries. Hungary has an explicit Bolar provision in its patent law and Poland has a prospective exemption, while in Slovenia early working by generic companies would not constitute patent infringement although there is no specific provision in law.

The intensity of negotiations around SPCs and Bolar reflect, in part, the pressures from industry. The "innovative" industry in the EU favours strong patent protection with maximum duration SPCs having retro-active validity and no Bolar exemptions. The "generic" industry, which is especially strong in the majority of candidate countries, would ideally oppose SPCs but cherishes the freedom to conduct trials prior to patent expiry. Strictly speaking, up to now, Bolar provisions have not formed part of the *acquis communautaire*, that is are not covered in any EU Treaty, Regulation, Directive, Decision or European Court of Justice (ECJ) judgement, and the nature of experimental testing is left to the discretion of individual EU countries. As it currently stands, no EU Member State explicitly provides such a possibility in its national legislation, although the issue has been addressed by case law in Germany, the Netherlands, Italy and Portugal. The European Commission has been pushing for the abolition of Bolar exemptions in acceding countries, arguing that this is required by the WTO. In response, the generic industry has pointed out that a WTO panel ruling has upheld the right to undertake research prior to patent expiry (EGMA 2003). The current situation seems to be that candidate countries should all implement an SPC (not retro-actively), but can maintain Bolar provisions if they are already in place.

Three further issues have attracted attention in recent years. The first is regulatory data protection. An increasing number of central and eastern European countries are moving towards requiring the full dossier of data for marketing authorizations, before they have introduced a data exclusivity period. An exclusivity period similar to that prevailing in the other EU Member States (six or ten years) seems to be the current consensus. Recent changes in EU pharmaceutical legislation, agreed upon on 2 June 2003, are certain to impact on the duration of the market exclusivity period and have implications for the early entrance of generic medicines. In particular, the period of data protection for medicines, authorized under the mandatory centralized procedure, should be ten years with the possibility to extend this by one year if the producer can demonstrate that the medicine in question can be used for a new treatment. For medicines authorized under the de-centralized procedure or under the optional centralized procedure, the period would also be ten years with the possibility for generic medicines to launch their application for marketing authorization two years before the expiry of this ten year period (CEC 2003). Second, regarding compulsory licensing, national laws on the working of a patent should meet the TRIPs provisions in each candidate country. If a product is being manufactured elsewhere and imported into the country, this should be sufficiently "working" to prevent compulsory licences being granted to local companies.

Finally, and very importantly, the debate around parallel trade is intensifying. Within the EU, the principle of regional exhaustion applies, namely, once a product has been legitimately put on the market in one Member State, it cannot be prevented from being re-sold in another Member State, even if the product is protected by the exclusivity granted by a patent or other intellectual property right in the latter state. Industry argues that accession of many relatively poor countries will stimulate parallel trade, but parallel traders say that these fears are exaggerated. Recent evidence from WHO (Eldridge et al. 2000) suggests that price differentials between east and west may be minimal after all, and at times prices may be higher in eastern Europe.

Nonetheless, the Spanish and Portuguese experience has defined the current tough stance vis-à-vis candidate countries. On 3 March 2000, the Council of Ministers agreed to take a "common position" in the enlargement talks whereby candidate countries should agree to provide a "specific mechanism". Under this mechanism the holder of a patent or an SPC filed in a Member State at a time when a product patent or SPC could not be obtained in the candidate country, could rely on the rights granted by that patent or SPC to prevent the import and marketing of that product in the Member State where the product enjoys patent or SPC protection. This implies that a proprietary company could litigate to prevent the parallel trade of specific products that were patented in the EU, but not fully protected in the candidate countries at the time of accession and candidate countries potentially agree to a free trade derogation, the duration of which is subject to intense negotiation. Slovenia, in its new industrial property legislation, adopted at the end of 2000, gives further protection to patent holders. The new law says that "a pharmaceutical product or substance which was not protected by a patent in Slovenia could only be exported from Slovenia with the consent of the holder of that patent". Estonia, Malta and Cyprus have provisionally agreed to similar language. The issue is of course controversial and it is likely to remain so for some time to come.

Regulatory issues

Regulatory authorities in candidate countries have organized themselves under the Collaboration Agreement of Drug Regulatory Authorities in EU Associated Countries and are in regular contact with the regulatory authorities in the EU. Eudranet has been extended to the regulatory authorities in the region and experts from the region have also been participating in the expert committees of the EU regulatory system. Although drug legislation in the candidate countries has been modernized through adoption of the *acquis communautaire*, enforcement has yet to be strengthened.

The PERF initiative

To bridge the gap between east and west, in July 1999 the European Commission set up the Pan-European Regulatory Forum (PERF) for both regulators in the EU and the candidate countries to identify practical arrangements for implementing EU pharmaceutical legislation ahead of the next enlargement. The formal agenda includes discussions on how a system of pharmaco-vigilance would work in an enlarged Union. It also includes discussions on how the prospective EU Member States will assess quality, safety and efficacy in dossiers of human and veterinary products, implement European Directives for products already on their national markets and make decisions on new products more transparent. Separate groups are also looking at ways of promoting good manufacturing practice and making greater use of electronic databases and information technology.

Dossier updates

Dossier updates have been a contentious issue in the accession talks. The Commission argues that candidate countries must make marketing authorizations for existing products comply with current European law on the day of accession, or withdraw them from the market. The accession states say the timetable for dossier updates is too tight and five have asked for a transitional arrangement (Cyprus to 2005, Slovenia and Malta to 2007, and Poland and Lithuania to 2008). Candidate countries also argue they are being treated more harshly than current EU members, which have had more time to conduct similar exercises.

A solution to the problem of updating pharmaceutical dossiers lies in EU Directive (99/83/EC) on "well-established medicinal use" which includes an abridged procedure for updating pharmaceutical dossiers. The Directive could be a valuable tool in dealing with dossier updates. In principle, it would make it possible for regulators to use bibliographic references to satisfy requirements for pharmacological and toxicological information. A full quality dossier would, however, still be required. For products long on the market, which for some reason do not have a full dossier and do not come under the scope of the generic essential similarity requirement, it would be possible to use the established Directive to show that the requirements for safety, quality and efficacy are being met.

The European Union centralized procedure in eastern Europe

Since 1 January 1999 central and eastern European regulatory agencies have been experimenting with an entirely new procedure for vetting medicines. It is an abbreviated form of the EU's own centralized procedure involving the use of the European Medicines Evaluation Agency's (EMEA) scientific assessments to speed medicine approvals. The procedure is initiated by the relevant company, is voluntary, and has been implemented under an agreement among CADREAC (Collaboration Agreement between Drug Regulatory Agencies in EU Associated Countries) agencies.[1] Between January 1999 and April 2000, CADREAC member agencies had handled 211 procedures relating to 54 EU marketing authorizations. There were 130 positive decisions in this period. For legal reasons, the agencies can only issue national marketing authorizations. Yet, significantly, the products generally have the same summary of product characteristics (SmPC) as those in the EU.

Because the abbreviated centralized procedure has worked so well, CADREAC is now considering extending the procedure to products approved before 1 January 1999 and it is considering introducing a simplified system for vetting products approved in the EU under mutual recognition. In doing so, it would build on the experience of the Czech Republic and Slovakia, which have been running pilot mutual recognition projects since spring 2000.

The procedure is voluntary and must be initiated by companies, but it has benefited the central and eastern European regulators by reducing their workload. Under the procedure, pharmaceutical companies give regulators access to EMEA and European Commission information on a product, namely the assessment report and summary of product characteristics, thus helping them to shorten the approval time.

Despite CADREAC's experience with the centralized procedure, and its future involvement with mutual recognition, it has not been formally included in the European Commission's 2001 review of its regulatory procedures. The 2001 review is being conducted by the Commission in consultation with companies, EU regulators and professional organizations. Its purpose is to update the regulatory procedures to take account of changes in technology and medical practice. These updates will be carried out via administrative and legal measures, with the legal measures probably not taking effect before 2004.

In anticipation of enlargement, CADREAC is also trying to move towards common pharmaco-vigilance procedures, including how to format and deliver adverse drug reaction (ADR) reports and how to encourage more spontaneous ADR reporting.

The European Union mutual recognition process in central and eastern Europe

Support has also been provided for a simplified procedure for reviewing pharmaceutical products approved through the EU's mutual recognition procedure (MRP). The simplified MRP could be applied to reviews of new chemical entities (NCEs) or to generics. Individual countries would decide how to use it, but it is expected many authorities would seize the opportunity to speed up generic approvals. In a parallel move, Slovakia launched its own pilot procedure for shortened MRP reviews on 1 April 2000. The Czech Republic started a pilot procedure in March 2000.

Within the EU, the MRP is the only way generic companies can gain approval for their products in more than one national market at a time. While CADREAC members broadly support the concept of simplifying regulatory reviews, there is concern in some agencies that multinationals could use the procedures to jump the regulatory queue. Hungary has said regulators need to guard against letting the procedures overtake applications from companies seeking national marketing authorizations.

Concluding remarks on regulation

The candidate countries have now introduced legislation incorporating the elements of the *acquis communautaire* on pharmaceuticals such as packaging, labelling, advertising, pharmaco-vigilance, inspections, good manufacturing practice (GMP), good clinical practice (GCP) and transparency, as well as authorization procedures. Yet as this review has shown, there is still work to be done on intellectual property and regulatory issues. The focus of those involved is now on the detail. Importantly, there seems to be some divergence between the setting up of the institutional framework and its practical implementation. It is nevertheless critical that the institutional framework is in place before or upon accession, as failure to do so may lead to safety concerns and can jeopardize access to essential medications by local populations. The enlarged EU needs to operate under similar broad rules to ensure fair play to business and access by patients.

Pricing of pharmaceutical products

Survey results

With the exception of Lithuania and Poland, where pricing and reimbursement are considered at the same stage, in all other surveyed countries pricing and reimbursement procedures are kept separate; in these countries a product has to be allocated a price before being considered for reimbursement. This, in a sense, implies that, for the majority of countries in the region, there exist two hurdles to arrive at a reimbursed price, although the price received at the first stage (pricing) is usually relatively high and subject to less regulatory scrutiny. The results of the survey on pricing are outlined below and summarized in Table 16.2.

Price setting for imported medicines

The pharmaceutical industry proposes its own prices in the majority of the countries surveyed, but none of its own prices in Romania and Slovenia. The pharmaceutical industry has freedom in price setting on imports only in the

Table 16.2 Pharmaceutical pricing

	Bulgaria	Czech Republic	Estonia	Hungary	Latvia	Lithuania	Poland	Romania	Slovakia	Slovenia
Pricing methodology for imported pharmaceutical products										
Free pricing			✗	✗	✗	✗				
Average pricing								✗		✗
Cost-plus		✗						✗		
Price negotiation						✗	✗	✗	✗	
Other									✗	
Combination approach								✗		
Pricing and reimbursement structure										
Together						✗	✗			
Separate	✗	✗	✗	✗	✗	✗		✗	✗	✗
Regulatory barriers										
Me-too pricing				✗						
Periodic price reduction						✗				
Pharmaceutical budget is fixed	✗			✗	✗	✗		✗		
Separate budgets for "expensive" products	✗			✗		✗				
Other			✗			✗	✗		✗	

Czech Republic. Even in this case, however, formal approval must be obtained from the authorities. Suggested prices are usually subject to negotiation and they by no means imply free pricing. Suggested prices may be accepted, although in several countries reimbursement status and inclusion into positive (reimbursement) lists may be subject to further renegotiation. Negotiations for price setting comprise international price comparisons, expected sales and their growth, and, sometimes, even cost structure of operations of a local subsidiary.

With the exception of the Czech Republic, in all other countries prices of imported medicines are automatically translated and published in local currency. Exchange rate instability therefore becomes an issue of paramount importance for pharmaceutical prices, especially when combined with the frequency of exchange rate translation. The frequency of doing so varies from semi-annual, to annual, to less frequent, although the criteria used to decide are not entirely clear. Except for Bulgaria, all countries that translate prices into local currency do so at least once a year.

Additional criteria for the pricing of imported medicines include price averaging or international price referencing. Indeed, in half of the countries in which the prices of pharmaceuticals are not set or proposed by the pharmaceutical industry, prices from a number of countries were averaged to represent the price in the country. The other half of the countries set their prices in accordance with the prices of another country, rather than an average of prices of various countries.

Pricing setting for locally produced pharmaceuticals

A variety of pricing methodologies apply to locally produced products. Hungary, Estonia and Latvia allow free pricing; in these countries, the Ministry of Health accepts the price proposed by the manufacturer. This can be seen as a measure indirectly promoting the interests of the local pharmaceutical industry. In Lithuania and Poland, a system of price negotiation applies. Finally, Slovenia sets prices through an average pricing rule with wealth adjustments, whereas Bulgaria and the Czech Republic use a cost-plus methodology, whereby manufacturers are required to submit cost data (manufacturing, advertising, Research and Development, distribution and so on) to the authorities and a mark-up is added on top of these data in order to arrive at the maximum "allowable" price in the Bulgarian market.

Cost containment measures and price revisions

If price revisions take place, they frequently do so at the manufacturers' request in half of the countries surveyed. These include Bulgaria, the Czech Republic, Latvia and Slovakia. It was reported that such revisions are granted in full as requested in Romania, whereas in Lithuania price revisions hardly ever meet the manufacturers' requests. Finally, price revisions of imported products include the effects of exchange rate depreciation in the Czech Republic, Slovakia and Slovenia.

Of the countries surveyed, Slovakia, Lithuania and Slovenia report the use of price freezes as a regular policy tool. Slovenia revealed that such freezes are typically in operation for over one year. The Governments of Romania and Lithuania use price cuts as a regular policy tool, whereas the Governments of Slovenia, Poland, and Lithuania are currently implementing or have already implemented price cuts in excess of 5%.

The survey also revealed a number of other regulatory barriers implemented by national decision-makers and aiming to contain rising drug costs by acting on the supply-side (intervention on price). Hungary is the only country in which the second or third product within a therapeutic class automatically receives a discounted price in relation to the first market entrant (me-too pricing). In Lithuania the Government fixes the price of a product for a period of time and then reduces the price after that period (periodic price reduction). Several candidate countries also have fixed pharmaceutical budgets. These include Bulgaria, Romania, Hungary, Lithuania and Latvia. In addition to a fixed global budget for pharmaceuticals, Bulgaria, Hungary and Lithuania have separate budgets for expensive products. Finally, all accession countries in the region will have to abolish their tariffs (should they exist) in their transactions with the rest of the EU upon accession and will have to adopt the Common External Tariff (CET) in their transactions with countries outside the enlarged EU. Our survey revealed that only Bulgaria and Romania applied tariffs on imported pharmaceutical finished products. National indirect taxes, like Value Added Tax (VAT), are levied on all or some drugs in every nation surveyed except Hungary, although this may be changing in the near future.

Implications of pricing policies

In the majority of surveyed countries, prices of imported (the majority) products are suggested by the industry, although this by no means implies free pricing. Free pricing may be allowed in some countries (for example the Baltic states), whereas in others health insurance organizations, or, indeed, the Ministry of Finance that approves all decisions, have the final say on the actual marketed prices. Proposed prices for imported pharmaceuticals are often submitted to competent pricing authorities together with prices from other countries, for an average to be set, or are taken by reference to a single other country. In most cases, other parameters are required, such as expected sales or even local operational costs. Still, policies on pharmaceutical pricing are very volatile and subject to frequent review. In April 2003, for example, the Government of Lithuania announced it would change its pricing policy and from then on it would apply the lowest price in Europe plus 5% as the domestic Lithuanian price.

With regard to locally produced pharmaceuticals, half of the countries surveyed reported free pricing, whereas in the remainder price negotiation prevails; negotiation can be on the basis of medical necessity, expected annual sales, or prices in a number of reference countries. With the exception of the Czech Republic, prices of all imported pharmaceuticals are automatically translated into local currency, with the price translation frequency varying. Exchange rate movements are therefore an important consideration in price setting, especially in countries where prices are translated into local currencies infrequently and exchange rate fluctuations are large.

Evidence on the operational environment in the region suggests that the application of various regulatory barriers (me-too pricing, periodic price reductions, fixed pharmaceutical budgets) and/or price cuts or freezes is less intense than it is in the majority of EU Member States. It is unknown whether this will change in the near future, particularly as the consequences of European Monetary Union, with its targets of fiscal deficits, need to be observed, but indications from two candidate countries (Poland and Hungary) suggest that it might. Indeed, nearly all countries in the region are willing to experiment with measures that have been tried previously in current EU Member States.

Among countries in the region, Bulgaria, Romania and Slovenia have reported tariffs being imposed on finished imported products. This is, however, likely to disappear in the near future due to the single market requirements, especially in Slovenia, and be replaced by the common external tariff for products imported from outside the EU. All countries except Hungary impose indirect taxes of some sort (for example VAT) on medicines consumed.

Countries in the region may also treat imported and locally produced products differently, thereby arriving at different regulatory practices which may be perceived to be discriminatory and not necessarily in accordance with the *acquis communautaire*. If this continues to happen among candidate countries, it will certainly constitute a breach of accession treaties and is likely to attract swift action by the European Commission.

Finally, candidate countries will have to take on board developments arising from ongoing discussions about how to strengthen the competitiveness of the European pharmaceutical industry while at the same time bringing benefits to patients (Commission of the European Communities 2003).

Reimbursement

Survey results

This section of the survey covers reimbursement policy, namely, the way products are paid for by health insurance funds, the establishment of reimbursement levels and the methodologies used, the extent of generic prescribing and cost-sharing policies. The results of this part of the survey are summarized in Table 16.3 and Table 16.4.

Limited lists

Other than Latvia that has neither a positive nor a negative list, all of the countries have a positive list for pharmaceutical reimbursement. This means that only products included in this list can be reimbursed. It is therefore critical that companies wishing to have their products reimbursed must get them onto the positive list. In addition to a positive list, Lithuania and Slovenia have a negative pharmaceutical reimbursement list. Latvia, without a positive or a negative list, is rather unique as 75% of the drugs consumed on its territory are not reimbursed, but obtained by patients on an out-of-pocket basis. Coverage is therefore a serious issue for Latvia, although extending it in the near future is not likely to occur.

Reimbursement criteria

Each country weighs several factors when deciding whether or not to include a new product in the positive reimbursement list. Each of the respondents considered safety, efficacy, quality and other clinical criteria. Every country except Romania included new drugs with a proven therapeutic benefit over existing therapies on the positive list. With the exception of Romania and the Czech Republic, each country takes cost effectiveness and other economic variables, such as budget impact analysis, into account. This is surprising at first glance as local expertise in cost effectiveness analysis is extremely limited, but several countries have shown a willingness to introduce this tool into their decision-making process, requesting manufacturers to submit pharmaco-economic evidence and allowing studies conducted abroad to be submitted, with the exception perhaps of Estonia that requires local adaptation. Several countries in the region have drafted their own pharmaco-economic guidelines in order to aid submissions by interested parties. Poland and Hungary have been at the forefront of this activity, but the Polish guidelines are not used widely. The three Baltic countries (Estonia, Latvia, Lithuania) have also drafted their own set of guidelines, which are actively used by the decision-making community. In adopting pharmaco-economic guidelines, candidate countries have taken on board the experience of other EU Member States, particularly Finland, the Netherlands and NICE in England and Wales.

Most countries also require budget impact analysis when deliberating whether to include a drug on the positive reimbursement list. This aims to identify precisely the likely beneficiaries from certain interventions and restrict the extension of the benefit to those categories of patients that are likely to benefit most. Finally, Poland is the only country that explicitly considers industrial policy criteria, such as investment by the pharmaceutical company in question, when deciding whether to add a medicine to its positive list.

Setting a reimbursement price

Countries use different methodologies to determine the reimbursement price. Most of the countries surveyed considered medical necessity but also budget impact analysis and cost effectiveness criteria, and drew on information on prices in other countries. All respondents except for the Czech Republic tend to reimburse fully breakthrough products that add considerable therapeutic benefit. Bulgaria, Slovenia, Hungary and Latvia reimburse products that fall into a defined class of diseases or conditions at 100%, regardless of price. The Czech Republic is the only country in which the price agreed with the manufacturer is favourable and affordable with health insurance; in the opposite case, a lower reimbursement rate would have been set, even though the product is essential for treatment of life-threatening conditions.

Table 16.3 Reimbursement processes

	Bulgaria	Czech Republic	Estonia	Hungary	Latvia	Lithuania	Poland	Romania	Slovakia	Slovenia
Limited lists										
Positive list	x	x	x	x		x	x	x	x	x
Negative list						x				x
Neither					x					
Reimbursement criteria										
Clinical criteria	x	x	x	x	x	x	x	x	x	x
Proven therapeutic benefit over existing products	x	x	x	x	x	x	x		x	x
Economic criteria	x		x	x	x	x			x	x
Budget impact	x	x	x	x	x	x	x		x	
Favourable price requested by manufacturer										
Industrial policy criteria							x			
Other	x			x				x		
Setting a reimbursement price										
Medical necessity	x	x		x	x	x		x	x	
Proven therapeutic benefit over existing products				x	x			x	x	
Economic criteria	x	x		x	x	x			x	
Budget impact analysis				x	x		x			x
Industrial policy criteria				x	x		x		x	
Average prices from other countries		x				x	x			x
User price from another country										
Other			x						x	

Criteria for reimbursement exclusion

Quantity sold

Excessive price

High overall expenditure

Failure to make adequate provision for research

Low benefit–cost ratio

Old product

Low efficacy as demonstrated by newer products

Other

Not sure, because policy is uncertain and non-transparent

Basis of cluster system in reference pricing

Drugs containing an identical molecule clustered together

Drugs containing similar molecules clustered together

Other forms of clustering

No reference pricing system

Reference setting

Reference price set on basis of daily defined usage

Other basis for reference pricing

No reference pricing system

Reference pricing specifics

The lowest of the cluster

The average of the cluster

The average of the lowest two of the cluster

Other

Table 16.4 Duration of reimbursement negotiations

	Bulgaria	Czech Republic	Estonia	Hungary	Latvia	Lithuania	Poland	Romania	Slovakia	Slovenia
Usually 0–90 days	✗									
Usually 90–120 days		✗								
Usually 90–180 days							✗			
Usually far exceeds 180 days					✗	✗			✗	✗
Never less than 90 days		✗						✗		
Never less than 180 days			✗	✗		✗		✗	✗	

Formal grading of (new) products submitted for reimbursement

Slovakia is the only country reporting a formal rating of new products submitted for reimbursement depending on their innovative potential. This system gives highly innovative products a top mark and me-toos a lower grade. Although Bulgaria and Hungary do not have such a system yet, they anticipate having one in the near future.

Convening frequency by reimbursement committee

The committee that decides on reimbursement applications convenes on a semi-annual basis in Bulgaria and Slovenia. In the rest of the countries, such committees convene at least as frequently, but on an irregular basis.

Duration of reimbursement negotiations

The duration of reimbursement negotiations in participating countries spanned from fewer than 90 days to well over 180 days (Table 16.4). Bulgaria and Poland had the quickest negotiations, which generally did not exceed 90 days. Negotiations in Slovakia, Lithuania and Latvia typically took many more than 180 days. Indeed, more than half the countries reported they were above the negotiations threshold set out by the Transparency Directive.

Reimbursement exclusion

Each country surveyed has criteria to exclude or remove a product from the reimbursement list or award low reimbursement status. It is not clear what these criteria are in Bulgaria and Slovakia because the policy is deemed uncertain and/or non-transparent. Hungary, Lithuania, Romania and Slovenia generally remove drugs from the reimbursement list when a new and more effective product comes to market. The positive lists in Hungary, Lithuania and Slovenia do not include drugs with a low benefit–cost ratio. Estonia, Hungary, Latvia and Slovenia exclude drugs that would generate a high overall expenditure from the list. Excessive price can keep a drug off the reimbursement list in Estonia, Hungary, Latvia and Lithuania. Bulgaria, Hungary, Lithuania, Poland, Slovakia and Slovenia re-appraise their reimbursement register once a year, while Romania reviews its positive list biannually, Latvia re-evaluates its register less frequently still, and Estonia has not reconsidered its list in a long time.

Reference pricing

All countries surveyed have some form of reference pricing system in place. Each country with a reference pricing system clusters drugs containing identical molecules together. For example, all ranitidines are grouped together. In contrast, only Hungary and Poland cluster together drugs containing similar molecules or with similar effects. Poland also uses other forms of clustering. All respondents with a reference pricing system except Lithuania and Romania set prices on the basis of a daily defined dosage (DDD). Lithuania and Romania use other methodologies to set prices.

Bulgaria, Romania, Hungary, Slovakia, Poland and Latvia all set their reference prices in accordance with the lowest priced drug of the cluster. Hungary
also sets prices based on the average price in the cluster or the average of the
lowest two prices in the cluster. In-patent products are included in the reference
clusters of Lithuania, Romania and Slovakia. In contrast, in Bulgaria, Hungary,
Latvia and Poland, in-patent products are excluded from the clusters.

Co-payments

In all of the countries except for the Czech Republic, co-payments for prescription medicines involve a percentage of the value of the drug dispensed (co-
insurance). Patients with chronic illnesses are exempt from co-payments in
Bulgaria, Hungary and Poland. Based on their income, patients can be exempt
from co-payments in Hungary. Based on their age, they can be exempt in
Lithuania. The remaining countries, Romania, Slovakia and Slovenia, use other
criteria for exemptions.

Implications of reimbursement policies

Countries in the region use multiple criteria to determine product reimburs-
ability; among them clinical criteria as well as proof of therapeutic benefit are
the most commonly cited. Prices from other countries are also taken into consideration, very often explicitly (either through average pricing or through price
in another country becoming the reimbursed price). Economic criteria (in the
majority of cases impact on the health or pharmaceutical budget) are also
routinely used to assess overall product affordability; it can be judged that cost-
effectiveness criteria are not explicitly used when making decisions about
reimbursement, but they may be considered in the negotiation process.

Poland is the only country in the region that seems to be applying industrial
policy considerations in its reimbursement procedures (but mostly for local
companies). Overall, respondents did not feel that industrial policy considerations did apply in the reimbursement procedure, despite the region being host
to significant drug production facilities.

Only Slovakia seems to have developed a formal system of rating new products (definition of innovation) for reimbursement purposes; the six criteria presented resemble the French ASMR (Amélioration du Service Medical Rendu)
classification. Two countries (Bulgaria and Hungary) expect such criteria to be
introduced in the (near) future, whereas in all other countries, no definition of
innovation applies currently or is envisaged in the future.

The most commonly cited reasons for excluding products from reimbursement were low efficacy, as demonstrated by newer products, and low benefit–
cost ratio; high overall expenditure was also cited in several countries as a reason
for exclusion from reimbursement, whereas individual components (price or
volume) were cited less frequently.

In over half of the countries that responded, the duration of reimbursement
negotiations is either never less than 180 days or usually exceeds 180 days by far
(Table 16.4). This is a point that needs to be addressed urgently in terms of
transparency and compatibility with the European *acquis communautaire*. In

contrast, reimbursement negotiations last on average less than 90 days in Bulgaria and Poland.

Reference pricing is a popular reimbursement methodology prevailing in most of the countries in the region. The most frequently used clustering method is of the "generic" type (identical molecule clustering), although in Hungary and Poland similar molecules or molecules with comparable effects may be grouped together. The reference price is usually the lowest of the cluster, and reference price revisions are conducted annually in the majority of cases.

In half the countries health insurance funds routinely monitor the prescribing patterns of physicians, and in a further four countries monitoring is conducted when there is suspicion of over-prescribing; sanctions of some sort or another are said to be in place for those who over-prescribe, but their precise nature and the extent of enforcement is unclear in the countries involved. Little is known about the extent to which health insurance funds produce and disseminate league tables based on their monitoring activities, although piecemeal evidence suggests they do not. Several countries operate budgetary constraints on prescribing by physicians and more countries have predicted that these may be introduced in the future as means of effectively controlling prescribing behaviour and overall pharmaceutical spending. Generic prescribing is encouraged by government and health insurance funds in several countries in the region; nevertheless, none of the countries reviewed has a mandatory generic prescribing rule.

There does not seem to be a limitation on promotional spending by the pharmaceutical industry, but it was reported that constraints exist on hospitality provided to doctors by pharmaceutical companies in many countries, although the precise nature is unclear. Clearly the latter has an impact on the former. Direct to consumer advertising (DTCA) is, in principle, not allowed although a version may be allowed, for example if there is no mention of specific products but only awareness raising about a specific disease (as is the case in the Czech Republic).

Regressive margins and flat fees are the preferred method of pharmacy reimbursement, which theoretically promotes generic dispensing unless prescribing physicians request "dispense as written". The situation with generic substitution is very fragmented and with the exception of Hungary, countries in the region do not seem to have a policy that makes it compulsory. The most commonly used prescription cost sharing methodology is co-insurance (proportion of the value of the drug dispensed), although significant exemptions apply either due to chronic illness, poverty status, or age, among others.

Nearly all countries in the region are in the process of developing clinical guidelines and some countries are using them already but the nature of implementation and enforcement is unclear and the consensus is that guidelines are rarely binding; only in Hungary and Lithuania must prescribing physicians observe them, and only in Lithuania and Romania do physicians incur penalties if they do not.

Finally, all respondent countries seem to have patient databases in place, either at prescriber or at pharmacy level, which are primarily used to monitor physician prescribing patterns and less so to conduct utilization reviews or monitor physician prescribing relative to diagnosis.

The challenges ahead for the candidate countries

As the previous sections revealed, accession eastwards presents significant challenges in the pharmaceutical sector for both existing Member States, and, most importantly, candidate countries. In particular, pharmaceutical policy extending prescription drug coverage and allowing wide access to medicines in "New Europe" citizens will be influenced by developments in three areas: first, the overall macroeconomic policy (particularly fiscal policy) and the economic pressures that the candidate countries face; second, health care reform and the need to reform financing and delivery of health care services; and third, the need to have a robust regulatory framework that would guarantee access to safe and essential medicines to citizens of the new accession countries. Governments, citizens, health care professionals and industry therefore need to take these factors into account when considering or demanding reforms in the organization and delivery of health services.

In terms of macroeconomics, the link between health care financing and fiscal policy has been documented elsewhere (Kanavos and McKee 1998). It would be fair to argue that the candidate countries will face a significant economic shock posed by integration, as indeed was the case with some of the current Member States at the time of accession. The amplitude and the depth of this shock, also potentially manifesting itself in a deterioration in the terms of trade in some cases, will certainly require fiscal prudence, which is known to impact on health care financing, particularly as it concerns capital investment. Rapidly growing economies are better positioned to invest in their health care systems and accelerate reform, particularly capital investment in health care.

Macroeconomic policy, however, is only one of the parameters at play. Decision-makers in an enlarged Europe face critical challenges to their health care systems that require continued attention. These challenges relate to the following: first, on the demand-side: containing rising costs of health care, while at the same time maintaining and enhancing quality of care and instituting change. Second, on the supply-side, try to increase the pool of available resources for health care services; it is no secret that, with the exception of Slovenia, health spending per head is significantly lower in an enlarged Europe than in the current EU Member States. This may be in part due to significant differences in prices of input factors between countries in the region and current EU Member States, but if one looks at health spending as a proportion of GDP, a similar picture emerges, whereby an enlarged Europe spends significantly less on health as a proportion of its national income than the current EU. This presents an enlarged Europe with two policy dilemmas: first, if differences in relative prices of inputs are significant, then the terms of trade will not be in the region's favour; this is the case with pharmaceutical products and high prices for imported products may make them unaffordable for payers, whether these are statutory health insurance systems or individual patients; in the latter case, of course, there are potentially significant negative implications for access to effective treatments. Second, increases in investment levels are not easy to materialize, particularly if the collection of contributions is constrained by evasive attitudes, or, simply, by structural issues such as the inability to collect contributions on a sustainable basis from self-employed individuals or those employed in the primary sector. Third, there is a significant issue with health care reform and capital investment. Understandably, the majority of countries in the region will need to continue to invest in upgrading their infrastructure, but this is pretty much a linear function of economic growth.

Finally, the conduct of drug policy presents huge challenges for all stakeholders in an enlarged Europe in the following aspects: first, the need to continue to implement robust regulatory practices that ensure availability of safe and efficacious drugs, good manufacturing practices (GMP), and observing standards through frequent inspections. Second, how to ensure adequate intellectual property rights protection, whether this is through product patents, patent term extensions or marketing exclusivity rights. While understandably all candidate countries have progressed significantly in ensuring this, it remains to be tested how the implementation of this framework will work out in national courts if and when patent litigation occurs. Third, how to guarantee speedy access to new treatments (transparency) and ensure that regulatory actions are not in breach of the *acquis communautaire*, particularly as regards transparency. Lengthy reimbursement negotiations, or indeed serious delays in approval times are likely to attract legal action by European institutions. Fourth, candidate countries face an increasingly "militant" environment in the pharmaceutical sector from industrial interests. Despite the limited competence of European institutions on health and drug policy, parts of the *acquis communautaire* and European-level jurisprudence can be used to challenge the validity of and render illegal national regulatory interventions. In this respect, lessons can be learnt from a recent (12 June 2003) case, where the ECJ condemned Finland for discriminating against new products by placing them on a two year special reimbursement list before deciding on their reimbursement status, thus being judged as violating the provisions of the transparency Directive. The ruling means that Finland will have to abandon a policy that has been in operation in its territory for several years. Fifth, how to extend access and coverage to citizens that currently have to pay fully out-of-pocket for their drugs. The Latvian experience, where only 25% of the €103 million pharmaceutical market is covered by statutory health insurance, is indicative in this respect, as only drugs for chronic illnesses are covered, whereas for the remainder of the prescription drug market, patients have to pay fully out-of-pocket. Sixth, the survey on pricing and reimbursement showed that methodologies in all candidate countries display striking similarities with several of the methods used in current EU Member States. While this in itself is not negative, what remains to be seen is the determination of decision-makers in an enlarged Europe to avoid making ad hoc decisions on drug policy and thereby compromising its effectiveness. Seventh, an enlarged Europe will continue to face international prices for imported drugs. Industry has been quite successful in achieving high prices for its products in the majority of the countries in the region, as some studies have found, and this is an achievement it will not relinquish easily for all future products. Additionally, past successes often set a precedent for the future. The fear of parallel trade is likely to exacerbate this and under no circumstances will new products be launched in an enlarged Europe below the average European price in order to fend off any parallel export activities from these countries. This makes the task of negotiating prices with industry tougher and is exacerbated by the fact that all the enlarged European countries (with the sole exception of Poland) are small in size and have limited negotiating power.

Like so many other issues covered in this book, the situation is dynamic and, at the time of writing, a major review of pharmaceutical legislation is in the co-decision process (Commission of the European Communities (CEC) 2003). This includes several proposals that, if adopted before May 2004, will make important changes to existing regulations that will have immediate effect to candidate countries on accession. First, the EMEA's centralized approval procedures would be extended to cover drugs used to treat cancer, AIDS, neuro-degenerative diseases and diabetes. The choice of a centralized procedure or a decentralized one, using national systems with mutual recognition, would remain for other medicines. Second, data protection would be standardized at ten years for medicines authorized under the mandatory centralized procedures, with the possibility of extending this by one year if the manufacturer can show that the product in question can be used for a new indication. Medicines authorized under the optional centralized or the decentralized procedures would also be covered by data protection for ten years, with the possibility of generic manufacturers launching an application for market authorization two years before the expiry of the ten year period.

Conclusions

Regulation and intellectual property

Countries in the region have upgraded their regulations to comply with EU legislation on regulatory practices and appear confident that they can participate in the centralized procedures and systems of mutual recognition upon accession. With regards to intellectual property, there is currently sufficient patent protection at product rather than process level, although this is not retroactive. SPCs have been introduced as part of the *acquis communautaire* but in certain cases, their implementation will commence with accession and are not retro-active either. Several countries have explicitly maintained Bolar provisions in their legislation; this does not contravene European legislation, which has taken steps to introduce it anyway in due course.

Pharmaceutical pricing

Free pricing for pharmaceuticals is less frequent nowadays and agreement must be reached to arrive at a mutually agreeable price on the market. Candidate countries are applying significant price restrictions which are very often modelled on policies practised in current EU Member States. Despite the increasing incidence of price controls, price cuts and price freezes for products reimbursed by statutory health insurance, it appears that price levels for new medicines are high and at times high enough not to threaten parallel exports from "east" to "west". Parallel exports from the east are in any case not allowed if the same product was not covered by patent in the east at the time of its introduction in the west. However, after accession it is envisaged that parallel exports may take off within the region itself.

Reimbursement of pharmaceuticals

Many similarities exist in reimbursement policies between candidate countries and current EU countries. Reference pricing, for identical molecules, is a favourite reimbursement policy, whereas some countries in the region are experimenting with other forms of product clustering. The use of economic evidence is increasing in the region; this concerns not only the drafting of pharmaco-economic guidelines, but, increasingly, the requirement to submit a pharmaco-economic study as part of a reimbursement application. In this respect, candidate countries present another similar trend compared with current EU Member States, although it is not entirely certain that the expertise exists on a grand scale to make good use of this policy tool. Reimbursement negotiations often last longer than the Transparency Directive stipulates, an element which may attract punitive action in the years to come. Delaying access to market/reimbursement was often seen as a means of preventing additional drug costs to health insurance. Such policies may no longer be possible in future.

The candidate countries seem to be more active on the supply-side (controlling prices of medicines) rather than actively implementing demand- or quasi demand-side policies. The former seek to control prescribing or dispensing behaviour via a combination of incentives and/or disincentives. Although experiments are currently under way in some countries, this may be an area of attention in the forthcoming years, although it would require investment and close monitoring from health insurance organizations. Quasi demand-side policies on the other hand, link pricing with overall consumption levels (volume). However, given the small size of most of these countries (with the sole exception of Poland), it is unlikely that price–volume agreements can provide a viable alternative to increasing overall drug expenditures.

Acknowledgements

The author gratefully acknowledges the support of the Commonwealth Fund through the Harkness Fellowship programme. The views presented here are those of the author and not those of the Commonwealth Fund, its director, officers or staff.

Note

1 CADREAC consists of regulators from Bulgaria, the Czech Republic, Estonia, Hungary, Latvia, Lithuania, Poland, Romania, Slovakia, Slovenia, Cyprus and Turkey.

References

Albreht, T., Lesen, M., Hindle, D. et al. (2002) *Health Care Systems in Transition: Slovenia*. Copenhagen: European Observatory on Health Care Systems.

Busse, R. (2000) *Health Care Systems in Transition: Czech Republic*. Copenhagen: European Observatory on Health Care Systems.

Commission of the European Communities (2003) Communication from the Commission to the Council, the European Parliament, the Economic and Social Committee and the Committee of the Regions. A stronger European-based pharmaceutical industry for the benefit of the patient – a call for action. COM(2003) 383 final. Brussels July 2003. Brussels.

Commission of the European Communities (CEC) (2003) Commission welcomes agreement by member states on pharmaceuticals reform, Press release, Brussels, 2 June 2003, http://pharmacos.eudra.org/F2/pharmacos/docs/Doc2003/June/ip03785.pdf, accessed 11 August 2003.

EGMA (2003) Pharmaceutical Intellectual Property Issues and Enlargement. http://www.egagenerics.com/facts_figures/eu_enlargement/bolar_enlargement.htm.

Eicher, H.G. (2003) Pharmacoeconomics and the "4th hurdle": drug reimbursement policies in Central and Eastern Europe, *International Journal of Clinical Pharmacology and Therapeutics*, 41(1):1–2.

Eldridge, G., de Joncheere, K. and Kanavos, P. (2000) Drug pricing and reimbursement of innovative products in five central and eastern European countries. Copenhagen: WHO Regional Office for Europe.

Freemantle, N., Behmane, D. and de Joncheere, K. (2001) Pricing and reimbursement of pharmaceuticals in the Baltic States, *Lancet*, 358(9278):260.

Gaal, P., Rekassy, B. and Healy, J. (1999) *Health Care Systems in Transition: Hungary*. Copenhagen: WHO Regional Office for Europe.

Hinkov, H., Koulaksuzov, S., Semerdjiev, I. and Healy, J. (1999) *Health Care Systems in Transition: Bulgaria*. Copenhagen: European Observatory on Health Care Systems.

Hlavacka, S. and Sckackova, D. (2000) *Health Care Systems in Transition: Slovakia*. Copenhagen: European Observatory on Health Care Systems.

Jesse, M. (2000) *Health Care Systems in Transition: Estonia*. Copenhagen: European Observatory on Health Care Systems.

Kanavos, P. (1999) Financing Pharmaceuticals in Transition Economies, *Croatian Medical Journal*, 40(2):244–59.

Kanavos, P. (2001) Overview of pricing and reimbursement systems in Europe. Brussels: Commission of the European Communities, DG III (Enterprise).

Kanavos, P. and McKee, M. (1998) Macroeconomic constraints and health challenges facing European health systems, in R.B. Saltman, J. Figueras and C. Sakellarides (eds) *Critical challenges for health care reform in Europe*. Buckingham: Open University Press.

Karaskevica, J. and Tragakes, E. (2001) *Health Care Systems in Transition: Latvia*. Copenhagen: European Observatory on Health Care Systems.

Karski, B. and Koronkiewicz, A. (2000) *Health Care Systems in Transition: Poland*. Copenhagen: European Observatory on Health Care Systems.

King, D. and Kanavos, P. (2002) Encouraging the use of generic medicines: implications for transition economies, *Croatian Medical Journal*, 43(4):262–9.

Mrazek, M. (2002) Comparative Approaches to Pharmaceutical Price Regulation in the European Union, *Croatian Medical Journal*, 43:453–61.

Petrova, G.I. (2001) Monitoring of national drug policies – regional comparison between Bulgaria, Romania, Macedonia, Bosnia Herzegovina, *Central European Journal of Public Health*, 9(4):205–13.

Vladescu, C., Radulescu, S. and Olsavsky, V. (2000) *Health Care Systems in Transition: Romania*. Copenhagen: European Observatory on Health Care Systems.

seventeen

Lessons from Spain: Accession, pharmaceuticals and intellectual property rights

Manuel Lobato

Introduction

The accession of Spain to the European Economic Community posed a particular problem in terms of intellectual property protection. Spain had at that time (1980–1986) an ineffective system of protection of intellectual property rights, especially in the pharmaceutical field. There were no product patents, Supplementary Protection Certificates (SPCs) or protection of dossier data. This system was in sharp contrast to the situation in other Member States. It was clear that the Spanish patent law had to be amended in order to meet the European standard of protection. The modifications were introduced gradually, and Spain took advantage of all possible delays in the introduction of the new provisions with the aim of protecting its domestic industry.

An understanding of the Spanish situation regarding intellectual property protection is useful in the context of the EU enlargement process, since candidate countries face similar problems, and effective intellectual property protection is now a prerequisite for EU accession.

The necessity of reform – the Spanish position during accession negotiations

It was clear that Spanish legislation had to be amended in order to meet European standards. Concerning intellectual property, the steps to be taken were set out in the Act of Accession. The Act also established protection for undisclosed product information, but Spain obtained a derogation until December 1992.

During accession negotiations Spain had great reservations about accepting European rules on intellectual property protection. Spain wanted to exhaust all possible forms of protection in order to delay the coming into force of a strong intellectual property system. Spain was successful in its aim, but in so doing, damaged its position on other chapters, in particular agriculture and fisheries. During its negotiations, Spain successfully delayed pharmaceutical, chemical and agrochemical product patent protection until October 1992. At the time of Spanish accession SPCs were not part of the *acquis communautaire*, so there were no negotiations on the subject. Later, when regulations were enacted on SPCs, Spain obtained a delay in implementation.

Protection of product data was postponed until December 1992, at which time Spain should have introduced a pharmaceutical regulatory system which would be consistent with Directive 65/65/EEC. However, Spain approved the provision later, in June 1993, which caused a problem in some specific cases of data protection that were pending in the courts.

The old and the new systems

In the process of the accession negotiations, between 1982 and 1985, it was evident that Spain did not provide the degree of protection of intellectual property rights afforded by other Member States. In the pharmaceutical sector national companies were relatively strong but undertook little innovative activity. These national companies depended heavily on old fashioned (often ineffective) medicines and on licences granted by research-based companies. To understand the main issues that arose from this situation it is first necessary to review the legal situation prior to Spanish accession in 1986.

Legislation on intellectual property protection in Spain was limited, and the enforcement of what legal provisions existed was weak. Patent law existed within the framework of a general Industrial Property Code (Industrial Property Statute of 1929), which had undergone almost no changes for six decades. The 1929 Statute was flawed in many respects, for instance, it allowed discoveries and business methods to be patented but prevented any product patents. The Spanish Patent Office was mainly a deposition office. Criminal sanctions for breaches of intellectual property rights were non-existent. Civil protection was very difficult to achieve and preliminary injunctions were, in practice, unavailable. Spain employed introduction patents (patents that protected the person who copied a patent lodged abroad and brought it to Spain) and blanket patents, whose sole objective was to provide legal safeguards for certain types of patent infringements.

As a consequence of this chaotic situation, intellectual property protection was a separate chapter in the Spanish negotiations on accession to the European Community. According to Protocol no. 8 of the Spanish Act of Accession, from the moment of accession Spain had to make its patent legislation compatible with the free movement of goods and with European standards of intellectual property protection, in particular, regarding contractual licences, compulsory licences and introduction patents. The Commission had a particular role to monitor the changes to Spanish legislation to achieve these goals. Spain was required to become a member of the European Patent Convention (EPC). Nevertheless Spain could profit from the provisions of Article 167 of the EPC, by which each Contracting State could reserve the application of product patents for pharmaceuticals and chemicals until 7 October 1992. Spain, in its declaration of accession, used this provision in order to delay chemical and pharmaceutical product patents in Spain coming into force. It was also a requirement that Spain would adhere to the Luxembourg Patent Convention, an obligation that had no effect because this Convention was eventually not ratified by European Governments.

Article 47 of the Spanish Act of Accession dealt with the problem of parallel imports of medicines. Parallel trade refers to the importation of an original product from one Member State to another by a person who has not been authorized by the patent holder, who had introduced this product in the European Community market. The *Merck v. Stephar* ruling of the European Court of Justice (ECJ) established that once a medicine (or indeed any product) is introduced into a market in any country of the European Community with the consent of the patent holder, it can then freely circulate to other countries. It is immaterial whether the product was introduced for the first time in a Member State where patent protection was not available. In this ruling, Merck sold a medicine in Italy, where any protection of medicinal products was excluded by the Italian Patent Law of the time, and a parallel importer then acquired them and sent them to another European Community Member State, where there was product patent protection. The ECJ declared this practice valid in spite of the lack of protection of the patent. So, free movement of goods prevailed over patent protection. This ruling aroused fear that Spanish accession would bring a huge alteration to the European pharmaceutical market. Medicines prices were controlled by the Spanish government at a level that was considered extremely low, particularly for some categories of medicines. If the *Merck v. Stephar* ruling was applied, then some believed it would lead to a collapse of the European market.

Article 47 of the Spanish Accession Act was drafted in order to avoid these consequences. This Article provided an exception to the free movement of goods as set out in the *Merck v. Stephar* ruling. According to Article 47 the patent holder in a European Community Member State could rely on a product patent to prevent parallel imports of medicines, agrochemicals and chemicals from Spain, even if the product was introduced in the Spanish market with its consent (by its licensees), for a period that would lapse three years after Spain had adopted full protection for medicines, agrochemicals and chemicals (which was on 7 October 1992). The reason for this additional three year period is that there was no pipeline protection. Old products which enjoyed patent protection in other European Community Member States did not benefit from product protection in Spain, hence a distortion of the European pharmaceutical market occurred. There were Member States in which no patent protection was available, such as Spain, Portugal and Greece, and where there were many medicines from diverse sources with the same active constituent. Only those medicines which were manufactured by the patent holder or with its consent could leave the Spanish (Portuguese or Greek) market when the three year period lapsed. The other medicines (copies, me-too products and so on) could only circulate within the Spanish (or Portuguese or Greek) market. On the other hand, in Member States where there was only one legitimate source of the product, that of the patent holder, prices were naturally higher than in the previously mentioned ones. The scope of the three year protection delay was to mitigate the consequences of the different degrees of protection and prices at the European level.

The Spanish Government consistently adopted a very conservative attitude towards the modernization of its intellectual property legislation, especially in the pharmaceutical field. In negotiations, Spain obtained all possible extensions (for example with the EPC) in order to delay protection. Only urgent measures were accepted, such as the approval of a new Patent Law, which was approved in the year of accession (1986). The delay in introducing product patent protection for chemicals, medicines and agrochemicals was the maximum afforded by the EPC. Even after accession, Spain maintained a mistrustful position against everything that appeared to provide protection of intellectual property. Thus, Spain was the only Member State that, unsuccessfully, challenged the Council Regulation on SPCs for Medicines (Regulation 1768/92), arguing that intellectual property matters were of the exclusive competence of Member States, so that the Council could only legislate in this field where there was unanimity of Member States (Article 308, former Article 235 of the Rome Treaty). Spain also obtained a moratorium on the application of SPCs until January 1998, while in other Member States this supplementary protection was afforded from 1982.

Impact of the new intellectual property rules on the health system

The protection afforded by the 1986 Patent Law as to medicines actually had a limited impact on the health system. As previously noted, Spain did not accept pipeline protection so the new protection afforded by the law did not extend to old products (which lacked the requirement for patenting of novelty). As to new products, only patent applications filed after October 1992, when the patent law came into force, could benefit from the new legal environment. But new products filed on this date would not be available on the market until up to ten or twelve years had lapsed. Consequently, these patents would only appear in the Spanish market after 2002. Furthermore, increasing restrictions on reimbursement meant that many new products would not be financed by the National Health System (such as drugs like Sildenafil for impotence, and others). The coming into force of the SPC had an even weaker effect, because it came into force in January 1998, so its real effects will not emerge until 2007 (Lobato 1994).

Nevertheless, Spanish pharmaceutical expenditure rose consistently during this period. The 1999 report of Farmaindustria (the association of national and multinational manufacturers) shows that public health care expenditure in 1982 was 973 billion pesetas, in 1986 (the date of accession to the European

Community) it was 1520.5 billion pesetas, and in 1997 it was 4604.6 billion pesetas (Farmaindustria (Spanish Pharmaceutical Industry) 1999). Subsequent years show a continuing increase in expenditure. While overall publicly financed health care expenditure increased at a rate of 7.5% per annum in the last decade, publicly financed pharmaceutical expenditure increased at a rate of 10.6% per annum (Whitaker et al. 2002).

An obvious explanation for the rise in health care expenditure was the expansion of the system to provide universal coverage, which came into effect in the 1980s, combined with the growing needs of an ageing population and expenditure to make up for decades of underinvestment in staff and facilities. However, increased expenditure also reflected the cost of new drugs (drugs approved after Spanish accession to the European Community), which were relatively high compared to the pre-accession period, as they tended to be comparable with prices in other European countries. In 1988 more than a fifth of marketed medicines had received authorization in the previous five years. Although the total number of products with authorizations remained almost constant, with 8088 (prescription and over the counter) medicines in 1994 and 8024 in 1998, the cost profile of the newer products was quite different. This situation had an obvious impact on expenditure (Farmaindustria (Spanish Pharmaceutical Industry) 1999:49).

The net effect was that the share of publicly financed health expenditure accounted for by pharmaceuticals increased from 15% at the time of Spanish accession to 20% in 1998 (Whitaker et al. 2002). This proportion is higher than in other Member States. In response to rising costs, the Spanish Government established a reference pricing system in 1999 (Zammit-Lucia and Dasgupta 1995). In this model, the reference group comprised medicines with the same active constituent and the same dosage. This led to falls of at least 10% in prices. Reference pricing also required harmonization of description of product characteristics (the technical file that sets out the properties and indications for each product) for all products within a cluster. Older medicines had to adapt to the requirements, in terms of bioequivalency, of the new clusters.

In conclusion, with roughly the same number of approved medicines, costs rose, as the newer medicines were more expensive, in part reflecting a general trend of harmonization in pharmaceutical prices across Europe. These new medicines were not protected by product patents. A product patent entitles the patent holder to prevent a third party from manufacturing or using the patented item irrespective of the process by which the item is produced. Process patents only protected these new medicines. Thus, it was perfectly legal to identify alternative manufacturing processes for active constituent of the medicine.

Yet, prices remained relatively high, since most products were licensed, with few generics or copies. Spanish licensees bought the manufactured product from the patent holder and agreed a price for the medicine with the Spanish authorities that was generally very close to that of the patent holder. There is now a policy to promote generics, which are typically priced at 25% less than the reference price. However, the impact of generics remains relatively small, amounting to only 2.5% of total public pharmaceutical expenditure (Whitaker et al. 2002:55).

Pharmaceutical law

Before 1986 mechanisms for authorization of medicines were unsatisfactory. The main regulatory provision was an administrative Decree of 1973, which, obviously, did not take into account Directive 65/65/EEC. This provision was very vague and allowed a considerable margin of discretion for health authorities in dealing with pharmaceutical authorization. The possibility of challenging a decision by a health authority was non-existent, because courts held that technical decisions of the administration were not subject to their decisions. There was no data protection, leading to delays in many innovative products being launched in Spain, in order to avoid the disclosure of information contained in the authorization dossier. As a result of this situation it became possible to find in Spanish markets a mix of original products, imitations, false generics (with no proof of bioequivalence) and licensed products. The reform of the Pharmaceutical Law introduced the EC Directives (Real Decreto 767/1993) into Spain. The new legislation had consequences for the determination of prices (transparency Directive) and dossier data protection. The new rules meant a greater legal certainty as they limited administrative discretion.

One important issue was parallel trade. Parallel trade was prohibited until October 1995. It was seen as harmful to the Spanish National Health System, because it sometimes led to shortages of products in Spain. It was, however, a lucrative business for those involved in it, but few, if any, benefits accrued to the consumer in other Member States. Consequently, in December 1999, the Spanish Government permitted double pricing of medicines. This clearly had implications in terms of competition law. It is also important as an indicator of a change of attitude by the Spanish Authorities in terms of pharmaceutical issues.

The structure of the industry

The years following accession saw changes in the structure of the domestic industry. In 1991 there were 310 pharmaceutical companies (defined as owners of at least one marketing authorization). This rose to 374 in 1998, falling to 359 in 2000 (Farmaindustria 2001). Prior to accession many of these companies were small and inefficient. Some succeeded in finding niches (generics, cosmetics, homeopathic medicines and so on) but others vanished as they were unable to compete. Overall, however, the readjustment has been very gradual and the overall effect has been that delays that Spain asked for made it more difficult to achieve much needed industry reconfiguration.

The reservations about adopting strong intellectual property protection has led to an unwillingness by research-based companies to invest in Spain. The more innovative Spanish companies concentrated on obtaining licence agreements with patent holders. Instead of developing their research and development capacity (which would have required a critical mass, with mergers and acquisitions between Spanish companies), national companies have concentrated on marketing existing products. Neither has this situation benefited the health care system, which has seen its prices continue to grow, in part reflecting high levels of expenditure on marketing and other promotional activities.

The new approach to intellectual property

Spain has now changed its earlier reservations about intellectual property and currently the authorities advocate a strong regime of protection. The new patent system examines all applications in terms of novelty, activity and industrial application. This system was fully implemented in December 2003. Since November 2001 Spain is an International Preliminary Examination Authority in the Patent Cooperation Treaty, and hopes to be the Reference Office for Spanish and Portuguese-speaking countries.

National and multinational companies have initiated new relationships, including some joint ventures. There are growing links between universities and research-based companies. Biotechnology, in particular, is seeing increased investments, with research contracts made between national and transnational companies and university teams. A special regulation to protect inventions made by government scientists (either at the Spanish Consejo Superior de Investigaciones Científicas, Spanish National Scientific Council or at the public universities) was implemented in early 2002. As a part of its 2000–2003 Science Plan, the Spanish Government has launched the Action Profarma Plan, an ambitious project with fiscal incentives for pharmaceutical research carried out in Spain (Farmaindustria 2001).

There are also discussions between Farmaindustria and the Spanish authorities to establish a new type of relationship. It has been proposed that the amount that Farmaindustria is required to return to the state if cost caps for pharmaceutical expenditure are exceeded should be invested in research and development. A preliminary agreement in this regard was signed at the end of 2001. Parallel trade has remained a concern and the new approach by the Spanish authorities has been welcomed by Farmaindustria.

Conclusion

The new system has brought benefits to the pharmaceutical industry, whether national or multinational, who are clearly the major beneficiaries of the new system. They made considerable profits, driven largely by the coincident expansion of the Spanish National Health System, although these were later reined in as the Government introduced ever stricter cost controls. Some Spanish companies fared badly because they relied on the persistence of the old system and their portfolios were based on obsolete medicines, many of which were excluded by the National Health System when it introduced a negative list in 1993. The other winners in this situation were patients, who had greater access to new medicines. The reforms created a new system that was much more conducive to innovation, with tangible increases in Spanish research and development.

Mistrust of intellectual property regulation can be seen to have been short-sighted, as well as being incompatible with international obligations. Spain is an example of a country that originally showed a clear reticence to implement intellectual property protection, but that has changed its mind on this subject as it did not obtain any benefit from having less protection than other European Community Member States.

In summary, while a reluctance to reform intellectual property protection may seem attractive in the short term, it is ultimately unavoidable, and it is likely to work to the advantage of candidate countries.

References

Farmaindustria (Spanish Pharmaceutical Industry) (2001) *La industria farmacéutica en cifras*. Madrid, Spain.

Farmaindustria (Spanish Pharmaceutical Industry) (1999) La industria farmacéutica en cifras. Madrid, Spain.

Lobato, M. (1994) *El nuevo marco legal de las patentes químicas y farmacéuticas*. Madrid, Spain: Civitas.

Whitaker, D., Sánchez, P. and (NERA), N. E. R. A. (2002) *Diagnóstico y perspectiva del gasto farmacéutico en España*. Madrid, Spain: Farmaindustria.

Zammit-Lucia, J. and Dasgupta, R. (1995) Reference pricing. The European Experience, Paper No 10. *Health Policy Review*.

eighteen

Looking beyond the new borders: Stability Pact countries of south-east Europe and accession and health

Ivana Bozicevic and Stjepan Orešković

The chapter begins with an overview of the development of the relationship between the EU and the five countries of south-east Europe that are not yet candidate countries for EU accession but are members of the Stability Pact (Albania, Bosnia and Herzegovina, Croatia, Serbia and Montenegro and The former Yugoslav Republic of Macedonia). It will then describe the structure and aims of the Stability Pact and explore how health issues are addressed within its framework. Finally, it will outline challenges and opportunities that the Stability Pact brings to these countries in terms of their potential accession to the EU.

In April 1997, the European General Affairs Council proposed a regional approach for the western Balkans, aiming to develop further relations with Albania, Bosnia and Herzegovina, Croatia, Serbia and Montenegro and The former Yugoslav Republic of Macedonia. Two years later the EU initiated the Stability Pact for south-eastern Europe[1] as a political declaration of commitment to strengthen peace, build respect for human rights and democracy, and foster post-conflict restoration and economic growth in the region. The Stability Pact partners are listed in Table 18.1.

In May 1999, the EU began a new phase in its relationship with the five countries of south-east Europe – Albania, Bosnia and Herzegovina, Croatia, Serbia and Montenegro and The former Yugoslav Republic of Macedonia – through the Stabilization and Association Process (SAP). The other two south-east European countries, Bulgaria and Romania, as EU candidate countries, are not

Table 18.1 Stability Pact partners

The countries of the region and their neighbours	Albania, Bosnia and Herzegovina, Bulgaria, Croatia, Czech Republic, Hungary, Poland, Republic of Moldova, Romania, Slovakia, Slovenia, Serbia and Montenegro, The former Yugoslav Republic of Macedonia, Turkey
The EU Member States and the European Commission	Austria, Belgium, Denmark, Germany, Greece, Finland, France, Italy, Luxembourg, Netherlands, Portugal, Spain, Sweden, Ireland, United Kingdom
Non-EU members of the G8	USA, Canada, Japan, Russian Federation
Other countries	Norway, Switzerland
International organizations	UN, OSCE, Council of Europe, UNHCR, NATO, OECD
International financial institutions	World Bank, International Monetary Fund, European Bank for Reconstruction and Development, European Investment Bank, Council of Europe
Regional initiatives	Black Sea Economic Cooperation, Central European Initiative, South-East European Cooperative Initiative, South-East Europe Cooperation Process

included in the SAP (http://www.stabilitypact.org). Kosovo, once an autonomous province of Yugoslavia, is a protectorate of the United Nations under international civil and military administration.

The SAP clearly recognizes these countries as potential candidates for EU accession and emphasizes the need for improved regional cooperation as a prerequisite for their membership. It offers them the prospect of gradual integration with European structures based on Stabilization and Association Agreements (SAAs), in the same way as the agreements with the current candidate countries in central and eastern Europe.

The Stability Pact acts through three working tables:

Working Table I – Human Rights and Democratization
Working Table II – Economic Reconstruction, Development and Cooperation
Working Table III – Security and Defence Issues

The first SAA was signed between the EU and The former Yugoslav Republic of Macedonia in April 2001, and subsequent ones with Croatia in October 2001 and Albania in January 2003. The SAA must be ratified by all EU Member States to enable the countries to achieve the status of candidates for EU membership (http://www.stabilitypact.org). The conclusion of the SAA represents the commitment to complete a formal association with the EU over a transition period. The minimum conditions that the countries must meet were defined on 29 April 1997, the main requirements being achievement of democratic, economic and institutional reforms.

The SAAs provide the general contractual relations between each of the countries and the European Commission and are adapted to the situation in each country, thus enabling some to pursue faster integration than others. The Agreement emphasizes respect for peace and stability and the development of political dialogue between the countries. The EU and its Member States have been the most important donors in the region since the transition from communism but, during the 1990s, financial support was mainly for crisis management and post-conflict reconstruction.

During the period 2000–2006, the EU's financial assistance for Albania, Bosnia and Herzegovina, Croatia, Serbia and Montenegro and The former Yugoslav Republic of Macedonia seeks to ensure long-term development and is administered through the CARDS (Community Assistance for Reconstruction, Development and Stabilization) programme. The aim of this programme is to support the objectives of the SAP, which includes: ethnic reconciliation and the return of refugees; judicial, economic and media reforms; democratic changes and administrative capacity building; and development of collaboration between countries receiving CARDS support and with EU Member States and candidate countries (European Commission 2001). In the countries that signed the Agreement, assistance also includes support for approximation of legislation to that of the EU in order to prepare them for effective participation in the integration process.

Trade liberalization is a major driving force towards closer links with the EU. A Memorandum of Understanding on intra-regional trade liberalization was signed by the Governments of Albania, Bosnia and Herzegovina, Bulgaria, Croatia, Romania, Serbia and Montenegro and The former Yugoslav Republic of Macedonia. It sought to complete a network of free trade agreements in the region by the end of 2002, allowing for at least 90% of goods to be exchanged free of tariffs and creating a market of up to 55 million consumers (Working Table II 2001). It is expected that the EU will gradually establish a free trade area with the countries that signed the SAA over the subsequent six years.

In the recent report on the SAP for south-east Europe, the Commission argues forcefully that ineffective functioning of the judiciary and inadequate implementation of the rule of law is regarded as the main impediment to the EU integration process in all of these countries. The health sector is rarely addressed explicitly, but issues mentioned in specific reports on the countries, such as environmental protection and trafficking of people and drugs and smuggling of tobacco are clearly matters of health concern (Stabilization and Association Process for South-East Europe 2003).

Thus the report on the SAP for Albania reports that the recommendations included in the 2002 SAP report have only been addressed partially and it identifies trafficking of people, drugs and weapons and low levels of environmental protection as some of the weaknesses that require further attention. It notes that Tirana seems to be one of the most polluted European cities. Waters remain highly polluted, due to inadequate sewage systems and water treatment facilities (Stabilization and Association Report 2003a).

The report on Bosnia and Herzegovina states that the health sector in both entities remains weak and faces inadequate funding. Parallel health systems exist within Bosnia and Herzegovina, and the 1998 Law on Health remains largely unimplemented. A state level environmental framework law is being developed but cannot be implemented without an effective environmental administration system. Awareness of environmental issues has increased – public attention has focused on the UN Environmental Programme study on depleted uranium and possible links with an increased incidence of childhood leukaemia. Basic drug supply has remained a matter of concern (Stabilization and Association Report 2003b).

Croatia continues to be the country that has made the greatest progress towards the status of candidate for EU accession and is working intensively to align its legislation to the *acquis*. The main challenge remains the need to strengthen law enforcement and address the lack of qualified legal staff. In 2002, the State Office for Standardization and Measurement became a full member of the International Laboratory Accreditation Cooperation (ILAC). The law on consumer protection has been adopted but the preparation of the new draft law on food safety and quality encountered delays. An agency for environmental protection is being established but the limited administrative capacity is of concern. Croatia also needs to do more to implement the National Plan on Combating Trafficking in Human Beings and the National Programme against Drug Abuse. The implementation of the CARDS programme effectively started in July 2002 and the Government has set up the necessary structures to manage EU assistance within individual ministries though there remains the scope for improvement of interministerial coordination (Stabilization and Association Report 2003c).

Under the auspices of the Sector for European Integration (SEI), work has started on a National Strategy for European Integration in The former Yugoslav Republic of Macedonia and a procedural manual for the harmonization of legislation has been prepared. As a priority in 2004 the report identifies the need for a comprehensive strategy to fight against corruption. Major efforts are needed to approximate the country's legislative system with the environmental *acquis*. Drug trafficking and abuse must also be more fully addressed (Stabilization and Association Report 2003d). The tragic assassination of the Serbian Prime Minister, Zoran Djindjic, in March 2003 is a remainder of the challenge to the Serbian Government posed by organized crime. In July 2002 the Commission stated that it would begin drafting the report on the feasibility of opening negotiations for an SAA when the Constitutional Charter and the Action Plan (especially the trade aspects) were in place. Cooperation has begun with the European Environment Agency. The report on Serbia and Montenegro is the only one that explicitly mentions the health sector, in terms of the need for the reorganization of the Ministry of Health, reflecting how the Serbian Government was without a Health Minister for almost a year, as well as the need to strengthen public health. Drug trafficking and abuse remains an issue of concern. Concrete steps towards improving statistics are also urgently required (Stabilization and Association Report 2003e).

The current socioeconomic situation in the region

When looking ahead to potential future accession to the EU, it is important to understand how these countries compare with the present candidate countries in central and eastern Europe. Yugoslavia adopted a unique model of communism, which was more open than in the countries of central and eastern Europe and the Soviet Union. In terms of health indicators, Yugoslavia was midway between western and eastern Europe (Watson 1995). Albania was also unique, remaining almost entirely isolated from developments in the rest of the world and maintaining a very traditional lifestyle. Its health indicators were significantly better than would be expected from its level of socioeconomic development, a difference thought to reflect a healthier lifestyle (Gjonca and Bobak 1994).

At the time when the wave of democratic changes were sweeping across eastern Europe, Yugoslavia was disintegrating into warfare, first in Croatia (1991–1995), followed by Bosnia and Herzegovina (1992–1996), Kosovo (1999) and finally The former Yugoslav Republic of Macedonia (2001) causing huge human suffering and economic losses. Democratic changes have been slower in materializing than in the current candidate countries. The consequences of conflict, exacerbated by economic collapse in the 1990s, are that the national incomes are substantially lower than in candidate countries, with rising levels of poverty and growing social and health inequalities. South-east Europe, with a combined population of 24.5 million, is now the poorest region in Europe, although quite heterogeneous in terms of socioeconomic development and levels of population health. GDP per head differs considerably across the countries, ranging in 2000 from US $1039 in Serbia and Montenegro to US $4153 in Croatia (World Bank 2000; WIIW Balkan Observatory 2003). In comparison with the central and eastern European countries, where the macroeconomic situation largely stabilized by the mid-1990s, most of the SEE countries are struggling to achieve economic growth and stability. The region's economic output in 2001 remained 12% below its 1990 level. In comparison, GDP of central and eastern European countries (Czech Republic, Hungary, Poland, Slovania, Slovenia) was in 2001 on average 19% higher than in 1990 (WIIW Balkan Observatory 2003).

Unemployment levels are considerably higher than in the central and eastern European countries and have been increasing worryingly since the beginning of the 1990s. In 1999 unemployment was 36% in The former Yugoslav Republic of Macedonia, 30% in Serbia and Montenegro and is believed to be even higher in Bosnia and Herzegovina. In Croatia it was 23% at the beginning of 2002. By the end of 2000 there were still 1.3 million refugees and internally displaced persons in the region, although the number has been decreasing since the mid-1990s (United Nations High Commissioner for Refugees 2000; European Commission 2001). It is estimated that 290000 persons from Bosnia and Herzegovina and Serbia and Montenegro have sought asylum in other parts of Europe since 1990. Between 1990 and 1999 over 300000 people left Albania and around 105000 left Croatia, mainly to western Europe and North America, although the official number of emigrants is likely to be an underestimate (Croatian Statistics Bureau 2000; World Bank 2000).

Health status in countries included in the Stabilization and Association Process

In terms of public health the countries of ex-Yugoslavia and Albania today represent probably the least explored region in Europe. Very little is known about the impact of the socioeconomic transition and wars on the health status of their populations and, in particular about the scale of emerging health inequalities. The quality of information on health indicators during the 1990s fell far short of standards in the EU. This is to some extent due to large-scale population movements caused by the wars, but also due to outdated data monitoring systems and inadequate capacity for data analysis in the countries themselves. For Bosnia and Herzegovina health data has not been sent to the WHO since 1991 (WHO 2001).

Figure 18.1 shows the life expectancy at birth for countries for which data is available. Since 1990 both the EU and the central and eastern European countries have experienced an increase in life expectancy. From 1995 to 1998 life expectancy at birth in Albania, Croatia and The former Yugoslav Republic of Macedonia decreased but afterwards showed signs of recovery and was in 2000 three to five years less than the EU average.

The available health data do, however, need to be interpreted with caution as there are many uncertainties about population estimates during the 1990s (Bozicevic et al. 2001; Sanjay et al. 2002). The censuses that were carried out in 2001 will, when fully analysed, provide a far more accurate picture of

Figure 18.1   Life expectancy in Albania, Bulgaria, Croatia, Romania, The former Yugoslav Republic of Macedonia, the EU and central and eastern European countries

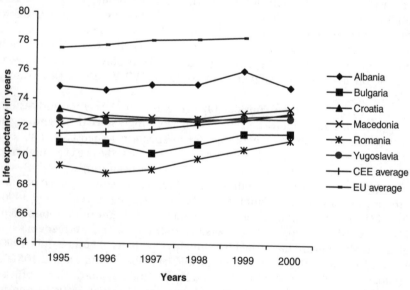

Source: WHO European Health for all database, 2003

population health outcomes in the region and will enable their assessment to be made in retrospect.

Infant mortality shows an improving trend since the early 1990s. In 1999 it ranged from 7.75 per 1000 in Croatia to 18.6 in Romania, compared to rates of 11.2 per 1000 in central and eastern Europe and 4.9 per 1000 in the EU.

The health sector and the Stability Pact

In the framework of the Stability Pact, the health sector is addressed through Working Table II and within the Initiative of Social Cohesion on the grounds that poor socioeconomic standards and inadequate social infrastructure can contribute to social and political instability in the region. The health sector was identified as one that required further development. As well as health issues, the initiative addresses social protection, housing, employment and labour market policies (Working Table II 2001).

There are also other initiatives within the framework of the Stability Pact that are relevant for the health sector. For example, Working Table I addresses issues of refugees and displaced persons, minority rights and building civil society. The anti-corruption initiative is also of great importance. Working Table II addresses environmental issues through the Regional Environmental Reconstruction Programme (RERP). Its priority areas are institutional strengthening and capacity building, environmental impact assessment, repair of environmental damage during the wars in the region and support to National and Local Environmental Action Plans (Task Force for Implementation of the Regional Environmental Reconstruction Programme for South-Eastern Europe 2001).

Partners in the Social Cohesion Initiative are, in addition to the Stability Pact beneficiary countries: Austria, Italy, France, Germany, Greece, Switzerland, Slovenia, the Council of Europe (and its Development Bank), the European Trade Union Confederation, the World Health Organization, the International Labour Organization, the International Organization of Employers, the Friedrich Ebert Foundation and the United Nations Development Programme. The Expert Sub-Group for Health is led on an informal basis by WHO and the Council of Europe. Its main aim is to assist governments in defining national priorities for the health sector, reducing health inequalities and modernizing legislative and regulatory frameworks (Working Table II 2001). It also aims to develop collaborative networks among the countries thus offering opportunities to exchange knowledge and experience.

The conflicts in the region, coupled with economic collapse, severely damaged health care infrastructure and disrupted the provision of health services. Wars caused immense human suffering. Medical care was provided in extremely difficult conditions with shortages of medical supplies, food and water on an everyday basis (Acheson 1993; Black 1993; Alderslade et al. 1996; Horton 1999; Spiegel and Salama 2000).

As with data on health, information of health care provision must be interpreted with caution. However, the picture is quite diverse across the region. The latest available data, from 1999, reports that the proportion of GDP spent on health care was 5.5% in The former Yugoslav Republic of Macedonia, 7% in Yugoslavia, 9% in Croatia, and only 3.1% in Albania in 1997, compared with the EU average of 8.5% (Nuri and Healy 1999; Vulic and Healy 1999; Hajioff 2000). Per capita real spending on health is considerably less than in the EU.

The governments in the region have expressed a commitment to improve health and social care in the region. At a meeting held in Dubrovnik, Croatia in September 2001, the health ministers from seven countries of south-east Europe (Albania, Bosnia and Herzegovina, Bulgaria, Croatia, The former Yugoslav Republic of Macedonia, Romania and Serbia and Montenegro) signed the Dubrovnik Pledge: Meeting the Health Needs of Vulnerable Populations in South-East Europe. In the declaration they recognize:

> the damaging effects on health of recent wars, continuing unrest and con-
> flict, as well as economic hardship faced by the populations of SEE during
> their countries' transition to market economies. We accept the challenge to
> play a key role in strengthening the fundamental human rights of our soci-
> eties and of vulnerable populations and individuals within them to effect-
> ive health care, social wellbeing and human development, in line with the
> principles of the World Health Organization and the Council of Europe.
> (WHO and Council of Europe 2001)

Improvement of the health status of vulnerable populations in the region is one of the most important aims of the Social Cohesion Initiative. Social and health inequalities were largely ignored during the communist period. Sadly, they still receive hardly any attention from health policy-makers. For example in Croatia, it is impossible to measure socioeconomic differentials in mortality as death certificates still do not contain an appropriate question that would address them.

Research in the countries of eastern Europe and the former Soviet Union show how a complex interaction between social and economic deprivation, low levels of social support and damaging lifestyles can contribute to health status deterioration, particularly of those who are already disadvantaged (Bobak et al. 1998; Marmot and Wilkinson 1999; McKee and Shkolnikov 2001). There has been some research on the health status of vulnerable groups in the countries of ex-Yugoslavia and Albania, largely on refugees (Weinberg and Simmods 1995; Lang 1997). However, there is a need for larger-scale studies that would explore the impact of increasing poverty and socioeconomic insecurity. There has been little thought of how health systems that are underfunded and increasingly market-driven will deal with the health and social needs of disadvantaged populations. The Task Force for Public Health Collaboration in South East Europe recently proposed Minimum Health Indicator Set for South-East Europe which contains 32 indicators from the WHO Health for All Database (Bardehle 2002). They do not, however, consider the impact on health outcomes according to income or social status. There is a clear need for more ambitious approaches to health measurement, taking advantage of newly available census data.

How do the Stability Pact Social Cohesion Initiative and the Stabilization and Association Process help prepare these countries for the prospect of European Union integration?

The Directorate-General for Employment and Social Affairs emphasized the importance of further developing the social policy sector in the SEE countries, as some areas addressed by the Social Cohesion Initiative like employment, pension reform and social dialogue are part of the *acquis communautaire* (Stability Pact Initiative for Social Cohesion 2002). The document "2½ Years of the Stability Pact" recognizes that the role of the EU in furthering approximation with European law in the SEE countries must be strengthened (Special Co-ordinator of the Stability Pact for South-East Europe 2001).

The Social Cohesion Initiative recognizes the importance of strengthening institutions and capacity building in the health and social sector areas. It is noted that "efficient institutions are indispensable to improve the performance of these sectors, harmonise labour legislation and employment policy with the EU and international standards". In the areas of health policy, it states that "relative legislation will be amended to comply with EU standards" (Working Table II 2001). It is expected that a Regional Monitoring Mechanism will be established to oversee how the reform processes in the countries complies with conditions for potential EU membership. It is also clear that there is a need to link the current reform processes in the health sector to the requirements of EU integration (Special Co-ordinator of the Stability Pact for South-East Europe 2001).

The SAA does not specifically mention health or health care. However, there are Articles within it that relate to it, such as the harmonization of legislation in the area of consumer protection, environment protection and work safety (Commission of the European Communities 2001).

The Social Cohesion Initiative provides financial assistance for a number of projects that are considered to reflect the priorities for public health and health care in Albania, Bosnia and Herzegovina, Bulgaria, Croatia, Romania, Serbia and Montenegro and The former Yugoslav Republic of Macedonia and that were proposed by the countries themselves within the framework of the Stability Pact Action Plan for Health (Annex 2 to the Initiative for Social Cohesion Action Plan 2001). At the end of January 2002, the Council of Europe provided a loan for a Croatian project "Capacity Building for Equal Access to High Quality Health Services", and approved projects proposed by Serbia and Montenegro on a Food Safety and Nutrition Services, on Strengthening of Community Mental Health Services proposed by Bosnia and Herzegovina and on Surveillance and Control of Communicable Diseases project proposed by Albania.

The links between these projects and the requirements of European integration are not very clear although the Action Plan for Health, within which these projects have been approved, aims to enable future compliance of the health sector in these countries with the *acquis communautaire*. It recognizes that "restructuring of public health functions and infrastructures can be achieved by reviewing, reformulating and harmonising health legislation and standards in line with international conventions and recommendations, as well as the *acquis communautaire* in all relevant public health areas". There are ongoing discussions that will hopefully clarify these issues and propose guidelines about how to link the projects within the Social Cohesion Initiative more explicitly with the requirements of the SAP.

Opportunities and challenges to improve health within the Stability Pact

The SAP is an instrument that enables the countries to achieve the status of candidate countries for EU membership. It brings both opportunities and challenges. In the mid-1990s, when most of the current candidate countries applied for EU membership, public health issues were less prominent at a European level than they are now. The lessons of the current accession process for health services and public health issues in the candidate countries in central and eastern Europe will be important for the next set of candidate countries. They can also provide the opportunity for the EU, the WHO and the SEE countries to develop a clearer strategy on health and accession.

Economic and social reforms are moving forward in the SEE countries and are a major requirement for European integration. The impact of policies in other sectors on health can be of particular relevance for the health sector in the SAP. The success of the initiative depends greatly on whether the institutional, research and management capacities in the health sector, and in particular with regard to public health, will be improved. However, fundraising for the health projects within the Social Cohesion Initiative has been rather slow, impeding implementation and the efficiency of the whole initiative.

Among the basic requirements for accession is access to comparable demographic and social data, which should provide an impetus for the countries to modernize their health statistics systems. Strengthening capacity for health data collection, analysis and monitoring would allow better identification of population health needs, planning and evaluation of health sector performance and identification of inequalities. Inadequate population health data is a major obstacle to evidence-based health policy in these countries. Investment in professional development of public health personnel is also of major importance. These countries urgently need skilled public health professionals who will be able to analyse, interpret and act on population health and health services data. Well-trained health managers and policy-makers are also needed to take forward the considerable amount of work related to health and the accession process.

The EU's integration process requires multisectoral and multiagency work to address challenges in areas such as agricultural policy, environmental health, safety at work and the free movement of patients and health professionals, as well as single market issues that have relevance for the health sector such as pharmaceuticals, food and technology (Special Co-ordinator of the Stability Pact for South-East Europe 2001). Some of the countries that have signed the SAA may become candidate countries by 2004, which will offer them further opportunities to participate in EU public health programmes. This can facilitate much needed enhancement of their public health research capacity. The Social Cohesion Initiative could use this opportunity to encourage countries to assess how their approved projects can be brought in in accordance with the EU's new public health strategy which puts the emphasis on three strands – setting up a comprehensive data system on the major determinants of health, strengthening communicable disease surveillance networks and developing policies for combating disease and promoting health (Annex 2 to the Initiative for Social Cohesion Action Plan 2001).

Building partnerships among beneficiary countries is a strong element of the Social Cohesion Initiative and may be its most ambitious part. The Initiative also identifies the need to involve NGOs and the public in the process of health policy-making, steps that will contribute to more democratic and transparent processes of decision-making in the health sector. Some of the projects, for example on food safety and communicable diseases surveillance, can be particularly beneficial in bringing health-related legislation in the countries in line with that of the EU.

In conclusion, the Stability Pact offers a new framework to help the countries in the region. The main aim of the Social Cohesion Initiative is to enable institutional strengthening and capacity building, recognizing that knowledge is a prerequisite for action. It also offers health professionals in the countries an opportunity to make the health sector more visible in the process of the EU integration. However, better links with the requirements of the SAP would more effectively support harmonization of health-related legislation to that of the *acquis communautaire*. Nevertheless, the success of this initiative depends greatly on the quality and the extent to which the capacities in the beneficiary countries will really be developed and on the breadth of vision of those who will be implementing the projects at country level.

Acknowledgements

We are grateful to Patrizia Mauro, Office of the Special Coordinator of the Stability Pact in Brussels for her comments and Maria Haralanova, Division for Country Support, WHO Regional Office for Europe for providing us with documents on the Social Cohesion Initiative.

Note

1 Albania, Bosnia and Herzegovina, Bulgaria, Croatia, Romania, Serbia, Montenegro and Kosovo, and The former Yugoslav Republic of Macedonia are commonly referred to in official documents as south-east European (SEE) countries.

References

Acheson, D. (1993) Health, humanitarian relief and survival in former Yugoslavia, *British Medical Journal*, 307:44–8.
Alderslade, R., Hess, G. and Larusdottir, J. (1996) Sustaining, protecting and promoting public health in Bosnia and Herzegovina, *World Health Statistics Quarterly*, 49(3–4):185–8.
Annex 2 to the Initiative for Social Cohesion Action Plan (2001) Action Plan for Health.

2001. Prepared for the 4th meeting of Working Table II of the Stability Pact, May. Tirana.

Bardehle, D. (2002) Minimum Health Indicator Set for South Eastern Europe, *Croatian Medical Journal 2002*, 43(2):170–3.

Black, M.E. (1993) Collapsing health care in Serbia and Montenegro, *British Medical Journal*, 307:1135–8.

Bobak, M., Pikhart, H., Hertzman, C., Rose, R. and Marmot, M. (1998) Socioeconomic factors, perceived control and self-reported health in Russia. A cross-sectional survey, *Social Science & Medicine*, 47:269–79.

Bozicevic, I., Orešković, S., Stevanovic, R. et al. (2001) What is happening to the health of the Croatian population, *Croatian Medical Journal*, 42(6):601–5.

Commission of the European Communities (2001) Proposal for a Council decision concerning the signature of the Stabilisation and Association Agreement between the European Communities and its Member States and the Republic of Croatia on behalf of the European Community. 9 July. 371 Final. Commission of the European Communities, Brussels.

Croatian Statistics Bureau (2000) *Croatian Statistics Yearbook 1999*. Zagreb.

European Commission (2001) CARDS Assistance Programme to the western Balkans. Regional Strategy paper 2002–2006. IP/01/464, October. Brussels: European Commission.

Gjonca, A. and Bobak, M. (1994) Albanian paradox, another example of protective effect of Mediterranean lifestyle?, *Lancet*, 350:1815–17.

Hajioff, S. (2000) *Health Care Systems in Transition: The former Yugoslav Republic of Macedonia*. Copenhagen: European Observatory on Health Care Systems.

Horton, R. (1999). Croatia and Bosnia: the imprints of war, *Lancet*, 353(9170):2139–44. http://www.stabilitypact.org Stability pact. 2002.

Lang, S. (1997) Abandoned elderly population, a new category of people suffering in war, *Journal of Public Health Medicine*, 19(4):476–7.

Marmot, M. and Wilkinson, R. (1999) *Social Determinants of Health*. Oxford: Oxford University Press.

McKee, M. and Shkolnikov, V. (2001) Understanding the toll of premature death among men in eastern Europe, *British Medical Journal*, 323(7320):1051–5.

Nuri, B. and Healy, J. (1999) *Health in Transition: Albania*. Copenhagen: European Observatory on Health Care Systems.

Sanjay, K., Black, M.E., Mandic, S. and Selimovic, N. (2002) Impact of the Bosnian conflict on the health of women and children, *Bulletin of the World Health Organization*, 80(1):75–6.

Special Co-ordinator of the Stability Pact for South-East Europe (2001) 2½ Years of Stability Pact: Lessons and Policy Recommendations. December.

Spiegel, P.B. and Salama, P. (2000) War and mortality in Kosovo, 1998–99: an epidemiological testimony, *Lancet*, 355:2204–9.

Stabilization and Association Process for South-East Europe (2003) Second Annual Report. Report from the Commission. Commission of the European Communities. 139. final. COM, Brussels.

Stabilization and Association Report (2003a) Albania. Commission staff working paper. SEC (2003) 339. Brussels: Commission of the European Communities.

Stabilization and Association Report (2003b) Bosnia and Herzegovina. Commission staff working paper. SEC 340. Brussels: Commission of the European Communities.

Stabilization and Association Report (2003c) Croatia. Commission staff working paper. Brussels: Commission of the European Communities.

Stabilization and Association Report (2003d) The former Yugoslav Republic of Macedonia Commission staff working paper. Brussels: Commission of the European Communities.

Stabilization and Association Report (2003e) Serbia and Montenegro. Commission staff working paper. Brussels: Commission of the European Communities.

Stability Pact Initiative for Social Cohesion (2002) Internal report on the Regional meeting of the Stability Pact Initiative for Social Cohesion. Paris.

Task Force for Implementation of the Regional Environmental Reconstruction Programme for South-Eastern Europe (2001) Report of the Third REReP Task Force meeting. September. Sarajevo.

United Nations High Commissioner for Refugees (2000) *The State of World's Refugees in 2000 – Fifty Years of Humanitarian Action*. Oxford: Oxford University Press.

Vulic, S. and Healy, J. (1999) *Health Care Systems in Transition: Croatia*. Copenhagen: European Observatory on Health Care Systems.

Watson, P. (1995) Explaining rising mortality among men in Eastern Europe, *Social Science & Medicine*, 41:923–34.

Weinberg, J. and Simmods, S. (1995) Public health, epidemiology and war, *Social Science & Medicine*, 40(12):1663–9.

WHO (2001) European Health for All Database, WHO Regional Office for Europe.

WHO and Council of Europe (2001) Health Ministers' Forum: "Health Development Action for South East Europe". The Dubrovnik Pledge: Meeting the Health Needs of the Vulnerable Populations in South East Europe. September. Copenhagen: WHO, Council of Europe.

WIIW Balkan Observatory (2003) The joint project of the Vienna Institute for International Economic Studies and the London School of Economics and Political Sciences. Available at: http://www.wiiw.ac.at/balkan/data.html. WIIW Balkan Observatory.

Working Table II (2001) Economic Reconstruction, Development and Co-operation. Initiative for Social Cohesion. Regional Conference. October. Bucharest.

World Bank (2000) The Road to Stability and Prosperity in South-Eastern Europe. A regional strategy paper. World Bank.

Index

Page numbers in *italics* refer to boxes and tables, those in **bold** indicate main discussion.

FUNDING HEALTH CARE
OPTIONS FOR EUROPE

Elias Mossialos, Anna Dixon, Josep Figueras and Joe Kutzin (eds)

The question of how to generate sufficient revenue to pay for health care has become a serious concern for nearly all European policy-makers. This book examines the advantages and disadvantages of funding arrangements currently in use across Europe. Adopting a cross-national, cross-disciplinary perspective, it assesses the relative merits of the main methods of raising resources including taxation; social, voluntary and supplemental forms of insurance; and self-pay including co-payments. Chapters written by leading health policy analysts review recent evidence and experience in both eastern and western Europe. The volume is introduced by a summary chapter which integrates conceptual issues in funding with an overview of the main advantages and disadvantages of each method of funding drawn from the expert chapters.

This is an important book for students of health policy, health economics, public policy and management, and for health managers and policy makers.

Contents
Funding health care – Financing health care – Social health insurance financing – Health financing reforms in central and eastern Europe and the former Soviet Union – Private health insurance and medical savings accounts – Voluntary health insurance in the European Union – User charges for health care – Informal health payments in central and eastern Europe and the former Soviet Union – Lessons on the sustainability of health care funding from low- and middle-income countries – Funding long-term care – Strategic resource allocation and funding decisions – Funding health care in Europe – Index.

328pp   0 335 20924 6 (Paperback)   0 335 20925 4 (Hardback)

HOSPITALS IN A CHANGING EUROPE

Martin McKee and Judith Healy (eds)

- What roles do hospitals play in the health care system and how are these roles changing?
- If hospitals are to optimize health gains and respond to public expectations, how should they be configured, managed and sustained?
- What lessons emerge from experiences of changing hospital systems across Europe?

Hospitals of the future will confront difficult challenges: new patterns of disease, rapidly evolving medical technologies, ageing populations and continuing budget constraints. This book explores the competing pressures facing policy-makers across Europe as they struggle to respond to these complex challenges. It argues that hospitals, as part of a larger health system, should focus on enhancing health outcomes while also responding to public expectations. Adopting a cross-national, cross-disciplinary perspective, the study assesses recent evidence on the factors driving hospital reform and the strategies used to improve organizational performance. It reviews the evidence from eastern as well as western Europe and combines academic research with real-world policy experience. It looks at the role of hospitals in enhancing health rather than simply processing patients. The book concludes that hospitals cannot be managed in isolation from society and the wider health system, and that policy-makers have a responsibility to define the broader health care goals that hospitals should strive to meet.

Hospitals in a Changing Europe synthesizes current evidence in a readable and accessible form for all practitioners, policy-makers, academics and graduate level students concerned with health reform.

Contents
Part one: The context of hospitals – *The significance of hospitals – The evolution of hospital systems – Pressures for change – The role and function of hospitals –* **Part two: External pressures upon hospitals** – *The hospital and the external environment – Are bigger hospitals better? – Investing in hospitals – Hospital payment mechanisms – Linking organizational structure to the external environment –* **Part three: Internal strategies for change** – *Improving performance within the hospital – The changing hospital workforce in Europe – Introducing new technologies – Optimizing clinical performance – Hospital organization and culture –* **Part four: Conclusions** – *Future hospitals – Index.*

320pp   0 335 20928 9 (Paperback)   0 335 20929 7 (Hardback)

REGULATING ENTREPRENEURIAL BEHAVIOUR IN EUROPEAN HEALTH CARE SYSTEMS

Richard B. Saltman, Reinhard Busse and Elias Mossialos (eds)

- What have been the major trends in entrepreneurial behaviour and regulation in European health care?
- To what degree do approaches to regulation and entrepreneurialism differ among subsectors and countries across Europe?
- What does the evidence show about successes and failures, and which successful options are open to policy-makers?

A wide range of entrepreneurial initiatives have been introduced within European health care systems during the last decade. While these initiatives promised more efficient management, they also triggered concerns about reduced equity and quality in service provision.

This book explores emerging regulatory strategies that seek to capture the benefits of entrepreneurial innovation without sacrificing the core policy objectives of a socially responsible health care system. It opens with an extended essay on current trends and evidence across health care subsectors and across countries, presenting a wide range of alternatives for policy-makers, and assessing their relative advantages and disadvantages. It then reviews entrepreneurialism and regulation in specific contexts (such as hospitals, primary health care, social services) and considers related issues including the impact of corruption and the potential lessons from deregulation of public utilities.

Regulating Entrepreneurial Behaviour in European Health Care Systems brings together the perspectives of politics, economics, management, medicine, public health and law and will be a valuable resource for students, academics, practitioners and policy-makers concerned with health policy and health reform.

Contents
Part one: Balancing regulation and entrepreneurialism in Europe's health sector – Theory and practice – *Part two: Conceptual issues* – Good and bad health sector regulation – What can we learn from the regulation of public utilities? – Accreditation and the regulation of quality in health services – Corruption as a challenge to effective regulation in the health sector – Where entrepreneurialism is growing – Regulating entrepreneurial behaviour in hospitals – Entrepreneurial behaviour in pharmaceutical markets and the effects of regulation – Regulating entrepreneurial behaviour in social care – Regulating the entrepreneurial behaviour of third-party payers in health care – Where entrepreneurialism is strong but not changing – The regulatory environment of general practice – Regulating entrepreneurial behaviour in oral health care services – Index.

256pp   0 335 20922 X (Paperback)   0 335 20923 8 (Hardback)

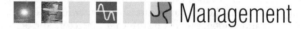
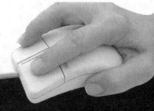